Foundations of Behavioral Health

Bruce Lubotsky Levin • Ardis Hanson
Editors

Foundations of Behavioral Health

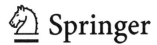 Springer

Editors
Bruce Lubotsky Levin
Department of Child and Family Studies
College of Behavioral and Community
Sciences
University of South Florida
Tampa, FL, USA

Behavioral Health Concentration
College of Public Health
University of South Florida
Tampa, FL, USA

Ardis Hanson
Research and Education Unit
Shimberg Health Sciences Library
University of South Florida
Tampa, FL, USA

ISBN 978-3-030-18433-9   ISBN 978-3-030-18435-3   (eBook)
https://doi.org/10.1007/978-3-030-18435-3

This Springer imprint is published by the registered company Springer Nature Switzerland AG
The registered company address is: Gewerbestrasse 11, 6330 Cham, Switzerland

Foundations of Behavioral Health is dedicated to the memory of Dr. Kevin Hennessy, who spent his career at the SAMHSA working with a variety of federal, state, and local stakeholders in the behavioral health services field throughout the United States.

Kevin helped conceptualize this textbook. We have yet to meet a more knowledgeable, friendly, energetic, and considerate person. He was a gifted person simply because he was a remarkable listener. He also possessed the unique yet rare ability to synthesize a comprehensive range of behavioral health issues in light of the relevant research literature. He knew the clinical (micro) aspects of behavioral health services as a licensed clinical psychologist, yet he was able to draw the macro-implications for services research, practice, and policy. Kevin was only 50 years young when he suddenly passed away.

Even though Kevin possessed all of these remarkable qualities, he was very humble, devoted to his family, and passed through life with amazing grace. Since our first telephone conversation about developing a textbook on behavioral health, we treasure the journey we experienced with Kevin. He was, and forever will remain, the most significant behavioral health professional who provided the scholarship and vision for Foundations of Behavioral Health. His tremendous guidance, energy, dedication, and innovative initiatives will be sorely missed by his family, colleagues, friends, and readers of this textbook.

Foreword

Even in the twenty-first century, the public health community continues to face formidable challenges. There is a need for more integrative and collaborative approaches in public health initiatives, considering the complex relationships among the social determinants of health within natural and built environments, population health and health-care systems, and economic, education, and social and community contexts. The continuing changes in the landscape of public health challenge our ability to reconceptualize our approach to how health-care professionals can contribute to health promotion, health education, and disease prevention efforts in communities constantly facing the globalization of communicable and noncommunicable diseases and environmental threats due to man-made and natural disasters.

With an ever-increasing global focus on integrative approaches to solve public health problems, it is essential that behavioral health professionals are seen and utilized as integral members of interdisciplinary and interprofessional health-care teams. While clinically trained behavioral health professionals come from a variety of academic preparations in psychiatry, psychology, counseling, social work, and pastoral counseling, there is also a need for these same behavioral health professionals to develop strong foundations in population health and behavioral health. An example of this interprofessional education and training is found within the University of South Florida College of Public Health, where a cadre of professionals are being educated in behavioral health (i.e., the study of alcohol, drug abuse, and mental disorders from a population perspective) within master's and doctoral degree programs. This group of professionals is uniquely positioned to educate the public on disease prevention, health promotion, and development and financing of effective service systems specifically in the behavioral health arena.

This tome features the work of scholars from the academic and professional fields of public health, medicine, behavioral health, social work, economics, criminology, health communication, and pharmacy and illustrates the benefits of an interdisciplinary approach to integrative population health and behavioral health-care delivery. In addition, it provides a global perspective of practice and policy in behavioral health. Each chapter concludes with a section entitled "Implications for

Behavioral Health." This section reminds the readers of the importance of the chapter topic for the larger fields of behavioral health and public health.

This text examines the critical relationships for understanding the importance of integrating population health and behavioral health services from a variety of lenses (national, regional, and global). Public health graduate students and professionals would greatly benefit from exploring the chapters in this volume considering the increase in complex comorbid disease clusters. In addition, behavioral health professionals would clearly better understand the nature of the important partnership between public health and behavioral health for improving and sustaining the health of populations at risk.

I am grateful to the coeditors and the authors for providing such an insightful, skills-focused, and practical learning tool and reference guide for the much-needed population- and systems-oriented behavioral health professionals of the future.

Donna J. Petersen
Senior Associate Vice President
USF Health, University of South Florida
Tampa, FL, USA

Dean and Professor
College of Public Health, University of South Florida
Tampa, FL, USA

Preface

Foundations of Behavioral Health is being completed in the midst of congressional debate over attempts to repeal the Patient Protection and Affordable Care Act (ACA) which was originally signed into law by Former President Barack Obama on 23 March 2010. However, debate over health-care reform is hardly new, with many attempts at health-care reform attempted during the previous (approximately) half century.

Nevertheless, there are three basic reasons this textbook has been developed. First, health care is one of the most basic and important issues in the United States; however, health care is still not a right. Second, there continues to be expanded discontent, as well as frustration, with health-care delivery systems in the United States, particularly with access to services, treatment costs, and service outcomes. Third, behavioral health (i.e., alcohol, drug abuse, and mental health) delivery systems are disjointed from other behavioral health delivery systems and isolated from health-care delivery systems.

Foundations of Behavioral Health examines the organization, financing, delivery, and outcomes of behavioral health services from both the United States and global perspectives. Our textbook covers many fundamental issues in behavioral health, including epidemiology, insurance and financing, health inequities, implementation sciences, lifespan issues, cultural competence, and policy, which also have implications for public health services and integrated health-care services. It also addresses topics of concern to health administrators, planners, policymakers, evaluators, and treatment professionals, including at-risk indigenous populations, individuals in the juvenile justice systems, individuals with intellectual and developmental disabilities, and individuals living in rural and frontier areas.

The development and organization of *Foundations of Behavioral Health* has been influenced by our work and experiences in teaching, research, and community service. Our efforts culminated in the establishment of the Behavioral Health Concentration (BHC) at the University of South Florida (USF) College of Public Health (COPH), a collaborative teaching initiative between the USF COPH and the USF College of Behavioral and Community Sciences. The BHC is only one of the several US-accredited schools/colleges of public health offering a concentration/

focus/specialization in alcohol, drug abuse, and mental disorders from a population or public health perspective. In addition, our involvement with editing *The Journal of Behavioral Health Services & Research (JBHS&R)* has kept us current with evidence-based practices and challenges in services delivery in behavioral health.

Based on our unique experiences, we are convinced that behavioral health services research and services delivery should be examined within a public health framework. Such a framework includes an interdisciplinary and interprofessional approach to studying behavioral health. Accordingly, the contributors to *Foundations of Behavioral Health* include a variety of nationally prominent academicians, researchers, and professionals. An important element of this text is that each chapter contributor understands how their expert knowledge is a part of the broader public health context in which their specialty exists.

These national experts have made it possible to provide an integrated textbook that can be used by graduate students in public health, behavioral health, social work, psychiatric nursing, psychology, psychiatry, applied medical anthropology, mental health counseling, criminology, medical sociology, and public administration. In addition, we have also designed *Foundations of Behavioral Health* as a reference and handbook for public health administrators, researchers, practitioners, and policymakers who work with mental health issues at the local, state, and/or national levels of the government.

Organization of the Textbook

Foundations of Behavioral Health is organized into three basic sections: (1) Overview (issues), (2) At-Risk Populations, and (3) Services Delivery. The Overview section of this textbook includes six chapters that provide information regarding the defining characteristics of behavioral health. Chapter 1, written by the editors of this volume, contains an introduction to behavioral health and examines social determinants of health and disease. In Chapter 2, Heslin provides a discussion of the epidemiology of behavioral health problems from a global perspective. In Chapter 3, Timko and Cucciare provide an overview of the substance use disorders as well as co-occurring disorders. Chapter 4, written by Samuel Zuvekas, discusses insurance and financing of behavioral health services. In Chapter 5, Massey and Vroom discuss the importance of implementation sciences in behavioral health. Finally, in Chapter 6, the volume editors discuss the challenges of behavioral health services research data.

The second part of *Foundations of Behavioral Health* contains six chapters exploring a variety of at-risk populations who are in need of behavioral health services. In Chap. 7, Weist and associates examine the delivery of behavioral health services to children and adolescents in school environments. Dembo and associates, in Chapter 8, discuss youth involved in juvenile justice systems in the United States. Chapter 9, written by Becker and Lynn, examines critical issues in women's behavioral health from an interdisciplinary public health perspective. In Chapter 10,

Baldwin and associates discuss the challenges faced by the American Indian and Alaskan native populations regarding behavioral health services. In Chapter 11, Cohen and Krajewski review the prevalence and impact of behavioral health services in older adult populations. Finally, in Chapter 12, Tasse and associates present an overview of behavioral health services for persons with intellectual and developmental disabilities.

The third major part of *Foundations of Behavioral Health* consists of five chapters on behavioral health services delivery. Chapter 13, written by Haack and associates, presents a general overview and rationale for integrating health and behavioral health services. The editors then present, in Chapter 14, the major issues in the delivery of behavioral health services for individuals living in rural and frontier areas. Chapter 15, written by Callejas and Hernandez, reframe the concept of cultural competence for the delivery of behavioral health services to culturally diverse populations. In Chapter 16, Ott provides an overview of the role of pharmacy services in behavioral health. Finally, in Chapter 17, the editors of this volume integrate the current trends in global behavioral health policy, systems, and services, examining the magnitude of the problem, from definitional and operational perspectives, with a focus on child and adolescent behavioral health.

As expected, it is impossible to include every possible topic in a single textbook devoted to behavioral health services. Nevertheless, *Foundations of Behavioral Health* emphasizes the critical importance of using an interdisciplinary public health approach to understand behavioral health issues from a public health framework.

Throughout the development and preparation of this *Foundations of Behavioral Health* textbook, there have been a number of individuals who have provided sage counsel, continuing support, and/or significant encouragement. We would like to extend our deep appreciation to Ms. Janet Kim of Springer for her many helpful suggestions during the copyediting and production stages of this new textbook. Finally, we are ultimately grateful to our families for their continuing love and immeasurable support during the very lengthy preparation of this *Foundations of Behavioral Health* textbook.

Tampa, FL, USA   Bruce Lubotsky Levin
Tampa, FL, USA   Ardis Hanson

Contents

The original version of this book was revised. The correction is available at
https://doi.org/10.1007/978-3-030-18435-3_18

Contributors

Julie A. Baldwin Northern Arizona University, Flagstaff, AZ, USA

Marion Ann Becker School of Social Work and Louis de la Parte Florida Mental Health Institute, University of South Florida, Tampa, FL, USA

Betty G. Brown Northern Arizona University, Flagstaff, AZ, USA

Linda M. Callejas Department of Child and Family Studies, College of Behavioral and Community Sciences, University of South Florida, Tampa, FL, USA

Richard Chapman University of South Florida, Tampa, FL, USA

Donna Cohen Department of Child and Family Studies, College of Behavioral and Community Sciences, University of South Florida, Tampa, FL, USA

Jennifer Cristiano Agency for Community Treatment Services, Inc., Tampa, FL, USA

Michael A. Cucciare Center for Mental Healthcare and Outcomes Research, Central Arkansas Veterans Healthcare System, North Little Rock, AR, USA

VA South Central (VISN 16) Mental Illness Research, Education, and Clinical Center, Central Arkansas Veterans Healthcare System, North Little Rock, AR, USA

Department of Psychiatry, University of Arkansas for Medical Sciences, Little Rock, AR, USA

Richard Dembo Criminology Department, University of South Florida, Tampa, FL, USA

Ralph J. DiClemente Emory University, Atlanta, GA, USA

New York University, New York, NY, USA

Emery R. Eaves Northern Arizona University, Flagstaff, AZ, USA

Katie Eklund School Psychology Program, University of Arizona, Tucson, AZ, USA

Kristan Elwell Northern Arizona University, Flagstaff, AZ, USA

Jennifer M. Erickson University of Washington Medical Center, Department of Psychiatry and Behavioral Sciences, Seattle, WA, USA

Jessica Faber Agency for Community Treatment Services, Inc., Tampa, FL, USA

Sara Haack University of Hawai'i John A. Burns School of Medicine, Department of Psychiatry, Honolulu, HI, USA

Ardis Hanson Research and Education Unit, Shimberg Health Sciences Library, University of South Florida, Tampa, FL, USA

Mario Hernandez Department of Child and Family Studies, College of Behavioral and Community Sciences, University of South Florida, Tampa, FL, USA

Kevin C. Heslin National Center for Health Statistics, Washington, DC, USA

George Washington University, Washington, DC, USA

Matthew Iles-Shih University of Washington Medical Center, Department of Psychiatry and Behavioral Sciences, Seattle, WA, USA

Andrew Krajewski Department of Sociology and Criminology, College of the Liberal Arts, Pennsylvania State University, State College, PA, USA

Bruce Lubotsky Levin Department of Child and Family Studies, College of Behavioral and Community Sciences, University of South Florida, Tampa, FL, USA

Behavioral Health Concentration, College of Public Health, University of South Florida, Tampa, FL, USA

Vickie Ann Lynn Department of Community and Family Health, College of Public Health, University of South Florida, Tampa, FL, USA

Oliver T. Massey Department of Child and Family Studies, College of Behavioral and Community Sciences, University of South Florida, Tampa, FL, USA

Lauren Meyer University of Arizona, Tucson, AZ, USA

Carol A. Ott Purdue University College of Pharmacy, Indianapolis, IN, USA

Eskenazi Health/Midtown Community Mental Health, Indianapolis, IN, USA

Elizabeth A. Perkins Department of Child & Family Studies, College of Behavioral and Community Sciences, University of South Florida, Tampa, FL, USA

Donna J. Petersen Senior Associate Vice President, USF Health, University of South Florida, Tampa, FL, USA

Dean and Professor, College of Public Health, University of South Florida, Tampa, FL, USA

Anna Ratzliff University of Washington Medical Center, Department of Psychiatry and Behavioral Sciences, Seattle, WA, USA

Tammy Jorgensen Smith College of Behavioral and Community Sciences, University of South Florida, Tampa, FL, USA

Joni Splett University of South Carolina, Columbia, SC, USA

Marc J. Tassé The Ohio State University, Columbus, OH, USA

Asha Terminello Agency for Community Treatment Services, Inc., Tampa, FL, USA

Christine Timko Center for Innovation to Implementation, Veterans Affairs (VA) Health Care System, Menlo Park, CA, USA

Department of Psychiatry and Behavioral Sciences, Stanford University School of Medicine, Stanford, CA, USA

Enya B. Vroom Department of Child and Family Studies, College of Behavioral and Community Sciences, University of South Florida, Tampa, FL, USA

Mark Weist University of South Carolina, Columbia, SC, USA

Heather J. Williamson Northern Arizona University, Flagstaff, AZ, USA

Samuel H. Zuvekas US Agency for Healthcare Research and Quality, Rockville, MD, USA

About the Editors

Bruce Lubotsky Levin, DrPH, MPH is associate professor at the Department of Child & Family Studies at the University of South Florida (USF) College of Behavioral and Community Sciences, and editor-in-chief of *The Journal of Behavioral Health Services & Research*. He is also associate professor and head, *Behavioral Health Concentration*, USF College of Public Health. He is co-PI and director of Curriculum, USF Institute for Translational Research in Adolescent Drug Abuse (NIH-NIDA grant), for the past 7 years and is coauthor and senior editor of nine other textbooks with Ardis Hanson, including *Introduction to Public Health for Pharmacists, Second Edition* (Oxford University Press, 2018); *Mental Health Informatics* (Oxford University Press, 2013); *Mental Health Services: A Public Health Perspective, Third Edition* (Oxford University Press, 2010); and *A Public Health Perspective of Women's Mental Health* (Springer, 2010). His research focus is the study of alcohol, drug abuse, and mental disorders from a public health or population perspective, translational research, behavioral health services research, and policy.

Ardis Hanson, PhD, MLIS is the assistant director of Research and Education at the Shimberg Health Sciences Library at the University of South Florida. She has over 25 years of experience as a research librarian and has published extensively in behavioral health services, policy, and research. Her research focus is on language and social interaction, that is, how language is used in everyday practice to negotiate claims and identities, particularly in how behavioral health policy is created.

Population-Based Behavioral Health

Bruce Lubotsky Levin and Ardis Hanson

Introduction

While the origins of epidemiology can be traced to John Snow and the 1854 cholera outbreak in England (Snow, 1855), C-EA Winslow, in 1920, provided one of the initial and most essential definitions of public health in the United States:

> Public health is the science and art of preventing disease, prolonging life, and promoting physical health and efficiency through organized community efforts... which will ensure to every individual a standard of living adequate for the maintenance of health... to enable every citizen to realize his [and her] birthright of health and longevity. (Winslow, 1920, pp. 6–7)

More than a century later, the Institute of Medicine's (IOM) Committee for the Study of the Future of Public Health published the book *The Future of Public Health*, which assessed public health programs and the coordination of services across US government agencies and within state and local health departments. The Committee defined the *substance* of public health as "organized community efforts aimed at the prevention of disease and promotion of health" (Institute of Medicine, 1988, p. 41). In addition, the Committee described the *mission* of public health as "the fulfillment of society's interest in assuring conditions in which people can be healthy" (Institute of Medicine, 1988, p. 40).

B. L. Levin (✉)
Department of Child and Family Studies, College of Behavioral and Community Sciences, University of South Florida, Tampa, FL, USA

Behavioral Health Concentration, College of Public Health, University of South Florida, Tampa, FL, USA
e-mail: Levin@usf.edu

A. Hanson
Research and Education Unit, Shimberg Health Sciences Library, University of South Florida, Tampa, FL, USA

© Springer Nature Switzerland AG 2020
B. L. Levin, A. Hanson (eds.), *Foundations of Behavioral Health*,
https://doi.org/10.1007/978-3-030-18435-3_1

1

Table 1 Ten essential public health services

Monitor health status to identify community health problems
Diagnose and investigate identified health problems and health hazards in the community
Inform, educate, and empower people about health issues
Mobilize community partnerships to identify and solve health problems
Develop policies and plans that support individual and community health efforts
Enforce laws and regulations that protect health and ensure safety
Link people to needed personal health services and assure the provision of health care
Assure a competent public health and personal health-care workforce
Assess effectiveness, accessibility, and quality of personal and population-based health
Research for new insights and innovative solutions to health problems

The three core functions of public health are (1) assessment, (2) policy development, and (3) quality assurance (IOM, 1988), and the ten essential public health services for these core public health functions (Public Health Functions Steering Committee, 1994) are shown in Table 1.

More recently, there are a growing number of major initiatives in public health which are of major importance nationally, including the integration of primary care and public health (Institute of Medicine, 2012b), living well with chronic illness (Institute of Medicine, 2012a), the social determinants of health (Stockman, Hayashi, & Campbell, 2015), women's behavioral health (National Academies of Sciences, Engineering, & Medicine, 2018b), and rural and frontier health (National Academies of Sciences, Engineering, & Medicine, 2018a).

A population-based approach emphasizes health promotion and disease prevention. It also involves formal activities by both the public and private sectors, working together to concentrate on sustaining the health of populations. This public health framework of iterative problem-solving includes a select number of phases, commencing with identification of the problem, assessing risks, and ascertaining protective factors. The next stage includes the development, implementation, and evaluation of interventions. The final phase in this iterative process is monitoring implementation in relation to the impact on policy and cost-effectiveness.

This first chapter highlights the concept of behavioral health within an overall framework of population or public health. It examines the burden of behavioral health problems on individuals, families, friends, and communities and the challenges within existing behavioral health delivery systems. It also emphasizes the importance of re-focusing behavioral health (the study of alcohol, drug abuse, and mental disorders from a population or public health perspective) on systems integration strategies, which incorporate technology, facilitate recovery, and promote prevention.

Behavioral Health

As we complete two decades of the twenty-first century, behavioral health problems (i.e., behavioral disorders), continue to be significant public health problems. The burden of disease from behavioral disorders is overwhelming and costly. The most recent Global Burden of Disease (GBD) study ranked mental and substance use disorders as the fifth leading cause of disability-adjusted life years (DALYs) and the leading cause of years lived with a disability globally (Whiteford, Ferrari, & Degenhardt, 2016). Mental and substance use disorders globally account for nearly one quarter of all years lived with a disability. In terms of lost economic output, the World Economic Forum estimates the amount to be approximately $16 trillion in US dollars over 20 years or the equivalent of 25% of the 2010 global gross domestic product (Bloom et al., 2011).

Globally, mental and substance use disorders are the leading cause of disability in children and adolescents. Although approximately 50% of all mental disorders develop by the age of 14, many individuals go untreated until adulthood (World Health Organization, 2014a). In terms of DALYs, these disorders ranked as the sixth leading cause of DALYs (5.7%, 55.5 million children), equivalent to 25% of all disabilities in children worldwide (Erskine et al., 2015).

The United States

Among comparable countries, the United States not only has the highest rate of death from mental and substance use disorders, but these disorders are the leading cause of disease burden for females and the third leading cause of disease burden for males (Murray et al., 2013).

Approximately one in five Americans (43 million) has a behavioral disorder during any given year, with anxiety disorders (e.g., phobias, panic disorder, and post-traumatic stress disorder) found to be the most prevalent behavioral disorders in adults. Of these 43 million, approximately ten million American adults (1 in 25) experience serious functional impairment due to mental or substance use disorders. These disorders are the single largest source of DALYs in the United States, representing nearly 14% of disability from all causes (Murray et al., 2013). These disabilities affect physical, social, and behavioral functioning across the lifespan.

Approximately one in five children and adolescents (ages 9–17) in the United States has a diagnosable behavioral disorder during any given year, with approximately 11% of children experiencing significant functional impairment and 5% of children experiencing extreme functional impairment (Adelman & Taylor, 2010). In addition, at any one time, between 10 and 15% of children and adolescents have symptoms of depression. In 2015, a significant increase in the national annual prevalence of major depressive episodes among adolescents aged 12–17 (8.2% in 2011 to 12.5% in 2015) was reported (SAMHSA, 2017). Substance use also increased. An estimated 2.2 million (8.8%) of adolescents (12–17) use illicit drugs and 5.8% of adolescents (an estimated 1.4 million adolescents) engaged in binge alcohol use (SAMHSA, 2017).

Financing of Care

Behavioral health care in America have evolved into a complicated array of uncoordinated and fragmented services, programs, and delivery systems, often creating significant problems in accessing needed services. The considerable gap between epidemiologic estimates of behavioral disorders and the actual number of individuals receiving care over the course of a lifetime strongly suggests many Americans have attempted to cope with their behavioral health problems without seeking treatment. They do not seek help, do not enter formal behavioral health-care delivery systems, or receive assistance through other health and/or social service systems, including (primary) health care, welfare, correctional, pastoral counseling, or long-term care delivery systems.

In addition, the historical reliance on the public sector for long-term care and on the private sector for acute care has contributed to the limited overall continuity of care for behavioral health services. While state and federal governments historically funded public behavioral health care, the financing systems for these services have increasingly been mixed, involving a multitude of public and private payers and providers of behavioral health care.

Globally, the direct and indirect economic costs of mental disorders are estimated at approximately $2.5 trillion in the United States (Trautmann, Rehm, & Wittchen, 2016). The indirect costs, estimated at $1.7 trillion in the United States, are more than double the direct costs ($0.8 trillion in the United States). This finding is in direct contrast to the costs of care for other physical diseases, such as cardiovascular diseases and cancer (Trautmann et al., 2016). In 2013, the United States spent $201 billion on individuals with behavioral disorders in the general population, individuals who were institutionalized, and active-duty military populations (Roehrig, 2016). In 2014, spending totaled $220 billion. Of this amount, mental health spending amounted to $186 billion (85% of overall spending), and substance use disorders spending amounted to $34 billion (15% of overall spending) (SAMHSA, 2016). See chapter "Financing of Behavioral Health Services: Insurance, Managed Care, and Reimbursement" in this volume for a more detailed discussion on insurance, financing, and managed behavioral health care in the United States.

Burden of Behavioral Disorders

In addition to the definition, substance, mission, and functions of public health in the preceding discussion, public health may also be viewed within the larger context of health. The World Health Organization not only defines health as "a state of complete physical, mental, and social well-being and not merely the absence of disease or infirmity"; it also affirms that "enjoyment of the highest attainable standard of health is one of the fundamental rights of every human being without distinction of race, religion, political belief, economic or social condition" (World Health Organization, 2006, p. 11). Thus, behavioral health may be conceptualized as an integral part of the overall health of individuals and populations, though different cultures and ethnicities vary in their definitions of what constitutes behavioral health.

Complexity of Systems

State mental hospitals historically were the primary location for providing care for people with serious behavioral health problems throughout the United States. With the introduction of deinstitutionalization and community mental health centers in America, these hospitals were downsized in terms of population and often eventually closed. Largely independent from public health systems, publicly funded behavioral health systems then developed into a variety of specialty (sector) services within a number of different organizational settings. Concerned about the continued fragmentation and lack of integration between public health and behavioral health services, the IOM Committee recommended the integration of health and behavioral health services, with a primary focus on disease prevention and health promotion (Institute of Medicine, 1988).

The de facto behavioral health systems in the United States are comprised of numerous behavioral health-care service components as well as social welfare, justice, and educational systems across both public and private sector services. Each sector exists in individual silos. Each has its own agencies, management, funding streams, and services. These sectors provide acute and long-term services across a variety of settings, including home-based, community-based, and institutionally based. In addition, care is provided across the specialty behavioral health sector, the general medical/primary care sector, and the voluntary care sector.

Influences on how this care is provided, accessed, organized, delivered, and financed come from professional licensing and accreditation organizations, managed care organizations, insurance companies, advocacy and regulatory agencies, and health-care policymaking groups (see chapter "Financing of Behavioral Health Services: Insurance, Managed Care, and Reimbursement" in this volume for a detailed discussion of insurance and financing of behavioral health services). In addition, other systems that provide behavioral health services may not have identification of behavioral disorders as a primary mission and fail to link patients with behavioral disorders to appropriate venues for care.

The provision of mental health and substance abuse services in both jails and prison serves as an example. The provision, utilization, and costs of these services are not uniformly accepted across the United States. Continuum of care post parole, probation, or reentry into the community is a common problem, as in a more community-based orientation to treatment and supportive services (see chapter "Behavioral Health and the Juvenile Justice System" in this volume for a more detailed discussion of mental health treatment in juvenile justice settings).

State and federal legislation, which influence the delivery of services, are often in conflict with each other. Legislative proviso language, regulatory and administrative requirements, and financial appropriation language also affect the eventual delivery of services, especially to vulnerable and underserved populations. Other factors that influence delivery of care include new practice models, such as integrated health and behavioral health services, as well as increasingly hybridized public and private sector provider networks. However, the continuing challenge for behavioral health is how to provide the best possible treatment, despite distinct service sectors, to improve the quality of life and long-term outcomes for persons with mental and substance use disorders.

System Transformation

Of the five goals of the President's New Freedom Commission on Mental Health (2003) to fundamentally transform the delivery of behavioral health services, technology remains as one of today's main priorities.

Technology is a critical factor in the delivery of care. Not only does it advance research in the development of evidence-based practices; it also is an effective e-channel in the diffusion, early adoption, and effective implementation of efficacious and effective practices. With a focus on improving service delivery and utilization, the ultimate goal of technology, from a public behavioral health perspective, is on disease prevention and health promotion. Technology also plays a significant role in workforce development, as the integration of electronic health records now include specific best practices and data for behavioral health treatment and practice. It also develops and expands the behavioral health knowledge base, providing longitudinal and comparative data to address disparities, trauma, acute care, and long-term consequences of medications (see chapter "Pharmacy Services in Behavioral Health" in this volume for more on pharmacology). Clearly, integrated information technology (e.g., electronic health records) and communication infrastructure (e.g., telehealth systems) are well worth the investment to improve the delivery of care across underserved and vulnerable populations.

In March of 2019, in what seems very hard to fathom, the Internet turned 30 years old. Since its inception, traditional communications media has transformed into remarkable technologic initiatives and amazing available hardware and software.

The emergence of simple machine transmission protocol, voice over Internet Protocol (VoIP), and Internet Protocol television (IPTV) have radically changed how we communicate, with streaming media, podcasting, and real-time webcams. Social media changes almost daily, with new mobile applications and platforms. The availability of platforms has also resulted in many organizations, no matter how large or small, having as well as using social media accounts to get their message out to the public.

Media advocacy plays a significant role in setting public agenda and influencing the direction of public opinion on health, behavioral health, and social issues. Agenda setting may (1) establish the importance of a topic for the public and/or (2) address what the public should think about a topic. Media stories often are coded and identified with an episodic or a thematic frame. Episodic frames focus on discrete events, people, and places; however, they often provide the least amount of statistical or contextual information, which would better inform the public. Thematic frames focus on contextualizing the issue within a broader framework. These frames work much better from an informational and sense-making perspective, especially when looking at rapid dissemination and discussion of research results.

Respondents to a survey by the National Collaborating Centre for Determinants of Health reported that social media played an important role in public health (Ndumbe-Eyoh & Mazzucco, 2016). Respondents used social media to report and address health inequities, discuss effective strategies to improve services delivery, and participate in policy analysis and advocacy (Ndumbe-Eyoh & Mazzucco, 2016). While organizational and government websites are more often seen as a primary and authoritative source of information, social media is increasingly seen as a close second.

A systematic review on the use of social media in public health and health promotion had mixed reviews on the effectiveness of social media to improve health outcomes or increase health equity. Welch et al. (2016) found that some social media interventions may be effective for selected at-risk populations (age, socioeconomic status, ethnicities, and place of residence). However, the lack of consistency in the design and implementation of social media interventions, in some cases, resulted in no change or worsened outcomes in study participants. In addition, privacy, confidentiality, and appropriateness of "fit" of intervention with populations were identified as significant challenges (Welch et al., 2016).

Social Determinants of Health, Sustainable Development Goals, and Healthy People

Since 2003, research continues to show how a small number of health risks account for the majority of the morbidity and mortality associated with disease, disability, and death. Although the top ten global health risks, which account for more than one third of all deaths, continue to change, the top ten health risks still account for the majority of deaths. The literature also suggests risk factors potentially can be reversed and that addressing these risk factors could also reduce societal inequities.

The Grand Challenges in the Global Mental Health Initiative identified mental, neurological, and substance use (MNS) disorders as being within its scope (i.e., depression, anxiety disorders, schizophrenia, bipolar disorders, alcohol and drug use disorders, mental disorders of childhood, migraines, dementias, and epilepsy) (Collins et al., 2011). In addition, the Grand Challenges in the Global Mental Health Initiative defined "global" to include cross-national influences on mental health, such as climate change or macroeconomic policies. Its goals are to (1) identify root causes, risk, and protective factors; (2) advance prevention and implementation of early interventions; (3) improve treatments and expand access to care; (4) raise awareness of the global burden; (5) build human resource capacity; and (6) transform health systems and policy responses. Each of its goals listed the top challenges for its area and provided a list of possible research questions (Collins et al., 2011).

Social Determinants of Health

Predating the Grand Challenges in the Global Mental Health Initiative, however, was the social determinants of health framework. Published in 1998 by the World Health Organization (WHO), as a response to the Health for All (HFA) policy on Europe, WHO focused on the effects on population health caused by the following areas: social and economic status, stress, early life, social exclusion, work, unemployment, social support, addiction, food, and transport (Wilkinson & Marmot, 1998). Tying together environmental, socioeconomic, political, cultural, and infrastructure influences on health was a continued global health emphasis through the decades, with successive reports building an evidence-based practice, determining how to evaluate progress, and creating a global consensus (De Castro Freire, Manoncourt, & Mukhopadhyay, 2009; Kelly et al., 2007; Ollila, 2011; World Health Assembly, 2009, 2011; World Health Organization, 2014b, 2016).

Sustainable Development Goals

The Millennium Development Goals (MDG), adopted by the United Nations General Assembly and WHO, had 8 goals with 21 targets, with a series of measurable health indicators and economic indicators for each target (United Nations General Assembly, 2000). The MDG resulted in numerous global and regional reports on existing infrastructures, policies, and population needs (Beattie, Brown, & Cass, 2015; Stuckler, Basu, & McKee, 2010; Thomsen et al., 2013; World Health Organization, 2010).

Fifteen years later, the United Nations General Assembly (2015) adopted its 2030 Development Agenda entitled "Transforming Our World: The 2030 Agenda for Sustainable Development." The Sustainable Development Goals (SDG) encompass 17 global goals, with 169 targets, which address social and economic development issues including poverty, hunger, health, education, global warming, gender equality, water, sanitation, energy, urbanization, environment, and social justice (Sustainable Development Solutions Network, 2015; World Health Organization, 2017). One major difference between the MDG and the SDG is their approaches. The MDG identified an individual goal and focused on addressing its effects, while the SDG emphasizes the interrelatedness of each of its goals to the other and attempts to deal with the causes of the problem.

The United States incorporated the WHO's definition of health in its *Healthy People* initiatives, which address national 10-year plans with identified objectives and indicators for improving the health of Americans. *Healthy People* addresses four main areas, (1) general health status, (2) health-related quality of life and well-being, (3) the social determinants of health, and (4) health disparities, with a focus on both individual-level and population-level determinants of health and interventions. Much like the SDG, *Healthy People* examines the relationship between health status and biology, individual behavior, health services, social factors, and policies (Secretary's Advisory Committee on National Health Promotion and Disease Prevention Objectives for 2030, 2018).

Healthy People

Healthy People's *2020* national objectives firmly embed behavioral health practice and practitioners into its national goals. Within the topic "Mental Health and Mental Disorders," the primary objectives are mental health status improvement and treatment expansion. However, across other topics, such as "Disability and Health," "Substance Abuse," "Educational and Community-Based Programs," and "Social Determinants of Health" (to name just a few), components of behavioral health are also found.

For *Healthy People 2030*, the Secretary's Advisory Committee (2018) set as one of its priorities the inclusion of the social determinants of health (SDH) as a crosscutting theme, maintaining the SDH as a separate topic area and applying SDH as a selection criteria for topic objectives. In addition, the focus is (1) reducing deaths, (2) reducing morbidity, (3) reducing disability, (4) reducing health disparity while increasing health equity, and (5) increasing well-being. Objectives cover three types: (1) core, (2) developmental, and (3) research.

Finally, each objective is viewed vis-à-vis its public health burden, the magnitude of the health disparity, the degree to which health equity would be achieved if the target were met, the degree to whether the objective is a sentinel or bellwether indicator, and, finally, the actionability of the objective.

Implications for Behavioral Health

A population approach to behavioral health focuses on health promotion and disease prevention to improve the health and mental health of populations. *Foundations Behavioral Health* uses a public health framework to examine behavioral health services and delivery issues in the United States as well as from a global perspective. The six chapters in the first section of the volume address an overview of basic issues in behavioral health services. The second section of the volume presents chapters examining the development of effective behavioral health services in specific at-risk populations. Finally, the last five chapters in the third section of this volume present critical issues in the delivery of behavioral health services.

There are significant consequences for failing to treat behavioral disorders, from a developmental or lifespan perspective, affecting children as they age into adolescence, adulthood, and old age. The societal effects are devastating, in terms of years of life lived with a disability, increased morbidity and mortality, and the burden of disease on individuals, families, and communities.

Nevertheless, a public health perspective allows one to examine and address the continued fragmentation and gaps in the care for children, adults, and the elderly; recovery issues surrounding unemployment, stigma, and disability for people with serious behavioral disorders; and the lack of a national priority for behavioral health and suicide prevention.

National initiatives, such as the President's New Freedom Commission (2003) and the Obama Administration's focus on reducing stigma, access to care, and the real possibility of recovery, show a paradigm shift from a "wicked problem," i.e., challenging and complex issues (Rittel & Martin, 1973), to an inclusive, community-centered approach.

References

Adelman, H. S., & Taylor, L. (2010). *Mental health in schools: Engaging learners, prevention problems, and improving schools*. Thousand Oaks, CA: Corwin Press.

Beattie, R. M., Brown, N. J., & Cass, H. (2015). Millennium Development Goals progress report. *Archives of Disease in Childhood, 100*(Suppl 1), S1. https://doi.org/10.1136/archdischild-2014-307933

Bloom, D. E., Cafiero, E. T., Jané-Llopis, E., Abrahams-Gessel, S., Bloom, L. R., Fathima, S., ... Weinstein, C. (2011, September). *The global economic burden of non-communicable diseases: A report by the World Economic Forum and the Harvard School of Public Health*. Geneva, Switzerland: World Economic Forum. http://www3.weforum.org/docs/WEF_Harvard_HE_GlobalEconomicBurdenNonCommunicableDiseases_2011.pdf

Collins, P. Y., Patel, V., Joestl, S. S., March, D., Insel, T. R., Daar, A. S., ... Stein, D. J. (2011). Grand challenges in global mental health. *Nature, 475*(7354), 27–30. https://doi.org/10.1038/475027a

De Castro Freire, S. B., Manoncourt, E., & Mukhopadhyay, A. (2009). IUHPE and social determinants of health: Setting an action agenda. *Global Health Promotion, 16*(Suppl 1), 89–92. https://doi.org/10.1177/1757975909103764

Erskine, H. E., Moffitt, T. E., Copeland, W. E., Costello, E. J., Ferrari, A. J., Patton, G., … Scott, J. G. (2015). A heavy burden on young minds: The global burden of mental and substance use disorders in children and youth. *Psychological Medicine, 45*(7), 1551–1563. https://doi.org/10.1017/s0033291714002888

Institute of Medicine. (1988). *The future of public health.* Washington, DC: National Academy Press.

Institute of Medicine. (2012a). *Living well with chronic illness: A call for public health action.* Washington, DC: The National Academies Press.

Institute of Medicine. (2012b). *Primary care and public health: Exploring integration to improve population health.* Washington, DC: The National Academies Press.

Kelly, M. P., Morgan, A., Bonnefoy, J., Butt, J., Bergman, V., Mackenbach, J., … Florezano, F. (2007, October). *Final report of the Measurement and Evidence Knowledge Network: The social determinants of health: Developing an evidence base for political action.* Geneva, Switzerland: World Health Organization (WHO) Commission on the Social Determinants of Health, Measurement and Evidence Knowledge Network.

Murray, C. J. L., Atkinson, C., Bhalla, K., Birbeck, G., Burstein, R., Chou, D., … Murray. (2013). The state of US health, 1990-2010: Burden of diseases, injuries, and risk factors. *JAMA, 310*(6), 591–608. https://doi.org/10.1001/jama.2013.13805

National Academies of Sciences, Engineering, & Medicine. (2018a). *Achieving rural health equity and well-being: Proceedings of a workshop.* Washington, DC: The National Academies Press.

National Academies of Sciences, Engineering, & Medicine. (2018b). *Women's mental health across the life course through a sex-gender lens: Proceedings of a workshop–in brief.* Washington, DC: The National Academies Press.

Ndumbe-Eyoh, S., & Mazzucco, A. (2016). Social media, knowledge translation, and action on the social determinants of health and health equity: A survey of public health practices. *Journal of Public Health Policy, 37*(Suppl 2), 249–259. https://doi.org/10.1057/s41271-016-0042-z

Ollila, E. (2011). Health in all policies: From rhetoric to action. *Scandinavian Journal of Public Health, 39*(6 Suppl), 11–18. https://doi.org/10.1177/1403494810379895

President's New Freedom Commission on Mental Health. (2003). *Achieving the promise: Transforming mental health care in America: Final report* (DHHS publication no.). Rockville, MD: U. S. Department of Health and Human Services. http://www.eric.ed.gov/PDFS/ED479836.pdf

Public Health Functions Steering Committee. (1994). *Public health in America.* Washington, DC: U. S. Public Health Service.

Rittel, H., & Martin, W. (1973). Dilemmas in a general theory of planning. *Policy Sciences, 4,* 155–169.

Roehrig, C. (2016). Mental disorders top the list of the most costly conditions in the United States: $201 billion. *Health Affairs, 35*(6), 1130–1135. https://doi.org/10.1377/hlthaff.2015.1659

Secretary's Advisory Committee on National Health Promotion and Disease Prevention Objectives for 2030. (2018). *Report #2: Recommendations for developing objectives, setting priorities, identifying data needs, and involving stakeholders for Healthy People 2030.* Washington, DC: Author. https://www.healthypeople.gov/sites/default/files/Advisory_Committee_Objectives_for_HP2030_Report.pdf

Snow, C. E. A. (1855). *On the mode of communication of cholera.* London, UK: John Churchill.

Stockman, J. K., Hayashi, H., & Campbell, J. C. (2015). Intimate partner violence and its health impact on ethnic minority women, including minorities and impoverished groups. *Journal of Women's Health, 24*(1), 62–79. https://doi.org/10.1089/jwh.2014.4879

Stuckler, D., Basu, S., & McKee, M. (2010). Drivers of inequality in Millennium Development Goal progress: A statistical analysis. *PLoS Medicine, 7*(3), e1000241. https://doi.org/10.1371/journal.pmed.1000241

Substance Abuse and Mental Health Services Administration. (2016). *Behavioral health spend-ing and use accounts, 1986–2014* (HHS Publication No. SMA-16-4975). Rockville, MD: Substance Abuse and Mental Health Services Administration. https://store.samhsa.gov/shin/content/SMA16-4975/SMA16-4975.pdf

Substance Abuse and Mental Health Services Administration. (2017). *Behavioral health barom-eter, United States, Volume 4: Indicators as measured through the 2015 National Survey on Drug Use and Health and National Survey of Substance Abuse Treatment Services* (HHS Publication No. SMA–17–BaroUS–16). Rockville, MD: Substance Abuse and Mental Health Services Administration. https://www.samhsa.gov/data/sites/default/files/National_BHBarometer_Volume_4.pdf

Sustainable Development Solutions Network. (2015, April 17). *Data for development: A needs assessment for SDG monitoring and statistical capacity development*. New York, NY: United Nations. http://unsdsn.org/wp-content/uploads/2015/04/Data-for-Development-Full-Report.pdf

Thomsen, S., Ng, N., Biao, X., Bondjers, G., Kusnanto, H., Liem, N. T., … Diwan, V. (2013). Bringing evidence to policy to achieve health-related MDGs for all: Justification and design of the EPI-4 project in China, India, Indonesia, and Vietnam. *Global Health Action, 6*, 19650. https://doi.org/10.3402/gha.v6i0.19650

Trautmann, S., Rehm, J., & Wittchen, H. U. (2016). The economic costs of mental disorders: Do our societies react appropriately to the burden of mental disorders? *EMBO Reports, 17*(9), 1245–1249. https://doi.org/10.15252/embr.201642951

United Nations General Assembly. (2000, September). *United Nations millennium declaration*. New York, NY: Author. http://www.un.org/millennium/declaration/ares552e.htm

United Nations General Assembly. (2015, October 21). *Resolution adopted by the General Assembly on 25 September 2015: 70/1. Transforming our world: The 2030 Agenda for Sustainable Development (A/RES/70/1)*. New York, NY: United Nations. http://www.un.org/ga/search/view_doc.asp?symbol=A/RES/70/1&Lang=E

Welch, V., Petkovic, J., Pardo Pardo, J., Rader, T., & Tugwell, P. (2016). Interactive social media interventions to promote health equity: An overview of reviews. *Health Promotion and Chronic Disease Prevention in Canada, 36*(4), 63–75.

Whiteford, H., Ferrari, A., & Degenhardt, L. (2016). Global Burden of Disease studies: Implications for mental and substance use disorders. *Health Affairs, 35*(6), 1114–1120. https://doi.org/10.1377/hlthaff.2016.0082

Wilkinson, R., & Marmot, M. G. (1998). *The solid facts: Social determinants of health*. Copenhagen, Denmark: Centre for Urban Health, World Health Organization.

Winslow, C. E. (1920). The untilled fields of public health. *Science, 51*(1306), 23–33. https://doi.org/10.1126/science.51.1306.23

World Health Assembly. (2009, May 22). *Reducing health inequities through action on the social determinants of health* (WHA62.14). Geneva, Switzerland: Author. http://apps.who.int/gb/ebwha/pdf_files/WHA62-REC1/WHA62_REC1-en-P2.pdf

World Health Assembly. (2011, October 21). *Rio political declaration on social determinants of health*. Rio de Janiero, Brazil: World Health Organization. https://www.who.int/sdhconfer-ence/declaration/Rio_political_declaration.pdf

World Health Organization. (2006). *Constitution of the World Health Organization*. Geneva, Switzerland: Author. https://www.who.int/governance/eb/who_constitution_en.pdf

World Health Organization. (2010). *Accelerating progress towards the health-related Millennium Development Goals*. Geneva, Switzerland: Author. http://www.who.int/topics/millennium_development_goals/MDG-NHPS_brochure_2010.pdf?ua=1

World Health Organization. (2014a). *Health for the world's adolescents: A second chance in the second decade*. Geneva, Switzerland: Author. http://www.who.int/maternal_child_adolescent/documents/second-decade/en/

World Health Organization. (2014b). Health in All Policies (HiAP) framework for country action. *Health Promotion International, 29*(Suppl 1), i19–i28. https://doi.org/10.1093/heapro/dau035

World Health Organization. (2016). *Global monitoring of action on the social determinants of health: A proposed framework and basket of core indicators [consultation paper].* Geneva, Switzerland: Author. https://www.who.int/social_determinants/consultation-paper-SDH-Action-Monitoring.pdf?ua=1

World Health Organization. (2017). *World health statistics 2017: Monitoring health for the SDGs.* Geneva, Switzerland: Author. http://apps.who.int/iris/bitstream/10665/255336/1/9789241565486-eng.pdf?ua=1

The Global Epidemiology of Mental and Substance Use Disorders

Kevin C. Heslin

Introduction

Mental and substance use disorders (MSUD) are a major cause of disability worldwide. In 2017, depressive disorders were the third leading cause of years lived with disability, ranking higher than 351 other diseases and injuries assessed for 195 countries and territories (GBD 2017 Disease and Injury Incidence and Prevalence Collaborators, 2018). Globally, an estimated 12.9% of the world's population had a mental disorder in 2017 (Institute for Health Metrics and Evaluation, 2018). By identifying countries with both a high burden of mental illness and relatively scarce treatment resources, multinational studies can inform decisions on technical support and assistance by specialized agencies such as the World Health Organization (WHO). From a public health perspective, cross-national comparisons may also elucidate the links between mental illness and the multiplicity of circumstances in which people around the world are born, grow up, live, work, and grow older, as well as the different systems of care that are available to deal with their illnesses over the course of their lives (WHO, 2008).

Multinational research on the epidemiology of MSUD can provide more than comparisons between discrete geographic areas. As countries become increasingly connected and interdependent, such studies may also show how population mental health is related to the movement of people, goods, information, and ideas across borders. Increasing activity between countries through trade, investment, and migration, often referred to as indicators of the process of "globalization," may have consequences for

---

The original version of this chapter was revised. The correction to this chapter is available at https://doi.org/10.1007/978-3-030-18435-3_18

K. C. Heslin (✉)
National Center for Health Statistics, Washington, DC, USA

George Washington University, Washington, DC, USA
e-mail: kevin_heslin@gwu.edu

population mental health by facilitating the exposure to new risk and protective factors, the diffusion of innovative treatments, and the exchange of health-related information (Deaton, 2015). For example, expanding markets for Western entertainment media and its promulgation of thin body-type ideals have likely contributed to the rise of eating disorders among young women in Africa (Eddy, Hennessey, & Thompson-Brenner, 2007) and Asian region countries (Pike & Dunne, 2015) in recent years.

Globally, the number of people seeking refuge from life-threatening circumstances in their countries of origin is the highest it has been since the early 1990s, at 21.3 million (Betts & Collier, 2017). Trauma-related disorders among refugees can be exacerbated by a range of adverse resettlement experiences in destination countries (Kinzie, 2007; Kirmayer, Lemelson, & Barad, 2007), from encounters with unfamiliar cultural practices to inhuman treatment in immigration detention centers and the forced separation of family members (U.S. Department of Homeland Security, 2017; Zucker & Greene, 2018).

International trade agreements can affect the availability and affordability of pharmaceuticals within countries. In the past, public officials have been compelled during trade negotiations to reform national policies on pharmaceutical marketing and pricing. For example, the USA has used trade talks to promote the removal of restrictions on direct-to-consumer advertising of pharmaceuticals in Australia and South Korea (Gleeson & Menkes, 2017), as well as the elimination of cost-containment measures such as therapeutic reference pricing in New Zealand (Gleeson, Lopert, & Reid, 2013). Because the availability of new psychopharmaceuticals and other treatments has often led to increases in the diagnosis of mental disorders that are appropriate for those treatments (Oppenheimer, 2014), this aspect of international trade could conceivably affect how frequently disorders are identified and treated. Repeated epidemiologic surveys have the potential to detect the impacts of evolving international trade relations on population mental health, as they are mediated through changes in policies affecting the accessibility and affordability of pharmaceuticals.

These developments provide the context for this overview of the global epidemiology of MSUD. The chapter reviews selected findings from the WHO World Mental Health (WMH) Survey Initiative and several other data sources on the prevalence and incidence of schizophrenia and psychotic-like experiences, depressive disorders, anxiety disorders, post-traumatic stress disorder (PTSD), eating disorders, attention deficit hyperactivity disorder (ADHD), personality disorders, and SUD. The chapter concludes with a review of the contribution of the epidemiology of MSUD to national mental health policy-making and a consideration of its potential to inform the work of international human rights organizations.

The World Health Organization (WHO) World Mental Health (WMH) Survey Initiative

The global statistics reviewed in this chapter are drawn largely from articles based on the WMH Survey Initiative, a cross-national epidemiologic research consortium of nationally or regionally representative surveys in 28 countries classified by the

World Bank income categories (World Bank, 2018). Using standardized survey measures, disorder classification systems, and field procedures in face-to-face interviews, the WMH Survey Initiative represents the largest and most systematic effort to date to minimize the methodologic limitations of previous cross-national studies (Fayyad et al., 2017; Kessler & Ustun, 2004). In each participating country, the WMH Survey Initiative assessed the presence of MSUD as defined by the *Diagnostic and Statistical Manual of Mental Disorders (DSM), Fourth Edition* (American Psychiatric Association, 2013), using the WHO Composite International Diagnostic Interview (CIDI) (Kessler et al., 2004). Methodologically, this coordinated approach has distinct advantages over the WHO Global Burden of Disease (GBD) studies, which draw largely from epidemiologic literature reviews and relatively isolated national studies (World Health Organization, 2005b).

In making cross-national comparisons, several features of the WMH Survey Initiative and other international studies should be kept in mind. Kessler et al. have acknowledged concerns about the cross-cultural validity of research diagnostic instruments such as the CIDI, noting that estimates of the prevalence of some disorders in developing countries are questionably low (Kessler et al., 2004; Kessler & Ustun, 2004; Kessler, Alonso, Chatterji, & He, 2014). It is possible that the social, religious, and/or legal contexts of some countries reduce the willingness of survey respondents to report thoughts, feelings, and behaviors potentially indicative of mental disorders or the use of substances (Degenhardt et al., 2017). Indeed, local cultural norms could influence whether psychiatric symptoms are even experienced in psychological or emotional terms, which could in turn affect whether respondents endorse the symptom descriptions included in survey instruments (Bhugra & Mastrogianni, 2004).

It is important to note that unexpected findings on the use of mental health specialty services by apparent non-cases in some WMH Survey Initiative studies may actually reflect appropriate service use by individuals with subthreshold symptoms or with disorders not assessed by the CIDI (Wang et al., 2007). Finally, country-level response rates in the WMH Survey Initiative varied widely, from 45.9% in France to 97.2% in the Medellin metropolitan area of Colombia. Cross-national comparisons could be biased to the extent that survey response rates are related to the prevalence of MSUD and service use, although the weighting of data by population sociodemographic distributions should reduce that bias in the final estimates (Kessler et al., 2010; Wang et al., 2007). In the next sections, the author will examine the descriptive epidemiology of a number of MSUD through a review of studies from the WMH Survey Initiative, the GBD studies, and several other data sources.

Schizophrenia and Psychotic-Like Experiences

Schizophrenia is a complex disorder characterized by the three main symptom domains of delusions, hallucinations, and disorganized speech and behavior, with a typical age of onset in late adolescence or early adulthood. Schizophrenia is relatively rare, and the costs of finding cases through population-based surveys are prohibitive. If the true prevalence of schizophrenia was 0.5% in the population, prevalence estimates for three age groups by two gender groups, with 30 respondents in the numerator of each of the resulting six cells, would require that 36,000 individuals be interviewed (Eaton, Chen, & Bromet, 2011).

Probably the most credible information on the epidemiology of schizophrenia comes from population-based registers that draw data from inpatient and outpatient facilities for an entire country, in which treatment for schizophrenia and other health conditions is free of charge. For example, the Danish Psychiatric Central Research Register contains information on every psychiatric admission since 1970, as well as outpatient treatment and emergency room contacts since 1995 (Mors, Perto, & Mortensen, 2011). The register contains unique identification numbers that permit linkages to the Danish Civil Registration System, an administrative register that contains individual-level data on all persons residing in Denmark, with updates on migration, births, and deaths made on a daily basis (Schmidt, Pedersen, & Sorensen, 2014). All Danish residents are required to notify the Danish authorities of changes in address, both within the country and when moving to or returning from another country. These daily updates on migration and vital status permit the calculation of person-time at risk for the denominators of incidence rates in epidemiologic studies.

Linking records from the Danish Psychiatric Central Register and the Danish Civil Registration System, Thorup, Waltoft, Pedersen, Mortensen, and Norderntoft (2007) used data on all individuals born in Denmark between 1934 and 1990 to estimate age- and gender-specific incidence rates of schizophrenia from ages 15 to 72 (Thorup et al., 2007). Both men and women had peak incidence rates at ages 22 and 23, although the rate for men at that age was twice as high as that for women (approximately 80 and 40 incident cases per 100,000 person-years, respectively). With increasing age, however, the direction of this gender difference reversed. Whereas men had significantly higher incidence rates in the age range of 17–40 years, women had higher rates in the 50-to-68-year-old age range. Comparing cumulative incidence, i.e., the percentage of all people who had received a diagnosis up to a given age, rates were higher for men than women at all ages. By age 72, cumulative incidence was approximately 35% higher among men than woman (1.59% and 1.17%, respectively).

Increasingly, schizophrenia is viewed as a neurodevelopmental disorder influenced by an array of environmental risk factors that can affect the brain during early development, including prenatal influenza exposure, obstetric complications, and maternal and intrauterine nutritional deficiencies (McGrath, Feron, Burne, Mackay-Sim, & Eyles, 2003; McGrath, Nunes, & Quitkin, 2003). Given the heterogeneity of these environmental risks, it is not surprising the literature shows considerable variation in prevalence and incidence estimates globally. Saha, Chant, Welham, and McGrath (2005) reviewed estimates of the prevalence of schizophrenia from 188 studies published between 1965 and 2002, based on data from 46 countries. The mean lifetime prevalence estimate across all countries was 0.43%, with variation by country ranging from 0.18% in the 10th percentile of estimates to 1.16% in the 90th percentile (Saha et al., 2005).

The study of environmental risk factors for schizophrenia has focused mainly on in utero exposures that could affect the developing brain. However, a variety of stressors throughout the life course can precipitate the onset of schizophrenia in vulnerable individuals. For example, refugees fleeing war, genocide, and other life-threatening circumstances in their countries of origin are at greater risk of mental disorders, including schizophrenia. A Swedish population registry-based study of post-migration onset of schizophrenia and other psychoses among refugee and non-refugee immigrants from sub-Saharan Africa, Asia, Eastern Europe, Russia, the Middle East, and North Africa was conducted by Hollander et al. (2016). They found that, compared with non-refugee immigrants, refugees had more than 60% greater risk of first-onset schizophrenia over the study follow-up period, in models accounting for age, sex, income, and residential population density (Hollander et al., 2016). It is important to note that increased prevalence of schizophrenia among migrants compared with nonmigrants may also be related to selective migration, i.e., the greater tendency for individuals with an existing predisposition or vulnerability to a mental disorder to migrate (Morgan, Charalambides, Hutchinson, & Murray, 2010). However, the need to flee life-threatening circumstances seems a more plausible explanation for the "selective" migration of refugees than does a pre-migration disposition to mental disorder.

Although schizophrenia is a low-prevalence disorder, it was ranked as the 12th most disabling condition in a list of 333 diseases and injuries in the GBD Study of 2016, a meta-analysis that generated age-standardized prevalence estimates of the disorder globally, as well as by region and country (GBD 2016 Disease and Injury Incidence and Prevalence Collaborators, 2017). Regionally, the highest age-standardized point prevalence was in the East Asian countries of China, North Korea, and Taiwan (0.42%). Investigating potential causes of the higher prevalence of schizophrenia in China, one study estimated the cumulative risk for the disorder among the cohort of individuals who would have been in utero in Anhui province at the time of the Great Chinese Famine of 1959–1961. For the cohort of live births from the famine years of 1960 and 1961, the cumulative risk of adult schizophrenia was twice as high as it was for those born in the period immediately before (1956–1958) and after (1962–1965) the famine, thus supporting the hypothesis that intrauterine nutritional deficiency increases the risk of schizophrenia (St Clair et al., 2005).

Gender differences in schizophrenia have been documented extensively. In the review by Saha et al. (2005), mean lifetime prevalence for men was approximately 8% higher than that for women (0.37% vs. 0.34%, respectively). By contrast, the incidence of schizophrenia was approximately 40% higher among men than women—with mean rates, respectively, of 16.2 vs. 11.3 per 100,000 population (Saha et al., 2005). It is possible that clinicians and psychiatric researchers overdiagnose schizophrenia in men at first contact, thereby biasing upward incidence estimates among men (Guloksuz & van Os, 2018). Alternatively, the greater gender difference in incidence than lifetime prevalence estimates could reflect either better outcomes or greater illness-related mortality among men; that is, men may exit the population of people with schizophrenia faster than do women through either remission or earlier death, which would decrease prevalence for men. However, a review of studies in developing countries found only mixed support for systematic differences in schizophrenia outcomes by gender. For example, studies in India and Ethiopia found that the course and outcomes of schizophrenia were better for women than men, whereas men in Colombia and Nigeria tended to have better outcomes than women (Cohen, Patel, Thara, & Gureje, 2008).

Gender comparisons of first-onset schizophrenia based on historical data are further complicated by modifications in diagnostic classification systems over time. Specifically, an age exclusion limiting the diagnosis of schizophrenia to individuals with first onset before age 45 was included in the DSM-III in 1980. Because of the well-replicated observation that men have an earlier age of onset of schizophrenia than do women, this age exclusion contributed to an excess of cases among men in lifetime prevalence estimates (Castle, Wessely, & Murray, 1993). By 1987, the DSM-III-R had removed this age exclusion while adding a new exclusion for patients with nonbizarre delusions without hallucinations—a change that was shown in one study to reduce the number of patients diagnosed with schizophrenia by 10% (Fenton, McGlashan, & Heinssen, 1988). Historically, concerns about the effects of diagnostic criteria on estimates of the incidence and prevalence of schizophrenia (overall and by gender) have not been limited to the DSM but have also included the Research Diagnostic Criteria, Schneider's First-Rank Symptoms, and other classification systems (Lewine, Burbach, & Meltzer, 1984).

Psychotic-Like Experiences

As a discrete diagnostic entity, schizophrenia increasingly is regarded in the literature as the only most severe, chronically debilitating endpoint of a broad spectrum of psychotic disorders. This includes schizophreniform disorder, delusional disorder, brief psychotic disorder, and—at the least severe end of the spectrum—a variety of psychotic-like experiences that do not necessarily indicate an underlying psychotic disorder (Guloksuz & van Os, 2018; Perala et al., 2007).

Although the scientific validity and clinical utility of the concept of a psychosis spectrum is a matter of ongoing debate, a number of epidemiologic studies have examined psychotic-like experiences and symptoms as points on a continuum rather than as indicators of discrete, mutually exclusive diagnostic categories (David, 2010; Kendler, Gallagher, Abelson, & Kessler, 1996; Lawrie, Hall, McIntosh, Owens, & Johnstone, 2010; McGrath et al., 2017; Nuevo et al., 2012; van Os, Hanssen, Bijl, & Ravelli, 2000). Psychotic-like experiences are apparently not rare, and their prevalence varies geographically, according to several cross-national studies.

In the 1970s, the International Pilot Study of Schizophrenia found no major cross-national differences in the prevalence of schizophrenia and other psychotic disorders across nine countries, but there was wide variation in the percentage of respondents reporting specific psychotic-like experiences. For example, auditory hallucinations had a prevalence of 9% in Washington, DC, and 46% in Cali, Colombia, whereas delusions had a prevalence of 11% in Moscow and 24% in

Taipei (International Pilot Study of Schizophrenia & World Health Organization, 1973; Sartorius, Shapiro, Kimura, & Barrett, 1972). More recently, Nuevo et al. (2012) reported variations across 52 countries in the prevalence of four separate psychotic-like experiences (delusional mood, delusions of reference and persecution, delusions of control, and visual and auditory hallucinations). Overall, 11.4% of study participants with no lifetime history of schizophrenia reported having had at least one of these experiences in the 12 months before the interview, reaching as high as 16.3% in South Africa among the high-/upper-middle-income countries and 45.8% in Nepal among the low-/lower-middle-income countries.

Schizophrenia and other non-affective psychoses were not assessed in the WMH Survey Initiative because results from validation studies suggested that these conditions have been overestimated in layperson interviews (Wang et al., 2007). However, data on psychotic-like experiences were collected that provided important information on the association of these phenomena with histories of childhood adversity and abuse. McGrath et al. (2017) found that among seven types of adverse childhood experiences related to maladaptive family functioning, childhood sexual abuse had the strongest independent association with subsequent onset of psychotic-like experiences during childhood (4–12 years old). Childhood sexual abuse was also associated with onset of psychotic experiences in adolescence (13–19 years old) and later adulthood (30 years and older).

Depressive Disorders

The term "depression" is used to refer to a wide range of mental states that are often self-limiting and do not require professional attention. To establish the diagnosis of major depressive disorder (MDD), five of nine symptoms, one of which must be depressed mood or loss of interest or pleasure, must be present during the same 2-week period (APA, 2013). The GBD Study reported a 4.4% worldwide prevalence of depressive disorders in 2015 (WHO, 2017). A 2017 study based on WMH Survey Initiative data from 21 countries reported a 4.6% estimate for 12-month prevalence of MDD (Thornicroft et al., 2017). This is closer to the GBD Study estimate (WHO, 2017) than an earlier WMH Survey Initiative article reporting a 12-month MDD prevalence of 5.5% in ten developed countries and 5.9% in seven developing countries (Kessler et al., 2010).

Use of Services

Major depressive disorder often begins in youth or middle age, and the resulting economic losses because of impairments in work, school, and other aspects of role functioning have made the accessibility and affordability of high-quality mental health services a critical public policy concern for developed and developing countries alike (Wells, Sturm, Sherbourne, & Meredith, 1999). The WMH Survey Initiative found the use of mental health services by people with MDD shows wide cross-national variation. The percentage of people with MDD in the previous 12 months who received any type of MDD treatment ranged from 5.9% in China to 33.2% in Peru among low-/middle-income countries and from 20.2% in Italy to 61.8% in Spain among high-income countries. Comparing all low-/middle-income countries with all high-income countries, the percentage of individuals with MDD receiving specific types of treatment was, respectively, 11.2% versus 22.6% for specialty psychiatric services, 8.6% versus 29.6% for general medical services, and 4.6% versus 7.4% for nonmedical services (Kessler et al., 2015).

A major barrier to the use of services for MDD is a lack of recognition of the need for treatment by affected individuals, which could in turn influence how symptoms are communicated to others who might be in a position to facilitate the use of services (Hanlon, Fekadu, & Patel, 2014). In a study of 12-month MDD from the WMH Survey Initiative, only one out of every three affected people (34.6%) in low-/lower-middle-income countries recognized they needed treatment; the corresponding statistic for the high-income countries was two out of every three affected people (64.9%) (Thornicroft et al., 2017). Combining responses from countries of all income levels, 71.1% of people with MDD who recognized a need for treatment made at least one visit to a service provider in the previous 12 months; unfortunately, only 41.0% of these service users received treatment that could be considered minimally adequate in terms of medications and/or healthcare provider visits. This potential quality-of-care problem was worse in low-/lower-middle-income countries, where only one out of every five service users (20.5%) received care that was minimally adequate (Thornicroft et al., 2017). Examining problems with quality of care for depression from the supply side, a seminal WHO study showed wide variation in the detection of depression by primary care physicians across 14 countries (Sartorius, Ustun, Lecrubier, & Wittchen, 1996). Overall, physicians detected only half of all cases, with sites in several countries being even lower than that: 19.3% in Nagasaki, Japan; 26.6% in Ibadan, Nigeria; and 28.4% in Ankara, Turkey (Lecrubier, 2001).

Functional Limitations and Age

The WMH Survey Initiative examined the role and other functional impairments that could reduce labor market participation among individuals with MDD. Because employment is the main source of household income and household spending, the functional impairments associated with MDD could conceivably affect economic growth (Frumkin, 2000). Therefore, it seems counterintuitive that younger respondents with MDD in developed countries fared far worse than did their counterparts in developing countries in terms of the mean number of days they were unable to work or fulfill other routine obligations in the past year. Specifically, the mean number of days "out of role" were up to twice as high for the three youngest age groups in the developed as compared with the developing countries (Kessler et al., 2010).

One explanation for the greater degree of MDD-related functional impairments among respondents in developed countries is the possible mental health risks associated with more affluent lifestyles ("affluenza"), which may provide relatively fewer opportunities for younger people to develop adaptive coping strategies and emotional resilience (Koplewicz, Gurian, & Williams, 2009). However, this interpretation of an association between higher income and functional impairments at the national level is questionable, because the prevalence of functional impairments in a developed country could be disproportionately concentrated among poorer residents. Rather than overall national income, functional impairments in MDD and other conditions could be related to greater income inequality, i.e., a more uneven distribution of income across the population (Picketty, 2015). According to a WMH Survey Initiative study, the poorest respondents in the high-income countries of France, Germany, New Zealand, and the USA had twice the odds of depression than their high-income compatriots—a difference that was not found between income groups in the low- to middle-income countries (Kessler & Bromet, 2013). Finding a strong positive association between income inequality and the prevalence of mental disorders among 12 high-income countries, Pickett and Wilkinson (2010) suggested that inequality increases status competition and insecurity to the detriment of social relationships and cultural institutions that foster mental health (Pickett & Wilkinson, 2010).

Epidemiologic surveys consistently report that the prevalence of depressive disorders decreases with age and is particularly low among individuals aged 65 and older. Findings from a WMH Survey Initiative study showed that an age-associated decrease in the prevalence of 12-month MDD was less common in developing than developed countries (Kessler et al., 2010). In fact, when the data from developing countries were aggregated, MDD prevalence was found to increase with age (from 5.3% among respondents aged 18–34 to 7.5% among respondents over age 64). By contrast, when the data from all of the developed countries were aggregated, MDD prevalence ranged from a high of 7.0% in the youngest age group (18–34 years old) to a low of 2.6% in the oldest (65 and older). Exceptions to this overall pattern among the participating developed countries were Italy, Israel, and Spain, where the prevalence of MDD did not change significantly with age. Among the developed countries, Israel had the highest prevalence of MDD among respondents aged 65 and older (6.6%), whereas Japan had the lowest (1.0%) (Kessler et al., 2010).

Comorbid Conditions

The presence of comorbid MSUD among people with depression can complicate clinical management, with potentially serious consequences in terms of disablement and suicidal ideation and behavior. One of the strongest predictors of such outcomes among people with MDD is comorbid anxiety disorders (Wu & Fang, 2014). In a WMH Survey Initiative study, 19.5% of respondents with comorbid 12-month MDD and anxiety disorder reported that they had "seriously thought about committing suicide" in the previous 12 months compared with 8.9% of respondents without comorbid anxiety (Kessler et al., 2015). Among high-income countries, the prevalence of suicidal ideation in respondents with comorbid 12-month MDD and anxiety disorder was highest in Japan (32.7%), and among low-/middle-income countries, the highest prevalence of suicidal ideation with these comorbid disorders was in Colombia and Nigeria (both 20.8%).

Bipolar Disorders

Bipolar and related disorders are a spectrum of conditions that historically have roots in the classic diagnostic constructs of manic depression and affective psychoses. The defining features of these disorders are episodes of elevated, expansive, or irritable mood (mania, hypomania) alternating with episodes of depression of varying lengths and degrees of intensity (APA, 2013). The WMH Survey Initiative provides information on the global prevalence of bipolar spectrum (BPS) conditions, an overarching category that encompasses the more specific diagnoses of bipolar I/II disorders as well as subthreshold bipolar cases.

Aggregated across 11 countries in the Americas, Europe, and Asia, the lifetime and 12-month prevalence of BPS among adults were 2.4% and 1.5%, respectively (Merikangas et al., 2011). Broken down to country-level estimates, the USA had the highest lifetime and 12-month prevalence (4.4% and 2.8%), whereas India had the lowest (0.1% and 0.1%). As with a number of other mental disorders, higher-income countries tended to have higher prevalence of BPS; however, there were some notable exceptions to that pattern in both directions. For example, the high-income country of Japan had relatively low lifetime prevalence of BPS (0.7%), whereas the low-income country of Colombia had relatively high lifetime prevalence (2.6%). The WMH Survey Initiative also showed that comorbidities are common in BPS. Specifically, anxiety disorders, SUD, and behavioral disorders (e.g., conduct disorder and intermittent explosive disorder) had lifetime prevalence estimates of 62.6%, 36.6%, and 44.8%, respectively, among respondents with BPS across all participating countries (Merikangas et al., 2011).

Use of Services

Despite the often-adverse effects of BPS on role functioning, the use of mental health services by adults with BPS is quite low. Across all countries represented in the study by Merikangas et al. (2011), less than half of individuals with lifetime BPS diagnoses reported any use of services in the mental health sector. In country-level estimates grouped by the World Bank income categories, mental health service use among respondents with BPS was 25.2% in low-/lower-middle-income countries, 33.9% in upper-middle-income countries, and 50.2% in high-income countries. Given that the severity of depressive episodes was found to be greater among people with BPS in the lower-income countries, the lower use of mental health services in these countries is a cause for concern (Merikangas et al., 2011).

Anxiety Disorders

An apprehensive anticipation of future threats characterized by varying degrees of fear, worry, or physical tension, anxiety in moderate levels may actually be adaptive by motivating individuals to prepare for situations involving a perceived increase in risk. Anxiety is a symptom found in nearly all mental disorders. When anxiety is the main symptom causing an individual clinically significant distress and impairment, the diagnosis of an anxiety disorder may be made. Anxiety disorders have been among the most prevalent mental disorders in community epidemiologic studies using modern diagnostic criteria (Horwath, Gould, & Weissman, 2011). This section describes cross-national findings on the epidemiology of generalized anxiety disorder (GAD), separation anxiety disorder, social anxiety disorder, and specific phobia.

Generalized Anxiety Disorders

The symptoms of GAD are common and relatively diffuse. Although symptoms are persistent and present "for more days than not" for at least 6 months (APA, 2013), the sense of apprehensive expectation characteristic of anxiety disorders may be relatively minimal, and there are no panic attacks. Further, patients are often not able to identify a specific object or event as the focal point of worry, as is the case with specific phobia. Therefore, GAD is often regarded in clinical practice as a residual diagnostic category for patients who do not meet the more specific criteria for other disorders (e.g., specific phobia, obsessive-compulsive disorder). A diagnosis of GAD involves the presence of excessive anxiety and worry that is difficult for the patient to control, accompanied by three or more of the following six symptoms for at least 6 months: restlessness, fatigue, difficulty concentrating, irritability, muscle tension, and sleep disturbance (APA, 2013).

Within countries, the prevalence of GAD tended to be higher among lower-income, less-educated population subgroups in a WMH Survey Initiative study (Ruscio et al., 2017). When the data were aggregated at the country level, however, high-income countries had a higher prevalence of GAD (5.0%) than did middle-income and low-income countries (2.8% and 1.6%, respectively). Similarly, the prevalence of severe role impairment related to GAD was greater among the higher-income countries, reaching approximately 80% among affected individuals in the Netherlands and Romania. By contrast, the course of the disorder was somewhat more chronic and unremitting in the lower-income countries, with 59.5% of lifetime cases also screening positive for GAD in the previous 12 months, compared with 56.1% in middle-income and 45.9% in high-income countries. This persistence of symptoms in the lower-income countries may be related to the relatively lower levels of treatment among individuals with 12-month GAD, particularly for specialty mental health and general medical services (Ruscio et al., 2017).

Separation Anxiety Disorder

Separation anxiety disorder is more common among children than among adults; however, it can have serious functional consequences for those adults who are affected. Because of the excessive fear or anxiety involved with anticipating or experiencing separation from major attachment figures (e.g., family members), adults with this disorder may entirely avoid situations such as working outside the home or travelling independently.

The lifetime prevalence of separation anxiety disorder among adults in the WMH Survey Initiative was fairly similar among countries grouped by World Bank income categories: 4.7% in the high-income group, 4.7% in upper-middle-income group, and 5.5% in low-/lower-middle-income group (Silove et al., 2015). The range of country-level prevalence estimates for the three income groups was also similar: from 1.2% (Spain) to 9.2% (USA) in the high-income group, 0.9% (Romania) to 7.7% (Brazil) in the upper-middle-income group, and 0.2% (Nigeria) to 9.8% (Colombia) in the low-/lower-middle-income group. However, what most distinguished the three World Bank income groups was the prevalence of severe role impairments in work, home management, social life, and personal relationships. The higher the income level, the greater the prevalence of impairments related to separation anxiety disorder: 41.4% (high income), 38.2% (upper-middle income), and 17.6% (low-/low-middle income).

The finding that adults with separation anxiety disorder in poorer countries had fewer impairments could be interpreted in light of known cultural differences in the belief that separation between family members is desirable or normal. Specifically, there is wide variation across counties concerning the age at which it is considered appropriate for individuals to move out of their parental home (APA, 2013). Multigenerational households are more common in countries that are less developed economically, particularly in rural areas with fewer wage labor opportunities, where adults can continue living and working on family farms (Ruggles & Heggeness, 2008). In such cases, the behavioral aspects of separation anxiety disorder could be compatible with local norms for social functioning.

Social Anxiety Disorder

Social anxiety disorder is a common and frequently disabling disorder characterized by excessive performance and interactional fears that cause substantial levels of distress and avoidance. In the WMH Survey Initiative, the lifetime prevalence of social anxiety disorder in 26 countries grouped by the World Bank income categories was highest for the high-income countries, at 5.5% (versus 2.9% for upper-middle-income and 1.6% for low-/lower-middle-income countries). Among all 26 countries, the USA had the highest lifetime prevalence, at 12.1% (Stein et al., 2017).

Comparing high- and lower-income countries, assessments of equity in the accessibility of mental health services can be based on the degree to which indicators of increased need such as functional impairments determine the use of services (Andersen & Davidson, 1996). In the WMH Survey Initiative study, functional impairments among people with 12-month social anxiety disorder were more common in the higher-income countries, with the Netherlands having the highest prevalence of impairments at work (56.8%) and home (41.9%). However, the use of specialty mental health services was related to increased levels of impairment only in the high-income countries, raising concerns about global equity in access to care. Specifically, 34.4% of the most functionally impaired respondents in the high-income countries used specialty mental health services, compared with 19.2% of their counterparts with mild impairment. By contrast, in the low-/lower-middle-income countries, specialty mental health service use among the most impaired respondents was actually lower than that among respondents with mild impairment (6.3% vs. 10.7%, respectively) (Stein et al., 2017).

Specific Phobia

A key feature of specific phobia is that the fear or anxiety experienced is restricted to the presence of a particular stimulus—most commonly animals, blood, features of the natural environment (e.g., heights, storms, water), and enclosed places such as elevators and airplanes (APA, 2013). In an analysis pooling WMH Survey Initiative data from 22 countries, Wardenaar, Lim, Al-Hamzawi, and Alonso (2018) reported that the lifetime and 12-month prevalence of specific phobia were 7.4% and 5.5%, respectively. Stratifying by income at the national level, lifetime prevalence was higher in the high-income (8.1%) and upper-middle-income (8.0%) countries than in low-/lower-middle-income (5.7%) countries. Within each of these three national income categories, however, the range of lifetime prevalence estimates was quite similar: from 3.4% (Japan and Poland) to 12.5% (USA) among the high-income countries, 3.8% (Romania) to 12.5% (Brazil) among the upper-middle-income countries, and 2.6% (China) to 12.5% (Colombia) among the low-/lower-middle-income countries (Wardenaar et al., 2018).

Use of Services

A substantial evidence base exists for the treatment of anxiety disorders, especially for selective serotonin reuptake inhibitors (SSRIs) and various types of cognitive behavioral therapy (CBT). Because SSRIs are available as low-cost generics and CBT is a time-limited intervention requiring relatively low levels of resources, the WHO has identified anxiety disorders as appropriate for scaling up interventions in resource-limited settings (Eaton, De Silva, Rojas, & Patel, 2014). Findings from the WMH Survey Initiative, however, suggest that considerable barriers to treatment for anxiety disorders exist across countries in all World Bank income categories and that the use of treatment of adequate quality are, in some lower-income countries, unfortunately low. Specifically, an analysis of data from 21 countries examined the use of any treatment for anxiety, as well as the use of "possibly adequate treatment." Treatment was defined broadly as a course of pharmacotherapy for at least 1 month with at least four medical doctor visits or as psychotherapy, complementary/alternative medicine, or nonmedical care (e.g., social work counseling in a nonmedical setting) for at least eight visits. Not surprisingly, the results showed an inverse relationship between country income and the percentage of respondents with 12-month anxiety disorders who received possibly adequate treatment: 13.8% of respondents in high-income countries, 7.1% in upper-middle-income countries, and 2.3% in lower-middle-income countries. Results at the country level were even more revealing. No respondents with 12-month anxiety disorders in Nigeria, for example, reported receiving possibly adequate treatment in the previous 12 months. Corresponding findings for Lebanon (an upper-middle-income country), Iraq, and Peru were, respectively, 1.3%, 1.7%, and 1.1% (Alonso et al., 2018).

Post-traumatic Stress Disorder

Formerly categorized as a type of anxiety disorder, post-traumatic stress disorder (PTSD) is a key diagnosis in the relatively recent DSM category of trauma- and stressor-related disorders (APA, 2013). A defining characteristic of PTSD and related conditions is previous exposure to a traumatic or stressful event, whether it was a single overwhelming event or a period of prolonged, repeated abuse. The distress following such events can often be characterized in terms of anxiety or fear, but what distinguishes PTSD and other trauma- and stressor-related disorders from anxiety disorders is the predominance of additional clinical features. These include anhedonia (loss of enjoyment in life experiences), dysphoria (feelings of depression, discontent, or indifference), dissociation (the splitting of thoughts from emotional significance), and outwardly angry or aggressive symptoms (APA, 2013). The risk of onset and severity of PTSD varies across cultural groups within and across countries and regions of the world. The variation reflects differences in the frequency of various types of traumatic events (e.g., genocide, car accidents), the ongoing sociocultural context (e.g., pervasive coverage of gun violence in news and entertainment media), pre-traumatic factors (childhood material deprivation), and other factors (e.g., acculturative stress among migrants).

Refugees fleeing armed conflict, persecution, and other types of potentially life-threatening traumatic events in their countries of origin are a key focus of concern in the field of global mental health, as these individuals are at greater risk of PTSD and other common mental disorders than are non-refugee migrants. For many survivors, exposure to such trauma is prolonged and disabling. Further, enduring economic problems, discrimination, and violence can reactivate symptoms of remitted disorders or precipitate the onset of new ones (Kinzie, 2007). Both pre- and post-migration onsets of PTSD among Latino and Asian refugee and non-refugee migrants to the USA were examined by Rasmussen, Crager, Baser, Chu, and Gany (2012) using the data from the National Latino and Asian American Study, a nationally representative household survey of Asian and Latino immigrants in the USA (Alegria et al., 2004). Compared with non-refugee migrants, refugees more often experienced traumatic events in their countries of origin, such as being an unarmed civilian in a war zone (5.0% vs. 32.1%), being a civilian exposed to ongoing terror (6.1% vs. 28.1%), seeing dead bodies or serious injuries in others (21.1% vs. 35.3%), and being exposed to a major natural disaster (19.1% vs. 26.2%). With these histories of trauma in their countries of origin, refugees more often reported pre-migration onset of PTSD than did non-refugee migrants. After immigrating to the USA, however, onset of PTSD did not differ between refugees and non-refugee migrants, suggesting that the common stressors of resettlement had mental health consequences for both groups (Rasmussen et al., 2012).

At the population level, war and genocide have often resulted in PTSD and related disorders among both combatants and civilians, with effects that can be permanently disabling (Kirmayer et al., 2007). A study using WMH Survey Initiative data examined the prevalence of several lifetime mental disorders among respondents who had been civilians in any of eight European countries or Japan during World War II. The intent of the study was to estimate the risk associated with having lived during that period in "a place where there was a war, revolution, military coup, or invasion" or "where there was ongoing terror of civilians for political, ethnic, religious, or other reasons." Aggregating responses across all participating countries, approximately 20% of respondents reported being civilians in a war zone/region of terror during the war, from 2.9% in Romania to 49.1% in Ukraine. Lifetime prevalence of MDD was 11.0% in the total sample and 17.3% among individuals who had been civilians in a war zone/region of terror. Although the war-/terror-exposed group did not have elevated risks for specific types of anxiety disorders compared with the unexposed group (at the time of the study, PTSD was still categorized as a DSM anxiety disorder), the prevalence of any lifetime anxiety disorder overall was 12.3% in the exposed group, compared with 8.6% in the total sample (Frounfelker et al., 2018).

Sexual assault is a global public health concern with the potential for a wide range of adverse health consequences, particularly the development of PTSD (Herman, 2015). Survey researchers assessing the relationship between various types of lifetime traumatic events and the risk of PTSD have typically asked respondents whether they have experienced each of several different lifetime traumatic events. To minimize response burden, respondents who have experienced multiple traumatic events have been asked further detailed questions about the single traumatic event that they considered the worst of all. However, this "worst event" method may overestimate the impact of a given type of traumatic event on PTSD risk among individuals with multiple lifetime traumas, because worst traumas are by definition atypical; such research would produce findings on the relationship between PTSD and the most severe experiences of sexual assault rather than sexual assault per se. For this reason, the WMH Survey Initiative randomly selected a single traumatic event from among a respondent's lifetime traumatic events for more detailed questions. An analysis of responses provided by women in 11 countries found that sexual assaults were reported by 12.1% of respondents overall, ranging from 1.8% in Spain to 26.1% in the USA. The prevalence of PTSD associated with randomly selected sexual assaults averaged 20.2% across participating countries, with a higher prevalence in the high-income (24.0%) than low-income (11.7%) countries. Because of the low prevalence of sexual assault among men in the WMH Survey Initiative sample, this analysis could focus on women only (Scott et al., 2018).

Eating Disorders

Cross-cultural research indicates that eating disorders such as binge-eating disorder, anorexia nervosa, and bulimia nervosa are more common in developed countries where food is generally abundant and the predominant body ideals emphasize thinness, particularly for girls and women. Binge-eating disorder is characterized by a perceived lack of control during recurrent eating episodes involving an amount of food that is larger than what most people would eat during a similar time period. The types of compensatory behaviors (e.g., vomiting, laxative use) that characterize bulimia nervosa do not accompany these episodes. The three essential features of anorexia nervosa are persistent restriction of energy intake, intense fear of becoming fat ("fat phobia"), or persistent behavior that interferes with weight gain, and distorted self-perception of body weight or shape (APA, 2013). Research from Hong Kong (Gordon, 2003) and India (Khandelwal, Sharan, & Saxena, 1995) has described cases of a variant form of anorexia nervosa among women in which fat phobia and distorted body image—key cognitive features among cases in the West—were largely absent. Such findings suggest that although eating disorders are not limited to Western cultures, their expression varies across countries in ways that reflect distinct cultural beliefs and practices.

Before the WMH Survey Initiative, few population-based data on eating disorders outside of the USA existed. Kessler et al. (2013) estimated the prevalence of binge-eating disorder and bulimia nervosa in one low-income, three upper-middle-income, and nine high-income countries. Sao Paolo, Brazil, had the highest prevalence of both binge-eating disorder (lifetime, 4.7%; 12 months, 1.8%) and bulimia nervosa (lifetime, 2.0%; 12 months, 0.9%) among the countries represented. At the other end of the range, Romania had zero prevalence of bulimia nervosa (both lifetime and 12 months) and the lowest prevalence of binge-eating disorder (lifetime, 0.2%; 12 months, 0.1%). Using the USA as the comparison group, speed of recovery from bulimia nervosa was more rapid in France and Portugal but less rapid in Italy and the Netherlands. By contrast, speed of recovery from binge-eating disorder was more rapid in the USA than in Colombia, France, Germany, Italy, and the Netherlands (Kessler et al., 2013).

Notably absent in this WMH Survey Initiative analysis were non-Western developing countries, which have been the focus of much work on the potential impacts of globalization on the growth of eating disorders. Increased exposure to thin body ideals in Western media is positively associated with symptoms of eating disorders in young women in Africa (Eddy et al., 2007) and Asian region countries (Pike & Dunne, 2015). An innovative study in Fiji found increased onset of dieting and self-induced vomiting among young ethnic Fijian women over a 3-year period during which television use was widely adopted within that county (Becker, Burwell, Gilman, Herzog, & Hamburg, 2002). Increases in the prevalence of eating disorders across developing and non-Western countries have coincided with rapid economic growth and widespread cultural transformations such as shifts in traditional family structures and gender roles (Pike & Dunne, 2015).

Attention Deficit Hyperactivity Disorder

The diagnosis of ADHD has been the focus of much clinical uncertainty and debate since regulatory approval of stimulant treatment for children first passed in the 1960s. Nevertheless, field trials have shown that the ADHD diagnosis can be made with high reliability (Faraone, 2011), based on assessment of the three main symptom dimensions of inattention, impulsivity, and hyperactivity.

Until two decades ago, diagnoses of ADHD were made primarily in the USA, Canada, and Australia. Traditionally, clinicians outside the USA have relied more often on the WHO International Classification of Diseases (ICD) than they have the DSM for diagnosis and treatment planning. In Europe, the diagnosis is called hyperkinetic disorder (HKD), as defined by the ICD, 10th edition. Diagnostic criteria for HKD criteria are more restrictive than those for ADHD, i.e., they require more symptoms, all of which must be present in more than one setting (e.g., both home and school). In recent years, with increased knowledge transfer enabled by the worldwide web and other information technology tools, the uptake of the DSM taxonomy by more clinicians outside of the USA is regarded as a key factor in the rising global prevalence of ADHD in adults (Conrad & Bergey, 2014).

Among the 20 WMH Survey Initiative surveys that assessed adult ADHD, the current prevalence among individuals aged 18–44 years was 2.8% (Fayyad et al., 2017). The prevalence of adult ADHD was higher in high-income (3.6%) and upper-middle-income (3.0%) countries than in low- and lower-middle-income countries (1.4%). Estimates ranged from 0.8% in Poland to 7.3% in France among the high-income countries; 0.6% in Romania to 5.9% in Sao Paolo, Brazil, among the upper-middle-income countries; and 0.6% in Iraq to 2.5% in Colombia among the low- and lower-middle-income countries (Fayyad et al., 2017).

Use of Services

The use of ADHD treatment by affected adults is quite low, even in high-income countries. Specifically, estimates of the percentage of respondents who received any ADHD-specific treatment were 0.0% in a number of countries, including the high-income countries of Belgium, France, Germany, Italy, Portugal, and the Murcia region of Spain (but 13.2% in the USA) and the upper-middle-income countries of Lebanon, Romania, and Medellin, Colombia (but 1.9% in both Mexico and Sao Paolo, Brazil). For all four of the low-/lower-middle-income countries represented in the analysis, the use of any ADHD-specific treatment by affected adults was 0.0%. These findings on low ADHD treatment use are a concern in light of reports of the substantial functional impairments associated with adult ADHD in terms of cognition, social interaction, mobility, and occupational functioning (Fayyad et al., 2017).

Personality Disorders

Personality disorders are diagnosed when maladaptive and relatively inflexible patterns of thinking, feeling, and behavior cause impairments across a wide range of situations, leading to repeated antagonistic, disruptive, and self-defeating experiences (APA, 2013). Cross-cultural assessment of personality disorders in both the clinical and research contexts should consider symptoms in light of various ethnic, cultural, and socioeconomic factors. For example, the kinds of cognitive and perceptual distortions that characterize schizotypal personality disorder may reflect culturally appropriate, non-pathological traits derived from long-standing religious beliefs and practices (APA, 2013). An additional caution is that, in many countries, the diagnosis of personality disorder reportedly has been used against socially vulnerable groups, especially young women, who do not conform to dominant culturally prescribed roles and forms of self-expression. Political dissidents are vulnerable to being diagnosed with a personality disorder and subsequently institutionalized when they take positions in opposition to national authorities (WHO, 2005a).

Personality disorders in the DSM are divided into three broad groupings or "clusters" based on descriptive similarities. Cluster A includes disorders that share odd and aloof features (paranoid, schizoid, and schizotypal personality disorders); Cluster B includes disorders with dramatic, impulsive, and erratic features (antisocial, borderline, histrionic, and narcissistic personality disorders); and Cluster C includes disorders with anxious and fearful features (avoidant, dependent, and obsessive-compulsive personality disorders) (Sadock, Sadock, & Ruiz, 2015). In an analysis of WMH Survey Initiative data by Huang et al. (2009), the prevalence of any personality disorder (all clusters combined) for the 13 participating countries was 6.1%. At the national or regional level, the prevalence of any personality disorder ranged from 2.4% in Western Europe (including Belgium, France, Germany, Italy, and Spain) to 7.9% in Colombia. For the three clusters of personality disorders, prevalence estimates based on combined data for all 13 countries were 3.6% for Cluster A, 1.5% for Cluster B, and 2.7% for Cluster C. Cluster A and B disorders were most prevalent in Colombia (5.3% and 2.1%, respectively), and Cluster C disorders were most prevalent in the USA (4.2%). Among the respondents with any personality disorder, there was wide geographic variation in the percentage reporting the use of professional services for "problems with emotions, nerves, or substance use" in the 12 months before the survey, with estimates ranging from 6.0% in Nigeria to 37.3% in the USA (Huang et al., 2009).

These findings from the WMH Survey Initiative represent the most comprehensive source of cross-national data on the prevalence of personality disorders; however, the investigators duly noted the concerns about the cross-cultural validity of the personality disorder screening instrument (Huang et al., 2009). In addition, only currently married individuals in a special "couples" subsample were screened for personality disorders in the participating Western European countries. To the extent that individuals with personality disorders may be less likely to become or remain married, this sampling approach specific to Western Europe may partly explain the relatively low prevalence estimates for that region.

Substance Use

A key feature of a variety of social interactions and cultural traditions, alcohol serves many purposes for the world's 2.3 billion drinkers (WHO, 2018). Progress in the economic development of a country can be accompanied by increases in both the availability of alcoholic beverages and the disposable income with which to purchase them, leading to greater consumption. One downside of this development is that harmful use is linked to over 200 serious and costly health problems, including alcoholic liver disease (e.g., hepatitis, cirrhosis), road injuries, cancers, and cardiovascular disease (Brick, 2008). The prevalence of heavy episodic or "binge" drinking is fairly equal across countries within the Americas, Southeast Asia, Eastern Mediterranean, and Western Pacific regions of the WHO. However, within the African region, heavy episodic drinking is more common in lower-income countries, whereas in the European region, it is more common in higher-income countries (WHO, 2018).

In an analysis of WMH Survey Initiative data from 17 countries, the vast majority of respondents reported lifetime alcohol use, with the lowest prevalence being in South Africa (40.6%) (Degenhardt et al., 2008). A consistent finding across countries was the substantial increase in the initiation of alcohol use that occurs between the ages of 15 and 21. For example, the percentage of respondents initiating alcohol use by the ages of 15 and 21 was, respectively, 29.0% and 77.5% in Mexico, 39.3% and 98.5% in Ukraine, and 50.1% and 93.1% in the USA. Notable for Germany is that fully 82.1% of respondents had initiated alcohol use by age 15 (and 97.8% by the age of 21). Although the majority of the WHO member states have some type of restriction on advertising to prevent early initiation of alcohol use, these efforts focus largely on national television and radio. Nearly half of member states report no advertising restrictions on the Internet and social media, suggesting that regulations in many countries lag behind technological advances in marketing to young people (WHO, 2018).

Cannabis is the most commonly used illicit substance globally, with an estimated 182 million nonmedical users aged 15–64 in 2013 (WHO, 2016). The United Nations Office on Drugs and Crime (2018, June) reports the highest prevalence of cannabis use in North America, Western Central Africa, and Oceania. Historically, countries have not collected and reported data on drug use in a uniform way. Because of the standardized methodology used in the WMH Survey Initiative, it is possible to make meaningful comparisons of the use of cannabis and other substances across countries. In each country participating in the WMH Survey Initiative, lifetime use of cannabis, cocaine, and tobacco was lower than that of alcohol, but estimates varied greatly across countries (Degenhardt et al., 2018). Specifically, lifetime use of cannabis ranged from 0.3% in the People's Republic of China to 42.4% in the USA, with the greatest percentage of respondents reporting the first use by age 15 in New Zealand (26.8%). Lifetime use of cocaine ranged from 0.0% in the People's Republic of China to 16.2% in the USA, with the greatest percentage of respondents reporting the first use by age 15 in the USA (2.5%). Lifetime use of tobacco ranged from 16.8% in Nigeria to 73.6% in the USA, with the greatest percentage of respondents reporting the first use by age 15 in Ukraine (46.0%).

Substance Use Disorders

An essential feature of SUD is that the affected individual continues to use the substance despite significant substance-related problems, which may include serious and sometimes fatal medical problems affecting multiple organ systems (APA, 2013). Additional diagnostic criteria include using a greater quantity of the substance than originally intended, repeated unsuccessful attempts to reduce or control use, and failure to fulfill major role obligations at work, school, or home because of continued use (APA, 2013). One of the greatest barriers to treatment for SUD is the denial or low recognition of these problems by affected individuals themselves, who may reject offers of help from friends, family members, and professionals (Connors, DiClemente, & Donovan, 2001). The stigmatization of people who misuse alcohol and drugs can also act as a deterrent to help-seeking and recovery. For example, a population-based survey of US adults found that respondents with alcohol use disorders were less likely to use health and social services for these conditions if they believed that most people were prejudiced against individuals who had ever received such services (Keyes et al., 2010).

An analysis of WMH Survey Initiative data from 26 countries found that 12-month prevalence of any SUD ranged from 0.2% in the low-/lower-middle-income country of Iraq to 6.6% in the low-/lower-middle-income country of Ukraine (Degenhardt et al., 2017). Although Iraq had the lowest prevalence of SUD, the percentage of respondents with disorders who recognized a need for treatment was actually highest there, at 61.5%, and lowest in the high-income country of Germany, at 12.8%. Among respondents across all countries who believed they needed treatment, 67.5% received it. Receipt of services ranged from a low of 26.5% in the low-/lower-middle-income country of Peru to a high of 95.4% in the low-/lower-middle-income country of Nigeria. However, receipt of SUD treatment of at least minimally adequate quality was, unfortunately, quite low among those who used any services in the previous 12 months. As noted above, Germany had the lowest percentage of respondents with 12-month disorders who perceived a need for treatment (12.8%), but 100% of those who received treatment in the previous 12 months had treatment that met the standards of minimally adequate quality—as did those who received treatment in Romania. Among all respondents with SUD, including both those who did and those who did not perceive a need for treatment, only 7.1% received at least minimally adequate treatment in the previous 12 months: 1.0% in low-/lower-middle-income countries, 4.3% in upper-middle-income countries, and 10.3% in high-income countries (Degenhardt et al., 2017).

Chronic misuse of alcohol and other substances may cause changes in brain chemistry that make one more susceptible to mental disorders. This "toxicity hypothesis" of MSUD comorbidity is supported by a WMH Survey Initiative study in 18 countries showing that the first onset of psychotic experiences was associated with temporally prior alcohol use disorders, extra-medical prescription drug use, and tobacco use, even after controlling for other temporally prior MSUD, as well as respondent age, sex, and country (Degenhardt et al., 2018). Conversely, psychotic experiences were also identified as risk factors (rather than outcomes) for the onset of disorders related to alcohol, nicotine, and other drugs—even after controlling for other temporally prior MSUD, as well as respondent age, sex, and country (Degenhardt et al., 2018). This finding is consistent with the "self-medication hypothesis" of MSUD comorbidity, which posits that individuals initiate substance use to relieve symptoms of mental disorders, eventually leading to development of comorbid SUD (McGrath et al., 2003).

Gender and the Evolving Epidemiology of Mental and Substance Use Disorders

Numerous epidemiologic studies have documented a higher prevalence of anxiety and mood disorders among women than men, as well as higher rates of SUD among men than women (Brady & Randall, 1999; Kuehner, 2003; Pigott, 1999). However, these gender differences may be narrowing over time, particularly in countries where opportunities for women in employment, participation in civic life, and access to sexual and reproductive health services have increased. With greater globalization in labor markets, these opportunities have likely played out differently for women in developed and developing countries. For women with caregiving responsibilities who work outside the home in low-paying jobs without childcare facilities, these increased employment opportunities could bring with them new sources of interpersonal stress, which could conceivably precipitate the onset of MSUD (Lewis & Araya, 2002).

Seedat et al. (2009) used WMH Survey Initiative data to examine gender differences in lifetime MSUD across birth cohorts within countries, as well as within birth cohorts across countries. Compared with older birth cohorts, the greater risk of MDD among women compared with men was less pronounced for more recent birth cohorts. The greater risk of intermittent explosive disorder and SUD among men compared with women also became less pronounced in younger cohorts. The 15 countries represented in the analysis were characterized in terms of a composite measure of "gender role traditionality" based on WMH survey data on education, income, age at marriage, and contraception use. The results showed that country-level decreases in the "gender role traditionality" measure were associated with a narrowing of the differences between women and men in MDD and SUD (Seedat et al., 2009).

Implications for Behavioral Health

Mental health policies and programs are essential tools for improving population health and reducing what is often referred to as "the mental health treatment gap," that is, the difference between the number of individuals in need of mental health services and those receiving them (Maulik, Daniels, McBain, & Morris, 2014). Across countries with considerably different healthcare systems, the WMH Survey Initiative showed that a substantial proportion of individuals with MSUD had not received any kind of mental health service in the previous 12 months, particularly in lower-income countries (Wang et al., 2007). A key challenge for the epidemiology of MSUD is overcoming obstacles to the translation of research findings into policy-relevant information that can be used by public officials to reduce these gaps.

To identify factors that influence the uptake of research findings into mental health policy-making, Weinberg et al. (2012) interviewed individuals involved in implementing the WMH Survey Initiative in 12 different countries. The authors concluded that the surveys generated strong interest among policy-makers within countries, especially when a member of the study team had established relationships with such officials through previous employment in government health agencies. For example, the interviewees from Australia and Israel stated that, because of these long-standing relationships, they were able to conduct tailored presentations on WMH survey findings to important government stakeholders. These same interviewees described how the WMH surveys and other sources of population health data played a role in advocating for expansions in public coverage of mental health services in their respective countries (Weinberg et al., 2012).

By funding epidemiologic MSUD surveys, government stakeholders can influence the selection of research topics in ways that advance important health policy objectives. In Northern Ireland, support of the WMH Survey Initiative enabled the Ministry of Health to promote a focus on the issue of PTSD in parts of the country affected by the "Troubles" of the 1970s to 1990s. Because the prevalence of PTSD in certain parts of Northern Ireland was considerably higher than that of other countries with recent histories of war, such as Israel and Lebanon, the Ministry funded a follow-up study of WMH Survey Initiative respondents who were young during the time of the Troubles to obtain more detailed information on their experiences of the conflict.

As another example of the use of epidemiologic data in policy-making, the WMH Survey Initiative study in France found that half of the respondents using antidepressant medication did not meet diagnostic criteria for a depressive disorder and a fifth of those taking antidepressants did so for less than 3 weeks (the minimum period believed to be needed for clinical effect). After the French House of Deputies learned of the potential misuse of antidepressants, they conducted an investigation using a variety of information sources, including findings from the country's WMH Survey Initiative study, and found that an unexpectedly high number of general practitioners in France were prescribing the medications (Weinberg et al., 2012).

As urgent as the need to reduce the mental health treatment gap is, an equally pressing issue for global mental health policy is identifying and eradicating the systematic abuse that many people with mental illness endure in various clinical, social, and legal contexts (Szmukler, 2014). In the introduction to the *Resource Book on Mental Health, Human Rights and Legislation*, the WHO (2005a) underscored the urgency of strengthening the human rights provisions of mental health legislation and reforming mental health treatment systems and practices worldwide:

> There are more than 450 million people with mental, neurological, or behavioral problems throughout the world. In many countries, they are among the most vulnerable and the least legally protected... In some communities, people with mental disorders are tied or chained to trees or logs. Others are incarcerated in prisons without having been accused of a crime. In many psychiatric institutions and hospitals, patients face gross violations of their rights. People are restrained with metal shackles, confined in caged beds, deprived of clothing, decent bedding, clean water or proper toilet facilities and are subject to abuse... people with mental disorders often face social isolation and severe stigmatization... including discrimination in education, employment, and housing. Some countries even prohibit people from voting, marrying, or having children.

The successful translation of WMH Survey Initiative results into national health policies raises the question of how epidemiologic research can inform efforts to promote and protect the human rights of people with mental illness worldwide. Because of various logistical and ethical obstacles to study implementation, the sampling frames of population-based surveys typically exclude hospitals, prisons, long-term care homes, and other facilities—i.e., the very settings where the use of involuntary placement, physical restraints, and forced seclusion can result in violations of international human rights laws. Nevertheless, data collection and analysis can further the goals of policies to eliminate the systematic abuse of people with mental illness and other disabilities. State signatories to the United Nations (UN) Convention on the Rights of Persons with Disabilities (CRPD) are obligated to ensure the monitoring of health and correctional facilities by independent bodies (Szmukler, Daw, & Callard, 2014). From a research perspective, the Government of Indonesia is a particularly noteworthy CRPD signatory, having made extensive use of data collected from both households and facilities in their efforts to eliminate the widespread practice of chaining individuals with mental disorders and other disabilities to long wooden planks (i.e., shackling). In Central Java, one official has asserted that "the target of zero shackling cases… can be achieved if data on victims can be gathered properly" through district-level community health centers (Collins, Tomlinson, Kakuma, Awuba, & Minas, 2014). Monitoring conducted by the nongovernmental organization Human Rights Watch indicates that these efforts have led to a promising reduction in shackling, but much work remains before the goal of eradication is reached (Human Rights Watch, 2018).

Working within logistical and ethical constraints on access to potential study respondents, one approach for epidemiologic studies relevant to these issues would be to elicit retrospective reports on conditions in health and correctional settings from former patients, residents, or convicts. In countries with population-based health registers, probability samples of former psychiatric inpatients could be drawn for patient experience surveys that include items on maltreatment. However, limited such studies may be, they could provide government stakeholders and international human rights organizations with useful information on conditions in some of the settings where people with mental illness are most vulnerable to harm.

References

Alegria, M., Takeuchi, D., Canino, G., Duan, N., Shrout, P., Meng, X. L., … Gong, F. (2004). Considering context, place and culture: the National Latino and Asian American Study. *International Journal of Methods in Psychiatric Research, 13*(4), 208–220.

Alonso, J., Liu, Z., Evans-Lacko, S., Sadikova, E., Sampson, N., Chatterji, S., … Thornicroft, G. (2018). Treatment gap for anxiety disorders is global: Results of the World Mental Health Surveys in 21 countries. *Depression and Anxiety, 35*(3), 195–208. https://doi.org/10.1002/da. 22711

American Psychiatric Association. (2013). *Diagnostic and statistical manual of mental disorders: DSM-5.* Arlington, VA: American Psychiatric Association.

Andersen, R. M., & Davidson, P. L. (1996). Measuring access and trends. In R. M. Andersen, T. H. Rice, & G. F. Kominski (Eds.), *Changing the U.S. health care system: Key issues in health services, policy, and management.* San Francisco: Jossey-Bass Publishers.

Becker, A. E., Burwell, R. A., Gilman, S. E., Herzog, D. B., & Hamburg, P. (2002). Eating behaviours and attitudes following prolonged exposure to television among ethnic Fijian adolescent girls. *British Journal of Psychiatry, 180,* 509–514. https://doi.org/10.1192/bjp.180.6.509

Betts, A., & Collier, P. (2017). *Refuge: Rethinking refugee policy in a changing world*. Oxford: Oxford University Press.

Bhugra, D., & Mastrogianni, A. (2004). Globalisation and mental disorders. Overview with relation to depression. *British Journal of Psychiatry, 184*, 10–20. https://doi.org/10.1192/bjp.184.1.10

Brady, K. T., & Randall, C. L. (1999). Gender differences in substance use disorders. *Psychiatric Clinics of North America, 22*(2), 241–251. https://doi.org/10.1016/S0193-953X(05)70074-5

Brick, J. (2008). *Handbook of the medical consequences of alcohol and drug abuse* (2nd ed.). New York, NY: Routledge.

Castle, D. J., Wessely, S., & Murray, R. M. (1993). Sex and schizophrenia: Effects of diagnostic stringency, and associations with premorbid variables. *British Journal of Psychiatry, 162*, 658–664. https://doi.org/10.1192/bjp.162.5.658

Cohen, A., Patel, V., Thara, R., & Gureje, O. (2008). Questioning an axiom: better prognosis for schizophrenia in the developing world? *Schizophrenia Bulletin, 34*(2), 229–244. https://doi.org/10.1093/schbul/sbm105

Collins, P. Y., Tomlinson, M., Kakuma, R., Awuba, J., & Minas, H. (2014). Research priorities, capacity, and networks in global mental health. In V. Patel, H. Minas, A. Cohen, & M. J. Prince (Eds.), *Global mental health: Principles and practice*. Oxford: Oxford University Press.

Connors, G. J., DiClemente, C. C., & Donovan, D. M. (2001). *Substance abuse treatment and the stages of change: Selecting and planning interventions*. New York: Guilford Press.

Conrad, P., & Bergey, M. R. (2014). The impending globalization of ADHD: notes on the expansion and growth of a medicalized disorder. *Social Science and Medicine, 122*, 31–43. https://doi.org/10.1016/j.socscimed.2014.10.019

David, A. S. (2010). Why we need more debate on whether psychotic symptoms lie on a continuum with normality. *Psychological Medicine, 40*, 1935–1942. https://doi.org/10.1017/S0033291710000188

Deaton, A. (2015). *The great escape: Health, wealth, and the origins of inequality*. Princeton, NJ: Princeton University Press.

Degenhardt, L., Chiu, W. T., Sampson, N., Kessler, R. C., Anthony, J. C., Angermeyer, M., … Wells, J. E. (2008). Toward a global view of alcohol, tobacco, cannabis, and cocaine use: findings from the WHO World Mental Health Surveys. *PLoS Medicine, 5*(7), e141. https://doi.org/10.1371/journal.pmed.0050141

Degenhardt, L., Glantz, M., Evans-Lacko, S., Sadikova, E., Sampson, N., Thornicroft, G., … Kessler, R. C. (2017). Estimating treatment coverage for people with substance use disorders: an analysis of data from the World Mental Health Surveys. *World Psychiatry, 16*(3), 299–307. https://doi.org/10.1002/wps.20457

Degenhardt, L., Saha, S., Lim, C. C. W., Aguilar-Gaxiola, S., Al-Hamzawi, A., Alonso, J., … McGrath, J. J. (2018). The associations between psychotic experiences and substance use and substance use disorders: Findings from the World Health Organization World Mental Health surveys. *Addiction, 113*(5), 924–934. https://doi.org/10.1111/add.14145

Eaton, J., De Silva, M., Rojas, G., & Patel, V. (2014). Scaling up services for mental health. In V. Patel, H. Minas, A. Cohen, & M. J. Prince (Eds.), *Global mental health: Principles and practice*. Oxford: Oxford University Press.

Eaton, W. W., Chen, C. Y., & Bromet, E. (2011). Epidemiology of schizophrenia. In M. T. Tsuang, M. Tohen, & P. B. Jones (Eds.), *Textbook in psychiatric epidemiology* (pp. 263–288). Chichester: Wiley.

Eddy, K. T., Hennessey, M., & Thompson-Brenner, H. (2007). Eating pathology in East African women: The role of media exposure and globalization. *Journal of Nervous and Mental Disease, 195*(3), 196–202. https://doi.org/10.1097/01.nmd.0000243922.49394.7d

Faraone, S. (2011). Epidemiology of attention deficit hyperactivity disorder. In M. T. Tsuang, M. Tohen, & P. B. Jones (Eds.), *Textbook in psychiatric epidemiology* (pp. 449–468). Chichester: Wiley.

Fayyad, J., Sampson, N. A., Hwang, I., Adamowski, T., Aguilar-Gaxiola, S., Al-Hamzawi, A., … Kessler, R. C. (2017). The descriptive epidemiology of DSM-IV Adult ADHD in the World

Health Organization World Mental Health Surveys. *ADHD Attention Deficit Hyperactivity Disorders, 9*(1), 47–65. https://doi.org/10.1007/s12402-016-0208-3

Fenton, W. S., McGlashan, T. H., & Heinssen, R. K. (1988). A comparison of DSM-III and DSM-III-R schizophrenia. *American Journal of Psychiatry, 145*(11), 1446–1449. https://doi.org/10.1176/ajp.145.11.1446

Frounfelker, R., Gilman, S. E., Betancourt, T. S., Aguilar-Gaxiola, S., Alonso, J., Bromet, E. J., ... Kessler, R. C. (2018). Civilians in World War II and DSM-IV mental disorders: results from the World Mental Health Survey Initiative. *Social Psychiatry and Psychiatric Epidemiology, 53*(2), 207–219. https://doi.org/10.1007/s00127-017-1452-3

Frumkin, N. (2000). *Guide to economic indicators*. London: M. E. Sharpe.

GBD 2016 Disease and Injury Incidence and Prevalence Collaborators. (2017). Global, regional, and national disability-adjusted life-years (DALYs) for 333 diseases and injuries and healthy life expectancy (HALE) for 195 countries and territories, 1990-2016: A systematic analysis for the Global Burden of Disease Study 2016. *Lancet, 390*(10100), 1260–1344. https://doi.org/10.1016/s0140-6736(17)32130-x

GBD 2017 Disease and Injury Incidence and Prevalence Collaborators. (2018). Global, regional, and national incidence, prevalence, and years lived with disability for 354 diseases and injuries for 195 countries and territories, 1990–2017: A systematic analysis for the Global Burden of Disease Study 2017. *Lancet, 392*, 1789–1858. https://doi.org/10.1016/S0140-6736(18)32279-7

Gleeson, D., Lopert, R., & Reid, P. (2013). How the Trans Pacific Partnership Agreement could undermine PHARMAC and threaten access to affordable medicines and health equity in New Zealand. *Health Policy, 112*(3), 227–233. https://doi.org/10.1016/j.healthpol.2013.07.021

Gleeson, D., & Menkes, D. B. (2017). Trade agreements and direct-to-consumer advertising of pharmaceuticals. *International Journal of Health Policy and Management, 7*(2), 98–100. https://doi.org/10.15171/ijhpm.2017.124

Gordon, R. A. (2003). Eating disorders east and west: A culture-bound syndrome unbound. In M. Nasser, M. Katzman, & R. Gordon (Eds.), *Eating disorders and cultures in transition* (pp. 1–16). New York, NY: Brunner-Routledge.

Guloksuz, S., & van Os, J. (2018). The slow death of the concept of schizophrenia and the painful birth of the psychosis spectrum. *Psychological Medicine, 48*(2), 229–244. https://doi.org/10.1017/s0033291717001775

Hanlon, C., Fekadu, A., & Patel, V. (2014). Interventions for mental disorders. In V. Patel, H. Minas, A. Cohen, & M. J. Prince (Eds.), *Global mental health: Principles and practice* (pp. 252–276). Oxford: Oxford University Press.

Herman, J. L. (2015). *Trauma and recovery: The aftermath of violence–from domestic abuse to political terror*. http://public.eblib.com/choice/publicfullrecord.aspx?p=2039735_0

Hollander, A. C., Dal, H., Lewis, G., Magnusson, C., Kirkbride, J. B., & Dalman, C. (2016). Refugee migration and risk of schizophrenia and other non-affective psychoses: Cohort study of 1.3 million people in Sweden. *BMJ, 352*, i1030. https://doi.org/10.1136/bmj.i1030

Horwath, E., Gould, F., & Weissman, M. M. (2011). Epidemiology of anxiety disorders. In M. T. Tsuang, M. Tohen, & P. B. Jones (Eds.), *Textbook in psychiatric epidemiology* (3rd ed., pp. 311–328). Chichester: Wiley.

Huang, Y., Kotov, R., de Girolamo, G., Preti, A., Angermeyer, M., Benjet, C., ... Kessler, R. C. (2009). DSM-IV personality disorders in the WHO World Mental Health Surveys. *British Journal of Psychiatry, 195*(1), 46–53. https://doi.org/10.1192/bjp.bp.108.058552

Human Rights Watch. (2018). *Indonesia: Shackling reduced, but persists. Oversight crucial to end abuse of people with disabilities*. Retrieved December 30, 2018, from https://www.hrw.org/news/2018/10/02/indonesia-shackling-reduced-persists

Institute for Health Metrics and Evaluation. (2018). *GBD results tool*. Retrieved December 29, 2018, from http://ghdx.healthdata.org/gbd-results-tool

International Pilot Study of Schizophrenia, & World Health Organization. (1973). *Report of the International Pilot Study of Schizophrenia* (WHO offset publication; no. 2). Geneva:

International Pilot Study of Schizophrenia. http://apps.who.int/iris/handle/10665/39405?loca le=es

Kendler, K. S., Gallagher, T. J., Abelson, J. M., & Kessler, R. C. (1996). Lifetime prevalence, demographic risk factors, and diagnostic validity of nonaffective psychosis as assessed in a US community sample. The National Comorbidity Survey. *Archives of General Psychiatry, 53*(11), 1022–1031. https://doi.org/10.1001/archpsyc.1996.01830110060007

Kessler, R. C., Abelson, J., Demler, O., Escobar, J. I., Gibbon, M., Guyer, M. E., … Zheng, H. (2004). Clinical calibration of DSM-IV diagnoses in the World Mental Health (WMH) version of the World Health Organization (WHO) Composite International Diagnostic Interview (WMHCIDI). *International Journal of Methods in Psychiatric Research, 13*(2), 122–139. https://doi.org/10.1002/mpr.169

Kessler, R. C., Alonso, J., Chatterji, S., & He, Y. (2014). The epidemiology and impact of mental disorders. In V. Patel, H. Minas, A. Cohen, & M. J. Prince (Eds.), *Global mental health: Principles and practice* (pp. 82–101). Oxford: Oxford University Press.

Kessler, R. C., Berglund, P. A., Chiu, W. T., Deitz, A. C., Hudson, J. I., Shahly, V., … Xavier, M. (2013). The prevalence and correlates of binge eating disorder in the World Health Organization World Mental Health Surveys. *Biological Psychiatry, 73*(9), 904–914. https://doi.org/10.1016/j.biopsych.2012.11.020

Kessler, R. C., Birnbaum, H. G., Shahly, V., Bromet, E., Hwang, I., McLaughlin, K. A., … Stein, D. J. (2010). Age differences in the prevalence and co-morbidity of DSM-IV major depressive episodes: results from the WHO World Mental Health Survey Initiative. *Depression and Anxiety, 27*(4), 351–364. https://doi.org/10.1002/da.20634

Kessler, R. C., & Bromet, E. (2013). The epidemiology of depression across cultures. *Annual Review of Public Health, 34*, 119–138. https://doi.org/10.1146/annurev-publhealth-031912-114409

Kessler, R. C., Sampson, N. A., Berglund, P., Gruber, M. J., Al-Hamzawi, A., Andrade, L., … Wilcox, M. A. (2015). Anxious and non-anxious major depressive disorder in the World Health Organization World Mental Health Surveys. *Epidemiology and Psychiatric Sciences, 24*(3), 210–226. https://doi.org/10.1017/s2045796015000189

Kessler, R. C., & Ustun, B. (2004). The World Mental Health (WMH) Survey Initiative version of the World Health Organization (WHO) Composite International Diagnostic Interview (CIDI). *International Journal of Methods in Psychiatric Research, 13*(2), 93–121. https://doi.org/10.1002/mpr.168

Keyes, K. M., Hatzenbuehler, M. L., McLaughlin, K. A., Link, B., Olfson, M., Grant, B. F., & Hasin, D. (2010). Stigma and treatment for alcohol use disorders in the United States. *American Journal of Epidemiology, 172*(12), 1364–1372. https://doi.org/10.1093/aje/kwq304

Khandelwal, S. K., Sharan, P., & Saxena, S. (1995). Eating disorders: an Indian perspective. *International Journal of Social Psychiatry, 41*(2), 132–146. https://doi.org/10.1177/002076409504100206

Kinzie, J. D. (2007). PTSD among traumatized refugees. In L. J. Kirmayer, R. Lemelson, & M. Barad (Eds.), *Understanding trauma: Integrating biological, clinical, and cultural perspectives* (pp. 194–206). Cambridge, UK: Cambridge University Press.

Kirmayer, L. J., Lemelson, R., & Barad, M. (2007). *Understanding trauma: Integrating biological, clinical, and cultural perspectives*. Cambridge: Cambridge University Press.

Koplewicz, H., Gurian, A., & Williams, K. (2009). The era of affluence and its discontents. *Journal of American Academy of Child and Adolescent Psychiatry, 48*, 1053–1055. https://doi.org/10.1097/CHI.0b013e3181b8be5c

Kuehner, C. (2003). Gender differences in unipolar depression: An update of epidemiologic findings and possible explanations. *Acta Psychiatrica Scandinavica, 108*(3), 163–174. https://doi.org/10.1034/j.1600-0447.2003.00204.x

Lawrie, S. M., Hall, J., McIntosh, A. M., Owens, D. G. C., & Johnstone, E. C. (2010). The 'continuum of psychosis': Scientifically unproven and clinically impractical. *British Journal of Psychiatry, 197*, 423–425. https://doi.org/10.1192/bjp.bp.109.072827

Lecrubier, Y. (2001). Prescribing patterns for depression and anxiety worldwide. *Journal of Clinical Psychiatry, 62*(*Suppl 13*), 31–36; discussion 37–38.

Lewine, R. R., Burbach, D., & Meltzer, H. Y. (1984). Effect of diagnostic criteria on the ratio of male to female schizophrenic patients. *American Journal of Psychiatry, 141*(1), 84–87. https://doi.org/10.1176/ajp.141.1.84

Lewis, G., & Araya, R. (2002). Globalization and mental health. In N. Sartorius, W. Gaebel, J. J. Lopez-Ibor, & M. Maj (Eds.), *Psychiatry in society* (pp. 57–78). New York, NY: Wiley.

Maulik, P. K., Daniels, A. M., McBain, R., & Morris, J. M. (2014). Global mental health resources. In W. Patil, I. H. Minas, A. Cohen, & M. Prince (Eds.), *Global mental health: Principles and practice* (pp. 167–192). Oxford: Oxford University Press.

McGrath, J. J., Feron, F. P., Burne, T. H., Mackay-Sim, A., & Eyles, D. W. (2003). The neurodevelopmental hypothesis of schizophrenia: A review of recent developments. *Annals of Medicine, 35*, 86–93. https://doi.org/10.1080/07853890310010005

McGrath, J. J., McLaughlin, K. A., Saha, S., Aguilar-Gaxiola, S., Al-Hamzawi, A., Alonso, J., … Kessler, R. C. (2017). The association between childhood adversities and subsequent first onset of psychotic experiences: A cross-national analysis of 23998 respondents from 17 countries. *Psychological Medicine, 47*(7), 1230–1245. https://doi.org/10.1017/s0033291716003263

McGrath, P. J., Nunes, E. V., & Quitkin, F. M. (2003). Current concepts in the treatment of depression in alcohol-dependent patients. In R. N. Rosenthal (Ed.), *Dual diagnosis* (pp. 75–90). London: Routledge.

Merikangas, K. R., Jin, R., He, J. P., Kessler, R. C., Lee, S., Sampson, N. A., … Zarkov, Z. (2011). Prevalence and correlates of bipolar spectrum disorder in the world mental health survey initiative. *Archives of General Psychiatry, 68*(3), 241–251. https://doi.org/10.1001/archgenpsychiatry.2011.12

Morgan, C., Charalambides, M., Hutchinson, G., & Murray, R. M. (2010). Migration, ethnicity, and psychosis: Toward a sociodevelopmental model. *Schizophrenia Bulletin, 36*(4), 655–664. https://doi.org/10.1093/schbul/sbq051

Mors, O., Perto, G. P., & Mortensen, P. B. (2011). The Danish psychiatric central research register. *Scandinavian Journal of Public Health, 39*(Suppl 7), 54–57. https://doi.org/10.1177/1403494810395825

Nuevo, R., Chatterji, S., Verdes, E., Naidoo, N., Arango, C., & Ayuso-Mateos, J. L. (2012). The continuum of psychotic symptoms in the general population: A cross-national study. *Schizophrenia Bulletin, 38*(3), 475–485. https://doi.org/10.1093/schbul/sbq099

Oppenheimer, C. (2014). Psychiatry of old age. In S. Bloch, S. A. Green, & J. Holmes (Eds.), *Psychiatry: Past, present, and prospect* (pp. 239–262). Oxford: Oxford University Press.

Perala, J., Suvisaari, J., Saarni, S. I., Kuoppasalmi, K., Isometsa, E., Pirkola, S., … Lonnqvist, J. (2007). Lifetime prevalence of psychotic and bipolar I disorders in a general population. *Archives of General Psychiatry, 64*(1), 19–28. https://doi.org/10.1001/archpsyc.64.1.19

Pickett, K. E., & Wilkinson, R. G. (2010). Inequality: An underacknowledged source of mental illness and distress. *British Journal of Psychiatry, 197*, 426–428. https://doi.org/10.1192/bjp.bp.109.072066

Picketty, T. (2015). *The economics of inequality*. Cambridge: Harvard University Press.

Pigott, T. A. (1999). Gender differences in the epidemiology and treatment of anxiety disorders. *Journal of Clinical Psychiatry, 60*(Suppl 18), 4–15.

Pike, K. M., & Dunne, P. E. (2015). The rise of eating disorders in Asia: A review. *Journal of Eating Disorders, 3*, 33. https://doi.org/10.1186/s40337-015-0070-2

Rasmussen, A., Crager, M., Baser, R. E., Chu, T., & Gany, F. (2012). Onset of posttraumatic stress disorder and major depression among refugees and voluntary migrants to the United States. *Journal of Traumatic Stress, 25*(6), 705–712. https://doi.org/10.1002/jts.21763

Ruggles, S., & Heggeness, M. (2008). Intergenerational coresidence in developing countries. *Population Development Review, 34*(2), 253–281. https://doi.org/10.1111/j.1728-4457.2008.00219.x

Ruscio, A. M., Hallion, L. S., Lim, C. C. W., Aguilar-Gaxiola, S., Al-Hamzawi, A., Alonso, J., ...
Scott, K. M. (2017). Cross-sectional comparison of the epidemiology of DSM-5 generalized
anxiety disorder across the globe. *JAMA Psychiatry, 74*(5), 465–475. https://doi.org/10.1001/
jamapsychiatry.2017.0056

Sadock, B. J., Sadock, V. A., & Ruiz, P. (2015). *Kaplan & Sadock's synopsis of psychiatry:
Behavioral sciences/clinical psychiatry*. Philadelphia, PA: Wolters Kluwer.

Saha, S., Chant, D., Welham, J., & McGrath, J. (2005). A systematic review of the prevalence of
schizophrenia. *PLoS Medicine, 2*(5), e141. https://doi.org/10.1371/journal.pmed.0020141

Sartorius, N., Shapiro, R., Kimura, M., & Barrett, K. (1972). WHO international pilot study of
schizophrenia. *Psychological Medicine, 2*(4), 422–425. https://doi.org/10.1017/S0033291700
045244

Sartorius, N., Ustun, T. B., Lecrubier, Y., & Wittchen, H. U. (1996). Depression comorbid with
anxiety: results from the WHO study on psychological disorders in primary health care. *British
Journal of Psychiatry, 168*(S30), 38–43. https://doi.org/10.1192/S0007125000298395

Schmidt, M., Pedersen, L., & Sorensen, H. T. (2014). The Danish Civil Registration System as a
tool in epidemiology. *European Journal of Epidemiology, 29*, 541–549. https://doi.org/10.1007/
s10654-014-9930-3

Scott, K. M., Koenen, K. C., King, A., Petukhova, M. V., Alonso, J., Bromet, E. J., ... Kessler,
R. C. (2018). Post-traumatic stress disorder associated with sexual assault among women in
the WHO World Mental Health Surveys. *Psychological Medicine, 48*(1), 155–167. https://doi.
org/10.1017/s0033291717001593

Seedat, S., Scott, K. M., Angermeyer, M. C., Berglund, P., Bromet, E. J., Brugha, T. S., ... Kessler,
R. C. (2009). Cross-national associations between gender and mental disorders in the World
Health Organization World Mental Health Surveys. *Archives of General Psychiatry, 66*(7),
785–795. https://doi.org/10.1001/archgenpsychiatry.2009.36

Silove, D., Alonso, J., Bromet, E., Gruber, M., Sampson, N., Scott, K., ... Kessler, R. C. (2015).
Pediatric-onset and adult-onset separation anxiety disorder across countries in the World Mental
Health Survey. *American Journal of Psychiatry, 172*(7), 647–656. https://doi.org/10.1176/appi.
ajp.2015.14091185

St Clair, D., Xu, M., Wang, P., Yu, Y., Fang, Y., Zhang, F., ... He, L. (2005). Rates of adult schizophrenia following prenatal exposure to the Chinese famine of 1959-1961. *JAMA, 294*(5), 557–
562. https://doi.org/10.1001/jama.294.5.557

Stein, D. J., Lim, C. C. W., Roest, A. M., de Jonge, P., Aguilar-Gaxiola, S., Al-Hamzawi, A., ...
Scott, K. M. (2017). The cross-national epidemiology of social anxiety disorder: Data from the
World Mental Health Survey Initiative. *BMC Medicine, 15*(1), 143. https://doi.org/10.1186/
s12916-017-0889-2

Szmukler, G. (2014). Fifty years of mental health legislation: Paternalism, bound and unbound. In
S. Bloch, S. A. Green, & J. Holmes (Eds.), *Psychiatry: Past, present, and prospect* (pp. 133–
153). Oxford: Oxford University Press.

Szmukler, G., Daw, R., & Callard, F. (2014). Mental health law and the UN Convention on the
rights of persons with disabilities. *International Journal of Law and Psychiatry, 37*(3), 245–
252. https://doi.org/10.1016/j.ijlp.2013.11.024

Thornicroft, G., Chatterji, S., Evans-Lacko, S., Gruber, M., Sampson, N., Aguilar-Gaxiola, S., ...
Kessler, R. C. (2017). Undertreatment of people with major depressive disorder in 21 countries.
British Journal of Psychiatry, 210(2), 119–124. https://doi.org/10.1192/bjp.bp.116.188078

Thorup, A., Waltoft, B. L., Pedersen, C. B., Mortensen, P. B., & Norderntoft, M. (2007). Young
males have a higher risk of developing schizophrenia: A Danish register study. *Psychological
Medicine, 37*, 479–484. https://doi.org/10.1017/S0033291707009944

U.S. Department of Homeland Security, Office of Inspector General. (2017). *Concerns about
ICE Detainee Treatment and Care at Detention Facilities* (OIG-18-32). Washington, D.C.:
Government Printing Office. https://www.oig.dhs.gov/sites/default/files/assets/2017-12/OIG-
18-32-Dec17.pdf

United Nations Office on Drugs and Crime. (2018, June). *Analysis of drug markets: Opiates, cocaine, cannabis, synthetic drugs* (World Drug Report, 2018). Vienna: United Nations Office on Drugs and Crime. https://www.unodc.org/wdr2018/prelaunch/WDR18_Booklet_3_DRUG_MARKETS.pdf

van Os, J., Hanssen, M., Bijl, R. V., & Ravelli, A. (2000). Strauss (1969) revisited: A psychosis continuum in the general population? *Schizophrenia Research, 45*(1–2), 11–20.

Wang, P. S., Aguilar-Gaxiola, S., Alonso, J., Angermeyer, M. C., Borges, G., Bromet, E. J., … Wells, J. E. (2007). Use of mental health services for anxiety, mood, and substance disorders in 17 countries in the WHO world mental health surveys. *Lancet, 370*(9590), 841–850. https://doi.org/10.1016/s0140-6736(07)61414-7

Wardenaar, K. J., Lim, C. C. W., Al-Hamzawi, A. O., & Alonso, J. (2018). The cross-national epidemiology of specific phobia in the World Mental Health Surveys – CORRIGENDUM. *Psychological Medicine, 48*(5), 878. https://doi.org/10.1017/s0033291717002975

Weinberg, L., Whiteford, H., de Almeida, J. C., Aguilar-Gaxiola, S., Levinson, D., O'Neill, S., & Kovess-Masfety, V. (2012). Translation of the World Mental Health Survey data to policies: An exploratory study of stakeholders' perceptions of how epidemiologic data can be utilized for policy in the field of mental health. *Public Health Reviews, 34*(2), 1–21. https://doi.org/10.1007/bf03391672

Wells, K. B., Sturm, R., Sherbourne, C. D., & Meredith, L. S. (1999). *Caring for depression.* Cambridge, MA: Harvard University Press.

World Bank. (2018). *Data: World Bank country and lending groups.* Washington, DC: The World Bank Group. https://datahelpdesk.worldbank.org/knowledgebase/articles/906519

World Health Organization. (2005a). *WHO resource book on mental health, human rights, and legislation.* Geneva: World Health Organization. https://www.paho.org/hr-ecourse-e/assets/_pdf/Module1/Lesson2/M1_L2_23.pdf

World Health Organization. (2005b). *The World Mental Health Survey Initiative* [Web page]. Geneva: World Health Organization. https://www.hcp.med.harvard.edu/wmh/

World Health Organization. (2008). *Closing the gap in a generation: Health equity through action on the social determinants of health.* Geneva: WHO. https://www.who.int/social_determinants/thecommission/finalreport/en/

World Health Organization. (2016). *The health and social effects of nonmedical cannabis use.* Geneva: World Health Organization. http://www.who.int/substance_abuse/publications/msb-cannabis.pdf

World Health Organization. (2017). *Depression and other common mental disorders: Global health estimates.* Geneva: World Health Organization. https://www.who.int/mental_health/management/depression/prevalence_global_health_estimates/en/

World Health Organization. (2018). *Global status report on alcohol and health.* Geneva: World Health Organization. https://www.who.int/substance_abuse/publications/global_alcohol_report/en/

Wu, Z., & Fang, Y. (2014). Comorbidity of depressive and anxiety disorders: Challenges in diagnosis and assessment. *Shanghai Archives of Psychiatry, 26*(4), 227–231. https://doi.org/10.3969/j.issn.1002-0829.2014.04.006

Zucker, H. A., & Greene, D. (2018). Potential child health consequences of the federal policy separating immigrant children from their parents. *JAMA, 320*(6), 541–542. https://doi.org/10.1001/jama.2018.10905

Behavioral Health Approaches to Preventing and Treating Substance Use Disorders

Christine Timko and Michael A. Cucciare

Introduction

Worldwide, the harmful use of alcohol results in 3.3 million deaths each year, and 31 million persons have drug use disorders (World Health Organization (WHO), 2014). Substance use disorders (SUDs) are common, have harmful effects on health and safety, and are a significant drain on our nation's economy. Annually, excessive drinking costs the United States $249 billion (Centers for Disease Control and Prevention, 2018), and illicit drug use $193 billion (National Drug Intelligence Center, 2011), in lost productivity, healthcare expenses, and law enforcement and criminal costs. Preventing SUDs is critical, and early intervention and treatment are essential to avoid their devastating impact and reduce their high costs to society.

In this chapter, we review the literature on behavioral approaches to preventing and treating SUDs. We focus mainly on alcohol and illicit drugs, rather than on addictions to nicotine and prescription drugs, or on solutions to the current opioid crisis (Meldrum, 2016). In addition, we focus on behavioral therapies rather than pharmacological interventions. We include a discussion of behavioral treatments for

C. Timko (✉)
Center for Innovation to Implementation, Veterans Affairs (VA) Health Care System, Menlo Park, CA, USA

Department of Psychiatry and Behavioral Sciences, Stanford University School of Medicine, Stanford, CA, USA
e-mail: Christine.Timko@va.gov

M. A. Cucciare
Center for Mental Healthcare and Outcomes Research, Central Arkansas Veterans Healthcare System, North Little Rock, AR, USA

VA South Central (VISN 16) Mental Illness Research, Education, and Clinical Center, Central Arkansas Veterans Healthcare System, North Little Rock, AR, USA

Department of Psychiatry, University of Arkansas for Medical Sciences, Little Rock, AR, USA

© Springer Nature Switzerland AG 2020
B. L. Levin, A. Hanson (eds.), *Foundations of Behavioral Health*, https://doi.org/10.1007/978-3-030-18435-3_3

individuals who have co-occurring substance use and other mental disorders. After reviewing the literature, we present critical issues related to behavioral strategies for SUD prevention and treatment, such as the need for better coordination of care within healthcare systems. We also discuss behavioral treatments for SUDs in the context of financing services delivery, by considering personalized care that begins with low-intensity options and can be intensified if indicated. Throughout this chapter, we point out gaps in knowledge for which more research is needed.

Review of the Literature

The risky use of substances covers a spectrum of behaviors (Office of the Surgeon General, 2016). Regarding alcohol use, for example, hazardous drinkers consume alcohol above recommended limits set by the National Institute on Alcohol Abuse and Alcoholism (NIAAA). Hazardous drinkers experience physical, social, or psychological harm associated with their alcohol use but do not necessarily meet criteria for an alcohol use disorder. SUDs are associated with repeated and negative physical, psychological, and social effects from alcohol and other drugs (Office of the Surgeon General, 2016). In the DSM-5, a diagnosis of an alcohol use disorder requires meeting 2 or more criteria, out of 11 (e.g., neglect major roles to drink or use, increased tolerance), within a 12-month period; a criteria count is an overall severity indicator. Furthermore, an alcohol use disorder diagnosis in DSM-5 requires specifying severity, with 2–3 symptoms indicating a mild, 4–5 symptoms a moderate, and 6 or more a severe disorder.

One approach to addressing the needs of people with the full spectrum of substance use-related behaviors is the Screening, Brief Intervention, and Referral to Treatment (SBIRT) model. SBIRT is a comprehensive, integrated, public health approach to the delivery of early intervention and referral to more intensive treatment services for people with a range of unhealthy substance use. Screening identifies people with unhealthy use and, when followed by the assessment of the severity of substance use, can identify potential treatment goals, such as reducing episodes of heavy consumption or abstinence.

Designed for individuals at risk of developing SUDs and those who have already developed them, SBIRT can be applied in many clinical care settings. Indeed, SBIRT has been adapted for use in emergency departments, primary care clinics, office- and clinic-based practices, and other community settings (e.g., employee assistance programs), thereby providing opportunities for early intervention with at-risk individuals using substances before more severe substance use develops and/ or consequences occur. As discussed below, SBIRT interventions can include the provision of brief treatment for those with less severe substance use and referral to specialized SUD treatment for those with a SUD (Agerwala & McCance-Katz, 2012). A large body of research on SBIRT for alcohol, illicit drugs, tobacco, and prescription drugs demonstrates that it yields improvements in health (Babor, Del Boca, & Bray, 2017; Babor et al., 2007).

Screening and Assessment

SBIRT begins with the introduction of systematic screening into routine care at medical facilities and other community settings where people with SUDs are seen. Screening is a preliminary procedure to evaluate the likelihood that an individual has a SUD or is at risk of negative consequences from the use of alcohol or other drugs. Although screening tests were initially developed to identify active cases of alcohol and drug dependence, the aim of screening has been expanded to cover the full spectrum ranging from risky substance use to dependence.

Because primary care is the point of access to SUD treatment for many people, universal screening for unhealthy alcohol use in primary care is recommended (USPSTF, 2014). The ten-item Alcohol Use Disorders Identification Test (AUDIT) is the most studied screening tool for detecting the severity of alcohol use in primary care settings (USPSTF, 2014). The AUDIT performs adequately to identify hazardous and problem drinking but may be too long to be integrated easily into many primary care settings. Accordingly, the first three questions of the AUDIT, which ask about alcohol consumption and are called the AUDIT-C, were demonstrated to be an effective screening test for past-year hazardous drinking and for active alcohol use disorders (Bradley et al., 2007). AUDIT-C cutoff scores for unhealthy alcohol use are 4 for men and 3 for women (Bradley et al., 2007) and for alcohol use disorders are 5 or 6 for men and 4 for women (Dawson, Grant, Stinson, & Zhou, 2005).

Until recently, there has been a lack of brief and valid screening instruments for substances other than alcohol or tobacco. The Alcohol, Smoking and Substance Involvement Screening Test (ASSIST) is used increasingly to assess substance use and related problems, although it may be too lengthy to be feasible in busy primary care settings (McNeely et al., 2014). Shorter assessments for assessing drug use include the Drug Abuse Screening Test-10 (DAST-10) which is used to assess past-year drug consequences and problem severity and has demonstrated sound psychometric properties (Yudko, Lozhkina, & Fouts, 2007). Scores range from 0 to 10; a score of ≥ 3 suggests drug use risk (French, Roebuck, McGeary, Chitwood, & McCoy, 2001; Voluse et al., 2012). There is also a single screening question to identify drug use accurately in primary care patients: "How many times in the past year have you used an illegal drug or used a prescription medication for nonmedical reasons?"(Smith, Schmidt, Allensworth-Davies, & Saitz, 2009). A response of >1 time is considered positive for drug use risk.

Brief Interventions

The assessment of substance use may lead to either of two different primary care strategies, based on whether patients have at-risk substance use or a SUD. Patients with at-risk substance use often receive brief interventions. Brief interventions refer to any time-limited effort to provide information or advice, increase motivation to avoid substance use, or teach behavior change skills that will reduce substance use as well as the chances of negative consequences (Babor et al., 2007). Brief interventions vary in length and content but typically involve 1–2 counseling sessions of up to 30 min each and may consist of personalized feedback on age- and gender-matched normative comparisons of substance use, self-reported consequences of use, and motivation to change substance use (Cucciare, Simpson, Hoggatt, Gifford, & Timko, 2013).

Research shows that among the most cost-effective and time-efficient interventions are brief motivational conversations between a healthcare professional and a patient using substances (Babor et al., 2017; Babor et al., 2007). Indeed, protocol-driven brief interventions have been shown to be effective for reducing alcohol intake, associated injury recidivism, driving under the influence, and other adverse consequences of alcohol and drug use (Babor et al., 2017; Madras et al., 2009; Wamsley, Satterfield, Curtis, Lundgren, & Satre, 2018). However, the literature documenting the effectiveness of brief interventions for illicit drug use is weaker than that for alcohol (Kim et al., 2017; Saitz et al., 2014). For patients identified through screening and assessment as having SUDs rather than risky use, brief interventions may be inadequate, and so referrals to specialized treatments should be provided (Kim et al., 2017).

Specialty Treatment

Patients with SUDs often need more intensive treatment in specialty settings than can be offered in primary care. Therefore, SBIRT incorporates referral to treatment as a critical feature. This may include referral to brief treatment, which involves the delivery of time-limited, structured therapy for a SUD by a trained clinician, and is typically delivered to those at higher risk or in the early stages of substance dependence. It generally involves two to six sessions of behavioral therapies, which are described below. However, although not discussed in this chapter, brief treatment may also include the ongoing management of SUDs in primary care settings with the use of pharmacotherapy (Fiellin et al., 2013). Here, we describe behavioral therapies that are considered evidence-based practices in SUD treatment programs. SUD specialty care is delivered in a continuum of program types, including standard outpatient, intensive outpatient, and residential care, which is often followed by outpatient aftercare. Within these programs, care is provided individually and in groups.

Motivational interviewing (MI), an extremely well-known approach, is a client-centered, semi-directive therapeutic style to enhance intrinsic readiness for change by helping individuals explore and resolve ambivalence toward making a life change. An evolution of Rogers' person-centered counseling approach, MI and related motivational enhancement therapies (METs) elicit the person's own motivations for making a change (Miller & Rollnick, 2002).

A meta-analysis of 32 clinical trials that focused on treating alcohol use disorder found that the average effect size (for effect sizes, 0.2–0.3 is small, 0.5 is medium, and 0.8 and higher is large) of MI was 0.41 posttreatment and 0.26 across all follow-up points (Hettema, Steele, & Miller, 2005). An additional 13 trials tested the effect of MI in addressing illicit drug use, with average effect sizes of 0.51 for early follow-ups and 0.29 for later follow-ups (Hettema et al., 2005). A subsequent meta-analysis confirmed that MI promotes durable reductions in use of a range of substances (Sayegh, Huey, Zara, & Jhaveri, 2017). However, the variable effectiveness of MI found in these meta-analyses across providers, populations, target problems, and settings suggests a need for additional research to understand and specify how MI exerts its effects.

Cognitive behavioral therapy (CBT), pioneered by Aaron Beck and by Albert Ellis, is a class of interventions sharing the premise that mental disorders and psychological distress are maintained by cognitive factors. To achieve the goal of symptom reduction, improvement in functioning, and remission of the disorder, the patient becomes an active participant in collaborative problem-solving to test and challenge the validity of maladaptive cognitions and modify maladaptive behavioral patterns. Similar to findings for MI, a review of meta-analyses of CBT for SUDs found that effect sizes of CBT ranged from small to medium. Specifically, CBT was highly effective for treating cannabis and nicotine dependence but less effective for treating opioid and alcohol dependence (Hofmann, Asnaani, Vonk, Sawyer, & Fang, 2012).

Contingency management (CM) is based on the principles of operant conditioning. It provides reinforcing or punitive consequences to achieve therapeutic goals, such as abstinence from substance use or increasing treatment attendance (Petry, Alessi, Olmstead, Rash, & Zajac, 2017; Rash, Stitzer, & Weinstock, 2017). For example, abstinence is often reinforced with escalating vouchers (e.g., $2.50 for an initial negative urinalysis, adding $1.50 for each consecutive one), with possible added bonuses, that can be exchanged for goods or services. If a urinalysis is positive, no voucher is given, and the value for the next negative urinalysis is reset to the initial level. Besides vouchers, other reinforcers are clinical privileges, cash, or employment.

Meta-analyses report medium effect sizes for CM in treating SUDs (Lussier, Heil, Mongeon, Badger, & Higgins, 2006; Prendergast, Podus, Finney, Greenwell, & Roll, 2006). In addition, a systematic evaluation found that CM combined with standard psychological interventions to treat cocaine dependence in particular increases abstinence and improves treatment retention and is also of benefit in pharmacotherapy trials (Schierenberg, van Amsterdam, van den Brink, & Goudriaan, 2012). Another review (Farronato, Dursteler-Macfarland, Wiesbeck, & Petitjean, 2013) concurred that positive, rapid, and enduring effects on cocaine use are reliably seen with CM interventions. However, the reviews also noted that it is unclear who should cover the extra expense of CM. In addition, the more recent meta-analyses (Sayegh et al., 2017) suggested that because CM is extrinsically focused, it may produce follow-up effects of reducing substance use mainly in the short term.

Twelve-Step Facilitation has grown because 12-step groups such as Alcoholics Anonymous represent a readily available and no-cost resource in SUD recovery. Individuals can become involved with 12-step programs before, during, or after SUD treatment and in the absence of any treatment. A considerable body of evidence in the behavioral health field indicates that earlier engagement in 12-step groups, more frequent meeting attendance, more involvement in 12-step practices (e.g., obtaining a sponsor, performing service at meetings), and a longer duration of participation are associated with better SUD outcomes (Kaskutas, Bond, & Avalos, 2009; Moos & Moos, 2006; Wendt, Hallgren, Daley, & Donovan, 2017). This kind of evidence prompted behavioral health researchers to implement active methods to encourage 12-step group participation during and after treatment.

Interventions to increase 12-step group participation are effective in doing so and thus contribute to positive SUD outcomes through their impact on increasing 12-step group attendance and involvement. These interventions include Twelve-Step Facilitation Therapy (Nowinski, Baker, Carroll, & National Institute on Alcohol Abuse and Alcoholism, 2007); Intensive Referral (Timko & DeBenedetti, 2007); STAGE-12, which stands for Stimulant (cocaine, methamphetamine) Abuser Groups to Engage in 12-Step (Donovan & Wells, 2007); Making AA Easier (MAAEZ; Kaskutas, Subbaraman, Witbrodt, & Zemore, 2009); and integrated Twelve-Step Facilitation for Adolescents (Kelly et al., 2017).

Mindfulness training also is considered a promising treatment for SUD. Mindfulness refers to maintaining awareness of thoughts, feelings, bodily sensations, and the surrounding environment and accepting thoughts and feelings without judging them. When practicing mindfulness, people focus on what they are sensing in the present moment rather than reconsidering the past or anticipating the future.

A systematic review examined methodological characteristics and findings of studies that evaluated mindfulness treatments for SUD (Li, Howard, Garland, McGovern, & Lazar, 2017). The review also included a meta-analysis of randomized controlled trials of mindfulness treatments for substance use. Results revealed significant small-to-large effects of mindfulness treatments in reducing the frequency and severity of substance use, intensity of cravings, and severity of stress. Although mindfulness treatment for substance use is a promising intervention, research is needed to examine the mechanisms by which mindfulness interventions exert their effects.

Acceptance and commitment therapy (ACT) is another form of behavioral therapy, developed in the late 1980s, that combines mindfulness strategies with the practice of acceptance. Its rationale is that by acknowledging and accepting negative thoughts and feelings, people can learn to observe them and develop new ways to relate to them. ACT helps people become more flexible psychologically, better understand their personal values, and connect more to the present moment. As applied to SUDs, patients learn more accepting and mindful ways of relating to inner experiences, rather than engaging in substance use (e.g., in response to cravings or to escape negative affect), while moving forward in building meaningful patterns of activity that are inconsistent with substance use. In addition, because of ACT's transdiagnostic approach, it can effectively target key psychological problems commonly comorbid with substance use.

A meta-analysis (Lee, An, Levin, & Twohig, 2015) provided evidence that ACT is likely at least as efficacious as active treatment comparisons such as CBT or 12-step therapy and that substance use abstinence may be better maintained at follow-up when treated with ACT over other active conditions. Thus, the results provide promising, although preliminary, support for ACT as a treatment for SUDs. Additionally, Lee et al. noted that, while not exclusive to ACT, novel delivery methods (e.g., telehealth, computer, and phone applications) of ACT are rapidly being explored and have shown promise. As for mindfulness interventions, further study is needed that examines mechanisms of change that affect substance use among patients receiving ACT.

Research on treating SUDs in specialty care settings with regard to each of these evidence-based approaches (MI, CBT, CM, 12-step facilitation, and mindfulness) has yet to establish the extent to which one approach may be more effective than another.

So far in this chapter, we have focused on use of these approaches in treating individuals with SUDs in the absence of other mental health disorders. We turn now to assessing and treating individuals with both SUDs and other mental health problems, due to the high frequency of co-occurring diagnoses found across healthcare settings.

Clients with Co-occurring Diagnoses: Assessment and Treatment

Population-based surveys indicate that over 8.4 million adults in the United States have co-occurring substance use and mental disorders (Center for Behavioral Health Statistics and Quality, 2015). Specifically, over 30% of people with mental illness, and over 50% of people with severe mental illness, will experience a SUD in their lifetime (Center for Behavioral Health Statistics and Quality, 2015). People diagnosed with SUDs have high rates of co-occurring psychotic disorders and other serious mental illnesses, such as schizophrenia, bipolar disorder, and severe major depression and PTSD (Mueser & Gingerich, 2013). Individuals with co-occurring SUD and other mental disorders tend to have greater symptom severity and poorer functioning, and treatment engagement and outcomes, compared to those without such comorbidity (Burns, Teesson, & O'Neill, 2005; Merikangas & Kalaydjian, 2007). Thus, the assessment and treatment of SUDs in people with mental disorders is a high priority in behavioral treatment settings.

Assessing SUDs in People with Mental Disorders

Mueser and Gingerich (2013) note that it is essential that all patients with mental disorders are accurately screened and comprehensively assessed for comorbid SUDs. In particular, it is important to assess for any level of substance use among patients with psychosis because they are often more sensitive to the effects of psychoactive substances and experience relatively greater adverse effects (Lubman & Sundram, 2003). Clinicians should be aware that people with severe mental illnesses are highly sensitive to the effects of even modest amounts of alcohol or drugs, such that even lower levels of use may indicate an active SUD. Standard screening instruments such as the AUDIT have good sensitivity and specificity in detecting probable SUDs among people with mental disorders.

Treatment Approaches for Patients with Co-occurring Disorders

The same strategies we have discussed for treating SUDs are recommended for clients with co-occurring disorders: enhance motivation; use CBT to teach more effective interpersonal and coping skills; use CM to reward abstinence; and encourage participation in 12-step groups as well as practicing mindfulness (Baker, Thornton, Hiles, Hides, & Lubman, 2012; Kelly, Daley, & Douaihy, 2012; Mueser & Gingerich, 2013; Timko, Sutkowi, Cronkite, Makin-Byrd, & Moos, 2011).

In particular, MI has robust support for establishing a therapeutic alliance between patients with co-occurring disorders and their treatment providers (Kelly et al., 2012). Randomized controlled trials comparing MI to educational treatment or treatment as usual for these patients have demonstrated significant reductions in favor of MI for alcohol and illicit drug use and psychiatric symptoms (Westra, Aviram, & Doell, 2011). However, with regard to comorbid SUD, among people with schizophrenia in particular, although there is an emerging supportive literature for MI, CBT, and CM, as well as family interventions, there is a particular lack of rigorously conducted randomized controlled trials (Cather et al., 2018).

Although sequential or parallel approaches can be appropriate for patients with co-occurring disorders, there has been recognition of their limitations. Integrated approaches, in which both conditions are addressed simultaneously within the same treatment, are most effective for patients with SUD mental health comorbidities (Lubman, King, & Castle, 2010; Mueser & Gingerich, 2013). For example, in the case of approaches for treating comorbid SUDs and PTSD, trauma-focused psychotherapy delivered in the context of SUD treatment is more effective than treatment as usual or minimal intervention in reducing PTSD and SUD symptoms (Roberts, Roberts, Jones, & Bisson, 2016). However, only 18% of SUD treatment programs meet the criteria for services that are capable of addressing the needs of patients with co-occurring disorders (Ford et al., 2018).

Beyond specific behavioral therapy approaches, principles of behavioral treatment for patients with co-occurring disorders are being established. These include adopting a low-stress and harm-reduction approach, supporting functional recovery (a worthwhile and meaningful life that is not centered on using substances), and engaging the individual's social network (Haverfield, Schmidt, Ilgen, & Timko, 2018).

Other principles emphasize that because there is no one-size-fits-all treatment, a flexible approach with the ability to apply specific components of care to particular individuals is required (Lubman et al., 2010). That is, patients with co-occurring disorders require creative combinations of behavioral therapy and pharmacological interventions to provide the most effective treatment (Kelly et al., 2012).

The need for flexibility of approach is prompted in part by the many combinations of substances and mental disorders implied by the term "co-occurring disorders." For example, the combination of cognitive behavioral therapy and motivational interviewing and a longer duration of care provide additional benefits for co-occurring SUD and depression in particular (Baker et al., 2012; Riper et al., 2014). But, for all patients with co-occurring disorders, it is vital for effective treatment to instill hope and the belief that recovery is possible among patients, family members, and other treatment providers (Mueser & Gingerich, 2013).

Although this brief review of the literature on behavioral approaches to preventing and treating SUDs shows that much has been accomplished, there remain critical issues that have yet to be adequately addressed. These include the coordination of SUD services and, in particular, how to effectively transition patients with SUDs from primary care to specialty care when needed and how to ensure that patients maintain routine primary care when they have an episode of specialty care. We turn to these critical issues next.

Presentation of Critical Issues

A critical issue for preventing and treating SUDs is the coordination of services encompassed by the SBIRT model: screening; brief intervention; referral; and treatment. In many communities, screening and brief intervention services are lacking, referral is fragmented and inconsistent, and specialized treatment services operate independently of primary care and the larger healthcare system(s). A key aspect of SBIRT is the coordination of its four components into a community's system of services that links a network of early intervention and referral activities, conducted in medical and social service settings, to specialized treatment programs (Babor et al., 2017; Babor et al., 2007). We focus on two aspects of better service coordination: (1) improving SUD patients' transitions from primary to specialty care and (2) from specialty to primary care.

Transitions from Primary to Specialty Care

Unhealthy substance use is common among patients presenting to primary care settings. As many as 22–50% of patients presenting to primary care report at least one symptom of hazardous alcohol use (Hawkins, Lapham, Kivlahan, & Bradley, 2010; McQuade, Levy, Yanek, Davis, & Liepman, 2000), while 18–44% meet the criteria for a lifetime or current alcohol use disorder (McQuade et al., 2000; Smith, Schmidt, Allensworth-Davies, & Saitz, 2010). Similarly high rates are reported of past-year or current use of an illicit substance for nonmedical reasons (35%), and current (13%) and lifetime (47%) drug use disorders, among persons presenting to primary care (Smith et al., 2010).

Substance use may complicate the treatment of chronic health conditions addressed in primary care, such as diabetes and hypertension (Timko, Kong, Vittorio, & Cucciare, 2016). Therefore, it is critical that primary care providers be prepared to identify and determine appropriate treatment options for patients presenting with substance use. Being proficient in these skills is consistent with the increasing use of patient-centered models of primary care that emphasize healthy lifestyle change and management of chronic health conditions. However, providers face considerable challenges in supporting the transition of patients with more severe substance use from primary care to SUD care settings.

Although strategies for detecting and treating risky substance use are increasingly being used in primary care, information about the availability of specialty SUD care treatment options is rarely provided to patients (Williams et al., 2012). For example, the Veterans Health Administration (VHA) implemented a model of detecting and providing brief intervention for unhealthy alcohol use in primary care and showed increased documentation of screening and identification of hazardous use, as well as delivery of education about safe drinking limits and potential health effects of harmful alcohol use (Bradley et al., 2006; Lapham et al., 2012). However, rates of referral to specialty SUD care remained low (Lapham et al., 2012), with studies finding only 10–14% of patients screening positive for hazardous alcohol use receiving information about alcohol-related care (Lapham et al., 2012; Williams et al., 2012).

Factors That Impact SUD Care Transitions

Patient, provider, and healthcare system characteristics may directly influence the transition practices that impact access to and engagement in specialty SUD care. In turn, access and engagement may be associated with better health outcomes such as reduced substance use, abstinence, and better psychological functioning and quality of life (Cucciare, Coleman, & Timko, 2015). Of potential barriers to primary care physicians' specialty care referrals, patient characteristics have the largest effects (Forrest, Nutting, von Schrader, Rohde, & Starfield, 2006).

Patient Factors

Patients' clinical characteristics such as the presence of a drug rather than alcohol use disorder, negative consequences of substance use, and comorbid mental disorders are associated with a higher likelihood of receiving specialty SUD care (Forrest et al., 2006; Glass et al., 2010; Ilgen et al., 2011). A common barrier to accessing specialty SUD care is that patients' previous treatment experiences were negative (Mowbray, Perron, Bohnert, Krentzman, & Vaughn, 2010; Perron et al., 2009). Additional barriers include specialty care being inconvenient, involving a long wait until the initial appointment, long travel distances to the site, and inflexible hours of treatment provision (Beardsley, Wish, Fitzelle, O'Grady, & Arria, 2003; Coulson, Ng, Geertsema, Dodd, & Berk, 2009; Hoffman, Ford, Choi, Gustafson, & McCarty, 2008; Laudet, Stanick, & Sands, 2009; McCarty, Gustafson, Capoccia, & Cotter, 2009; Mowbray et al., 2010; Perron et al., 2009; Pulford, Adams, & Sheridan, 2006). Other common barriers are lack of knowledge about the harmful effects of continued substance use, patients' belief that they can cope with substance use on their own or the problem will improve by itself, and embarrassment (Mowbray et al., 2010; Perron et al., 2009). Stigma is a significant barrier to accessing SUD treatment services; individuals may choose to conceal their substance use to avoid it (Livingston, Milne, Fang, & Amari, 2012; Woodhead, Timko, Han, & Cucciare, 2018).

Perceived need for SUD treatment and stronger beliefs in the benefits of SUD treatment are facilitators of treatment entry (Falck et al., 2007; Kleinman, Millery, Scimeca, & Polissar, 2002; Masson et al., 2013). However, only small proportions of individuals identified as having SUDs perceive a need for treatment (3–19%) (Hedden & Gfroerer, 2011; Oleski, Mota, Cox, & Sareen, 2010). Patients may have unrealistic expectations about the content or duration of care because they are not provided opportunities to express their care preferences; therefore, these preferences are not realized, to the extent possible, in patients' care planning (Coleman et al., 2003). Possibly, offering a menu of potential treatment options that take patient choice into account may be a way to increase rates of treatment entry (Bradley & Kivlahan, 2014; McCrady, Epstein, Cook, Jensen, & Ladd, 2011; McKay, 2009).

Resources facilitating the transition from primary to specialty SUD care are the patient's self-efficacy to obtain and engage in care, motivation to change, and social support, including family involvement (Ball, Carroll, Canning-Ball, & Rounsaville, 2006; Jackson, 2006; Kleinman et al., 2002; Palmer, Murphy, Piselli, & Ball, 2009; Stevens et al., 2008; Viggiano, Pincus, & Crystal, 2012; Weisner, Mertens, Tam, & Moore, 2001).

Provider Factors

Provider factors that may influence patients' transitions to SUD specialty care include providers' cultural competence (Masson et al., 2013) and knowledge about the availability and potential efficacy of SUD treatment options both within their care system and larger community. Referrals to SUD treatment may be infrequent because providers often view such treatment as a revolving door that does not deliver positive outcomes (Woodhead et al., 2018).

Studies confirm the stigmatizing attitudes of providers toward individuals who need SUD treatment, in that such patients are perceived as not being truly sick (due to the supposed self-inflicted nature of substance abuse and dependency), irresponsible, aggressive, untrustworthy, and difficult (Kelly & Westerhoff, 2010; Schomerus et al., 2011; Treloar & Holt, 2006). These perceptions are associated with less willingness to intervene with people in need of SUD-related care and a barrier to the provision of high-quality care (Lovi & Barr, 2009; Skinner, Roche, Freeman, & Addy, 2005). Healthcare staff's negative attitudes toward patients who would benefit from SUD treatment often translate into delays of patients seeking help (Kelly & Westerhoff, 2010).

Primary care clinicians need to be familiar with available treatment resources for their patients who have probable or diagnosed SUDs. Knowing about available treatment resources, including those tailored for special populations, such as patients with comorbid chronic health conditions, and having a clear plan to access services, will facilitate patients' access to care resources (Timko et al., 2016).

Providers also often lack training in SUD treatment generally and in transition practices more specifically (Childers & Arnold, 2012). Formal training in transitional care that includes learning to communicate with providers at specialty SUD care sites, and how to elicit and implement patient and family preferences into treatment plans, may also be critical for improving the care transition process. Training in the referral process should ensure that physicians obtain the skills necessary to expand their scope of practice when appropriate, determine when and why a patient should be referred, and identify the type of setting to which the patient should be sent (Forrest et al., 2006).

There are several strategies available that have potential for helping primary care providers facilitate the transition or linkage of patients between primary care and substance use-related help. For example, the SBIRT approach includes a referral to treatment component that is designed to help connect patients in need of more intensive substance use help to such care. This includes helping patients select an appropriate care option and navigate barriers to accessing such care. However, one recent review suggests that this component of SBIRT (as currently designed) may have limited effectiveness for achieving this goal (Glass et al., 2015), suggesting a need for research to inform how to improve this approach for the primary care setting.

More intensive approaches to linking patients engaging in unhealthy substance use to care include Strengths-Based Case Management which involves identifying patient strengths to facilitate linkage to care, encouraging collaborative care decision-making, identifying barriers to care and how to resolve them, and monitoring progress toward care linkage over time (Rapp et al., 2008; Strathdee et al., 2006). Although this approach has been shown to improve linkage of substance-using patients to care in community settings, it has not been tested in primary care indicating a need for research on its effectiveness in this setting.

System Factors

The context in which primary care is positioned, such as part of a larger healthcare system or as a stand-alone clinic, may impact the SUD care transition process. The likelihood of specialty referral is higher when the primary care physician is located within a practice of larger size and a health plan with gatekeeping arrangements (Forrest et al., 2006). Practices in which nurses and administrative staff can make referrals (with physician input), and in which physicians can make referrals based on telephone consultations with patients, have higher rates of referral than practices without these mechanisms (Forrest et al., 2006).

Formal relationships between care settings, and the availability of information systems such as electronic medical records that facilitate the sharing of critical information (e.g., care history) between care sites, will vary according to setting location and have implications for the ability to transition patients to SUD care options. For example, the availability of comprehensive medical records that contain all care received and recommended across care sites, contact information for all providers involved in patient care, and/or co-location of SUD or mental health services will likely offer greater opportunity for clinics to improve primary care to SUD care transitions.

Together, patient, provider, and system-level factors influence whether effective referrals are made to transition patients with more severe substance use from primary care clinics to SUD specialty treatment settings. Equally critical is the referral and transition process from specialty care "back to" primary care. We turn to this topic next.

Transitions from Specialty to Primary Care

Ensuring that patients leaving SUD specialty treatment begin or continue to obtain regular primary care may be associated with many important health benefits. Patients with SUDs who regularly access primary care may experience reductions in addiction severity (Friedmann, Zhang, Hendrickson, Stein, & Gerstein, 2003), higher abstinence rates (Weisner, Mertens, Parthasarathy, Moore, & Lu, 2001), and fewer hospitalizations (Laine et al., 2001). For example, detoxification patients who had a plan to see their primary care provider had a lower rate of short-term relapse than those who did not intend to see their physician (Griswold, Greene, Smith, Behrens, & Blondell, 2007). And patients in detoxification who received primary care had lower odds of drug use and alcohol intoxication 2 years later

(Saitz, Horton, Larson, Winter, & Samet, 2005). At the post-specialty care stage, primary care physicians can provide systematic medical and recovery checkups (El-Guebaly, 2012).

Despite the documented and potential health benefits of primary care, many patients with SUDs fail to receive it (Gurewich, Prottas, & Sirkin, 2014). Of about 6000 patients entering addiction treatment, 41% did not have a primary care physician, and small proportions of patients with SUDs obtained primary care subsequent to addiction treatment. For example, 56% of detoxification patients failed to receive primary care in the following 2 years (Saitz, Larson, Horton, Winter, & Samet, 2004). These findings are alarming because patients with SUDs who lack primary care are likely to incur an increased health burden. Of SUD patients without a primary care contact in the prior 2 years, 61% had experienced medical problems in the prior 30 days, 47% had one or more chronic health conditions, and 20% had two or more chronic health conditions, with asthma and high blood pressure being the most common (De Alba, Samet, & Saitz, 2004).

The increased burden of medical illness experienced by patients with SUDs not using primary care also translates into higher use of hospital and emergency department services. Eighty percent of SUD patients without a primary care physician reported at least one prior hospitalization due to a medical condition (De Alba et al., 2004). In addition, 47% of such patients reported one or more visits to an emergency department in the prior 6 months (Larson, Saitz, Horton, Lloyd-Travaglini, & Samet, 2006).

Together, these findings suggest that SUD treatment settings should actively facilitate the continuity of, or new transition to, primary care among their patients. Although addiction treatment settings have the potential to engage patients in primary care, they are not being successfully utilized to initiate primary care linkage in this patient population. Approaches for linking patients in addiction treatment settings to primary care vary in terms of the resources needed to implement them effectively. Here, we briefly describe three evidence-based approaches to promoting the use of primary care services among patients with SUDs. We present the approaches from the most to the least resource intensive.

Co-location of Primary Care and Specialty SUD Care

One method that has been shown to improve the linkage between SUD specialty treatment and primary care is co-location of the two care services, typically also integrating primary care into the addiction treatment program (Friedmann et al., 2003; Weisner, Mertens, Parthasarathy et al., 2001). However, integration involves more than simple co-location; rather, it covers the dimensions of program structure and milieu; assessment, treatment, and continuity of care; and staffing and training (McGovern, Lambert-Harris, Gotham, Claus, & Xie, 2014). Such an integrated approach may lead to improvements in substance use outcomes (Weisner, Mertens, Parthasarathy et al., 2001) and initial and longer-term use of outpatient medical care services in a wide variety of addiction treatment programs (Friedmann et al., 2003) and among SUD patients with chronic medical conditions (Saxon et al., 2006).

Facilitated Referral

Another method to ensure that patients begin or maintain engagement in primary care following discharge from SUD specialty treatment is facilitated referral (Saitz et al., 2005; Samet et al., 2003; Sweeney, Samet, Larson, & Saitz, 2004). This approach involves a social worker, nurse, physician, or other staff members in an addiction treatment setting serving in a case management role to help facilitate the linkage of patients to off-site primary care appointments (Samet et al., 2003; Sweeney et al., 2004). The provider first conducts a health evaluation that includes education about the importance and potential health benefits of receiving primary care. This is followed by facilitated referral to primary care including contacting the patient, and family and friends if necessary, by phone after discharge to provide reminders about upcoming primary care appointments, and to conduct appointment rescheduling if necessary (Samet et al., 2003; Sweeney et al., 2004). The initial appointment is made with special attention to the patient's preferences regarding the physician's gender, particular expertise, scheduling availability, and spoken languages. A detailed letter or email containing the patient's medical conditions is provided to the off-site primary care clinic to support the referral process.

Facilitated referral was associated with increased rates of primary care usage and reduced substance use compared to standard care among detoxification patients (Saitz et al., 2005; Samet et al., 2003). Although co-location and facilitated referral within addiction treatment settings can improve linkage to primary care and health outcomes, they are relatively resource intensive. For example, both approaches require the inclusion of dedicated staff and, in some instances, staff with specialized training in SUDs (Weisner, Mertens, Parthasarathy et al., 2001), who can provide primary care or referral services to promote the use of primary care.

Factors, such as limited addiction clinic finances, staff, staff training, and space, make the task of improving the accessibility and engagement of primary care services within addiction treatment settings an enormous challenge for providers and clinics (Saitz et al., 2005; Samet, Friedmann, & Saitz, 2001). It may be feasible for some well-resourced SUD clinics to adopt and implement a co-located primary care clinic or facilitated referral, but widespread adoption of these strategies will likely remain elusive. Rather, it may be more feasible for SUD specialty treatment settings to adopt components of these approaches. Components may include providing education to patients on the benefits of seeking primary care, available care options, and how to address insurance and coverage concerns, as well as implement follow-up procedures such as periodic reminders via telephone or other means (email, letter) to schedule or attend follow-up appointments. When addiction treatment settings do not have the resources to implement co-location or facilitated referral as packaged in empirical studies, they may choose to implement components of these intervention approaches with the hope that some portion of effects observed in more comprehensive packages will generalize to their setting and patient population.

Brief Counseling and Referral

A third option, in addition to co-location and facilitated referral, to improve the transition from specialty SUD care to primary care consists of brief approaches to counseling and referral within the addiction treatment program. For example, Project ASSERT was developed as a brief approach to facilitate referral to primary care and other services for patients with SUDs presenting to emergency departments (Bernstein, Bernstein, & Levenson, 1997; D'Onofrio & Degutis, 2010). This approach, delivered by case managers, could be adopted in addiction treatment settings. It includes the detection of SUDs, a brief counseling session based on the principles of MI, and linkage to primary care (Bernstein et al., 1997; D'Onofrio & Degutis, 2010).

The counseling session consists of establishing rapport, providing feedback and education about the importance of receiving primary care, and assessing readiness to accept a referral using a single-item "readiness ruler" (1–10, with 10 indicating readiness). Depending on the patient's response, counseling follows to either help facilitate the referral process or address ambivalence to receiving a referral. An evaluation of this approach found that 47% of the 1096 substance-using patients enrolled in the study received a referral to primary care. Although follow-up rates were low (22%), among those who did return for 60- and 90-day follow-ups and had received a referral, alcohol and drug use severity was reduced and satisfaction with the referral process was high (Bernstein et al., 1997; D'Onofrio & Degutis, 2010).

This approach may be promising, but the existing evidence is not yet sufficient for demonstrating effectiveness. Studies are needed to determine whether this approach is an effective method for transitioning SUD patients from addiction treatment to primary care.

Significance for Services Delivery, Financing, and Research

As we have noted, despite the prevalence of substance use problems, relatively few individuals with SUDs access any form of help. In 2015, only 10.8% of the 21.7 million people who needed substance use treatment received it (Lipari, Park-Lee, & Horn, 2016). In addition, when help is sought, it often occurs 10 or more years after the onset of symptoms of disorder.

As we have also noted, there are many barriers to help seeking, including the stigma of having substance-related problems, concern that treatment is ineffective or not private, and disinterest in abstinence goals. Many people using substances at unhealthy levels believe that their problems are not serious and will improve without help or prefer to handle problems on their own. Further, factors such as family and work responsibilities, the need for childcare and transportation, and the long distance to and costs of treatment discourage help seeking.

In this context of acknowledged barriers to SUD treatment, a variety of low-intensity interventions have been developed and implemented to effectively engage individuals and reduce substance use. These include telephone and internet-based interventions, which attract individuals who otherwise would not seek help. These strategies offer easier access and flexibility to individuals who use substances and circumvent some of the barriers to entry into traditional treatment. They also offer the potential for greater privacy, although strong encryption and other safeguards are needed to ensure that individuals' data remain private and confidential for technology-based interventions. Low-intensity interventions have been shown in research to benefit those who use alcohol harmfully as well as those with more severe alcohol use disorders. For example, a computer-delivered CBT for SUD is an effective adjunct to standard outpatient treatment and thus provides an important means of making CBT more broadly available (Carroll et al., 2009).

Low-intensity interventions can lead to subsequent help seeking and be a starting point for personalized SUD interventions. Innovative behavioral health approaches to SUDs use patient progress while in treatment to personalize interventions. SUD treatments can also incorporate tailoring based on patient characteristics and preferences assessed at intake to personalize care further.

In an effort to examine care that explicitly considered patient preferences, primary care patients who reported heavy drinking were randomly assigned to 12 months of personalized alcohol care management or usual care (Bradley et al., 2018). In the personalized intervention, nurse care managers offered outreach and engagement, repeated brief counseling using MI, and shared decision-making about treatment options and alcohol medications if desired, supported by an interdisciplinary team. The 12-month follow-up showed that a greater proportion of patients in the intervention group than in the usual care group received alcohol-related care. However, no significant differences in substance use outcomes were observed. In explaining these results, the authors noted that as part of the intervention, the trial allowed patients to select their own drinking goals (e.g., abstinence, drinking reduction). However, in light of their review of other related studies (Oslin et al., 2014; Watkins et al., 2017), the authors suggested that to be effective, alcohol interventions may need to include stronger recommendations for abstinence and the use of medications and also make evidence-based behavioral treatments available within the primary care setting.

Implications for Behavioral Health

There is potential to improve access to and coordination of SUD treatment and improved implementation of SBIRT, which we have reviewed in this chapter, as well as for more effective referrals and transitions across the spectrum of care, including primary and specialty care settings, which are critical to high-quality SUD treatment.

An important addition to the implementation of SBIRT are the set of services provided via electronic media and information technologies. Technology-based interventions (e.g., computer- and internet-based interventions, text messaging, interactive voice response, smartphone applications) are extending the reach of effective behavioral treatments for SUDs both in specialty substance use treatment and primary care settings (Tofighi, Abrantes, & Stein, 2018). Advances in technology-based interventions addressing SUDs have made possible increased abstinence with minimal disruption to healthcare staff members and clinical workflow (Tofighi et al., 2018). These interventions cover a range of services, including screening, assessment, and brief and specialized treatment.

As we have discussed, they can provide more accessible and less costly modes of treatment than traditional modalities; that is, they help people access treatment services who would not otherwise seek them because of barriers related to geography (living in remote areas, living in heavy traffic-congested areas, traveling or relocating away from home), shame and guilt, or stigma.

Technology-based help resources can be provided as a sole treatment modality or in combination with other treatment modalities (e.g., in-person MI or CBT) and be either dropped or added to if found ineffective for an individual patient. The help resources of 12-step groups (e.g., Alcoholics, Narcotics, or Cocaine Anonymous, Al-Anon Family Groups) and other mutual help group forums (SMART Recovery, Rational Recovery, Women for Sobriety) are available online.

Despite the promise of technological approaches, rigorous research should continue to establish their feasibility and effectiveness for SUD prevention and treatment. For technology-based interventions to reach their full potential to reduce the burden of SUDs, strategies are needed to facilitate their dissemination and implementation in primary and specialty care, addressing issues of provider adoption, financial reimbursement, integration, and patient engagement (Tofighi et al., 2018). By joining together, the behavioral research, clinical provider, and consumer communities have reason for great optimism in efforts to prevent and treat harms due to alcohol and drug use and addictions.

Acknowledgements Preparation of this chapter was supported by a Senior Research Career Scientist Award (RCS 00-001) to Dr. Timko by the Department of Veterans Affairs (VA) Health Services Research and Development (HSR&D) Service. Views expressed are the authors'.

References

Agerwala, S. M., & McCance-Katz, E. F. (2012). Integrating screening, brief intervention, and referral to treatment (SBIRT) into clinical practice settings: A brief review. *Journal of Psychoactive Drugs, 44*(4), 307–317. https://doi.org/10.1080/02791072.2012.720169

Babor, T. F., Del Boca, F., & Bray, J. W. (2017). Screening, Brief Intervention and Referral to Treatment: Implications of SAMHSA's SBIRT initiative for substance abuse policy and practice. *Addiction, 112*(Suppl 2), 110–117. https://doi.org/10.1111/add.13675

Babor, T. F., McRee, B. G., Kassebaum, P. A., Grimaldi, P. L., Ahmed, K., & Bray, J. (2007). Screening, Brief Intervention, and Referral to Treatment (SBIRT): Toward a public health approach to the management of substance abuse. *Substance Abuse, 28*(3), 7–30. https://doi.org/10.1300/J465v28n03_03

Baker, A. L., Thornton, L. K., Hiles, S., Hides, L., & Lubman, D. I. (2012). Psychological interventions for alcohol misuse among people with co-occurring depression or anxiety disorders: A systematic review. *Journal of Affective Disorders, 139*(3), 217–229. https://doi.org/10.1016/j.jad.2011.08.004

Ball, S. A., Carroll, K. M., Canning-Ball, M., & Rounsaville, B. J. (2006). Reasons for dropout from drug abuse treatment: Symptoms, personality, and motivation. *Addictive Behaviors, 31*(2), 320–330. https://doi.org/10.1016/j.addbeh.2005.05.013

Beardsley, K., Wish, E. D., Fitzelle, D. B., O'Grady, K., & Arria, A. M. (2003). Distance traveled to outpatient drug treatment and client retention. *Journal of Substance Abuse Treatment, 25*(4), 279–285. https://doi.org/10.1016/S0740-5472(03)00188-0

Bernstein, E., Bernstein, J., & Levenson, S. (1997). Project ASSERT: An ED-based intervention to increase access to primary care, preventive services, and the substance abuse treatment system. *Annals of Emergency Medicine, 30*(2), 181–189. https://doi.org/10.1016/S0196-0644(97)70140-9

Bradley, K. A., Bobb, J. F., Ludman, E. J., Chavez, L. J., Saxon, A. J., Merrill, J. O., … Kivlahan, D. R. (2018). Alcohol-related nurse care management in primary care: A randomized clinical trial. *JAMA Internal Medicine, 178*(5), 613–621. https://doi.org/10.1001/jamainternmed.2018.0388

Bradley, K. A., DeBenedetti, A. F., Volk, R. J., Williams, E. C., Frank, D., & Kivlahan, D. R. (2007). AUDIT-C as a brief screen for alcohol misuse in primary care. *Alcoholism, Clinical and Experimental Research, 31*(7), 1208–1217. https://doi.org/10.1111/j.1530-0277.2007.00403.x

Bradley, K. A., & Kivlahan, D. R. (2014). Bringing patient-centered care to patients with alcohol use disorders. *JAMA, 311*(18), 1861–1862. https://doi.org/10.1001/jama.2014.3629

Bradley, K. A., Williams, E. C., Achtmeyer, C. E., Volpp, B., Collins, B. J., & Kivlahan, D. R. (2006). Implementation of evidence-based alcohol screening in the Veterans Health Administration. *American Journal of Managed Care, 12*(10), 597–606. https://www.ajmc.com/journals/issue/2006/2006-10-vol12-n10/oct06-2375p597-606

Burns, L., Teesson, M., & O'Neill, K. (2005). The impact of comorbid anxiety and depression on alcohol treatment outcomes. *Addiction, 100*(6), 787–796. https://doi.org/10.1111/j.1360-0443.2005.001069.x

Carroll, K. M., Ball, S. A., Martino, S., Nich, C., Babuscio, T. A., & Rounsaville, B. J. (2009). Enduring effects of a computer-assisted training program for cognitive behavioral therapy: A 6-month follow-up of CBT4CBT. *Drug and Alcohol Dependence, 100*(1–2), 178–181. https://doi.org/10.1016/j.drugalcdep.2008.09.015

Cather, C., Brunette, M. F., Mueser, K. T., Babbin, S. F., Rosenheck, R., Correll, C. U., & Kalos-Meyer, P. (2018). Impact of comprehensive treatment for first episode psychosis on substance use outcomes: A randomized controlled trial. *Psychiatry Research, 268*, 303–311. https://doi.org/10.1016/j.psychres.2018.06.055

Center for Behavioral Health Statistics and Quality. (2015). *Behavioral health trends in the United States: Results from the 2014 National Survey on Drug Use and Health* (HHS Publication No. SMA 15-4927, NSDUH Series H-50). Rockville, MD: Substance Abuse Mental Health Services Administration (SAMHSA). http://purl.fdlp.gov/GPO/gpo68296

Centers for Disease Control and Prevention. (2018, July 13). *Excessive drinking is draining the US economy* [Web page]. Atlanta, GA: Author (CDC). https://www.cdc.gov/features/costsofdrinking/index.html

Childers, J. W., & Arnold, R. M. (2012). "I feel uncomfortable 'calling a patient out'": Educational needs of palliative medicine fellows in managing opioid misuse. *Journal of Pain and Symptom Management, 43*(2), 253–260. https://doi.org/10.1016/j.jpainsymman.2011.03.009

Coleman, D. L., Moran, E., Serfilippi, D., Mulinski, P., Rosenthal, R., Gordon, B., & Mogielnicki, R. P. (2003). Measuring physicians' productivity in a Veterans' Affairs Medical Center. *Academic Medicine, 78*(7), 682–689.

Coulson, C., Ng, F., Geertsema, M., Dodd, S., & Berk, M. (2009). Client-reported reasons for non-engagement in drug and alcohol treatment. *Drug and Alcohol Review, 28*(4), 372–378. https://doi.org/10.1111/j.1465-3362.2009.00054.x

Cucciare, M. A., Coleman, E. A., & Timko, C. (2015). A conceptual model to facilitate transitions from primary care to specialty substance use disorder care: A review of the literature. *Primary Health Care Research and Development, 16*(5), 492–505. https://doi.org/10.1017/S1463423614000164

Cucciare, M. A., Simpson, T., Hoggatt, K. J., Gifford, E., & Timko, C. (2013). Substance use among women veterans: Epidemiology to evidence-based treatment. *Journal of Addictive Diseases, 32*(2), 119–139. https://doi.org/10.1080/10550887.2013.795465

D'Onofrio, G., & Degutis, L. C. (2010). Integrating Project ASSERT: A screening, intervention, and referral to treatment program for unhealthy alcohol and drug use into an urban emergency department. *Academic Emergency Medicine, 17*(8), 903–911. https://doi.org/10.1111/j.1553-2712.2010.00824.x

Dawson, D. A., Grant, B. F., Stinson, F. S., & Zhou, Y. (2005). Effectiveness of the derived Alcohol Use Disorders Identification Test (AUDIT-C) in screening for alcohol use disorders and risk drinking in the US general population. *Alcoholism, Clinical and Experimental Research, 29*(5), 844–854. https://doi.org/10.1097/01.ALC.0000164374.32229.A2

De Alba, I., Samet, J. H., & Saitz, R. (2004). Burden of medical illness in drug- and alcohol-dependent persons without primary care. *American Journal on Addictions, 13*(1), 33–45. https://doi.org/10.1080/10550490490265307

Donovan, D. M., & Wells, E. A. (2007). 'Tweaking 12-Step': The potential role of 12-step self-help group involvement in methamphetamine recovery. *Addiction, 102*(Suppl 1), 121–129. https://doi.org/10.1111/j.1360-0443.2007.01773.x

El-Guebaly, N. (2012). The meanings of recovery from addiction: Evolution and promises. *Journal of Addiction Medicine, 6*(1), 1–9. https://doi.org/10.1097/ADM.0b013e31823ae540

Falck, R. S., Wang, J., Carlson, R. G., Krishnan, L. L., Leukefeld, C., & Booth, B. M. (2007). Perceived need for substance abuse treatment among illicit stimulant drug users in rural areas of Ohio, Arkansas, and Kentucky. *Drug and Alcohol Dependence, 91*(2–3), 107–114. https://doi.org/10.1016/j.drugalcdep.2007.05.015

Farronato, N. S., Dursteler-Macfarland, K. M., Wiesbeck, G. A., & Petitjean, S. A. (2013). A systematic review comparing cognitive-behavioral therapy and contingency management for cocaine dependence. *Journal of Addictive Diseases, 32*(3), 274–287. https://doi.org/10.1080/10550887.2013.824328

Fiellin, D. A., Barry, D. T., Sullivan, L. E., Cutter, C. J., Moore, B. A., O'Connor, P. G., & Schottenfeld, R. S. (2013). A randomized trial of cognitive behavioral therapy in primary care-based buprenorphine. *American Journal of Medicine, 126*(1), 74.e11–74.e77. https://doi.org/10.1016/j.amjmed.2012.07.005

Ford, J. H., 2nd, Osborne, E. L., Assefa, M. T., McIlvaine, A. M., King, A. M., Campbell, K., & McGovern, M. P. (2018). Using NIATx strategies to implement integrated services in routine care: A study protocol. *BMC Health Services Research, 18*(1), 431. https://doi.org/10.1186/s12913-018-3241-4

Forrest, C. B., Nutting, P. A., von Schrader, S., Rohde, C., & Starfield, B. (2006). Primary care physician specialty referral decision making: Patient, physician, and health care system determinants. *Medical Decision Making, 26*(1), 76–85. https://doi.org/10.1177/0272989x05284110

French, M. T., Roebuck, M. C., McGeary, K. A., Chitwood, D. D., & McCoy, C. B. (2001). Using the drug abuse screening test (DAST-10) to analyze health services utilization and cost for substance users in a community-based setting. *Substance Use and Misuse, 36*(6–7), 927–946. https://doi.org/10.1081/JA-100104096

Friedmann, P. D., Zhang, Z., Hendrickson, J., Stein, M. D., & Gerstein, D. R. (2003). Effect of primary medical care on addiction and medical severity in substance abuse treatment programs. *Journal of General Internal Medicine, 18*(1), 1–8. https://doi.org/10.1046/j.1525-1497.2003.10601.x

Glass, J. E., Hamilton, A. M., Powell, B. J., Perron, B. E., Brown, R. T., & Ilgen, M. A. (2015). Specialty substance use disorder services following brief alcohol intervention: A meta-analysis of randomized controlled trials. *Addiction, 110*(9), 1404–1415. https://doi.org/10.1111/add.12950

Glass, J. E., Perron, B. E., Ilgen, M. A., Chermack, S. T., Ratliff, S., & Zivin, K. (2010). Prevalence and correlates of specialty substance use disorder treatment for Department of Veterans Affairs Healthcare System patients with high alcohol consumption. *Drug and Alcohol Dependence, 112*(1–2), 150–155. https://doi.org/10.1016/j.drugalcdep.2010.06.003

Griswold, K. S., Greene, B., Smith, S. J., Behrens, T., & Blondell, R. D. (2007). Linkage to primary medical care following inpatient detoxification. *American Journal on Addictions, 16*(3), 183–186. https://doi.org/10.1080/10550490701375319

Gurewich, D., Prottas, J., & Sirkin, J. T. (2014). Managing care for patients with substance abuse disorders at community health centers. *Journal of Substance Abuse Treatment, 46*(2), 227–231. https://doi.org/10.1016/j.jsat.2013.06.013

Haverfield, M. C., Schmidt, E., Ilgen, M., & Timko, C. (2018). *Social support networks and symptom severity among patients with co-occurring mental health and substance use disorders*. Menlo Park, CA: U. S. Department of Veterans Affairs, Center for Innovation to Implementation.

Hawkins, E. J., Lapham, G. T., Kivlahan, D. R., & Bradley, K. A. (2010). Recognition and management of alcohol misuse in OEF/OIF and other veterans in the VA: A cross-sectional study. *Drug and Alcohol Dependence, 109*(1–3), 147–153. https://doi.org/10.1016/j.drugalcdep.2009.12.025

Hedden, S. L., & Gfroerer, J. C. (2011). Correlates of perceiving a need for treatment among adults with substance use disorder: Results from a national survey. *Addictive Behaviors, 36*(12), 1213–1222. https://doi.org/10.1016/j.addbeh.2011.07.026

Hettema, J., Steele, J., & Miller, W. R. (2005). Motivational interviewing. *Annual Review of Clinical Psychology, 1*, 91–111. https://doi.org/10.1146/annurev.clinpsy.1.102803.143833

Hoffman, K. A., Ford, J. H., 2nd, Choi, D., Gustafson, D. H., & McCarty, D. (2008). Replication and sustainability of improved access and retention within the Network for the Improvement of Addiction Treatment. *Drug and Alcohol Dependence, 98*(1–2), 63–69. https://doi.org/10.1016/j.drugalcdep.2008.04.016

Hofmann, S. G., Asnaani, A., Vonk, I. J., Sawyer, A. T., & Fang, A. (2012). The efficacy of cognitive behavioral therapy: A review of meta-analyses. *Cognitive Therapy and Research, 36*(5), 427–440. https://doi.org/10.1007/s10608-012-9476-1

Ilgen, M. A., Schulenberg, J., Kloska, D. D., Czyz, E., Johnston, L., & O'Malley, P. (2011). Prevalence and characteristics of substance abuse treatment utilization by U.S. adolescents: National data from 1987 to 2008. *Addictive Behaviors, 36*(12), 1349–1352. https://doi.org/10.1016/j.addbeh.2011.07.036

Jackson, T. (2006). Relationships between perceived close social support and health practices within community samples of American women and men. *Journal of Psychology, 140*(3), 229–246. https://doi.org/10.3200/jrlp.140.3.229-246

Kaskutas, L. A., Bond, J., & Avalos, L. A. (2009). 7-year trajectories of Alcoholics Anonymous attendance and associations with treatment. *Addictive Behaviors, 34*(12), 1029–1035. https://doi.org/10.1016/j.addbeh.2009.06.015

Kaskutas, L. A., Subbaraman, M. S., Witbrodt, J., & Zemore, S. E. (2009). Effectiveness of Making Alcoholics Anonymous Easier: A group format 12-step facilitation approach. *Journal of Substance Abuse Treatment, 37*(3), 228–239. https://doi.org/10.1016/j.jsat.2009.01.004

Kelly, J. F., Kaminer, Y., Kahler, C. W., Hoeppner, B., Yeterian, J., Cristello, J. V., & Timko, C. (2017). A pilot randomized clinical trial testing integrated 12-step facilitation (iTSF) treatment for adolescent substance use disorder. *Addiction, 112*(12), 2155–2166. https://doi.org/10.1111/add.13920

Kelly, J. F., & Westerhoff, C. M. (2010). Does it matter how we refer to individuals with substance-related conditions? A randomized study of two commonly used terms. *International Journal on Drug Policy, 21*(3), 202–207. https://doi.org/10.1016/j.drugpo.2009.10.010

Kelly, T. M., Daley, D. C., & Douaihy, A. B. (2012). Treatment of substance abusing patients with comorbid psychiatric disorders. *Addictive Behaviors, 37*(1), 11–24. https://doi.org/10.1016/j.addbeh.2011.09.010

Kim, T. W., Bernstein, J., Cheng, D. M., Lloyd-Travaglini, C., Samet, J. H., Palfai, T. P., & Saitz, R. (2017). Receipt of addiction treatment as a consequence of a brief intervention for drug use in primary care: A randomized trial. *Addiction, 112*(5), 818–827. https://doi.org/10.1111/add.13701

Kleinman, B. P., Millery, M., Scimeca, M., & Polissar, N. L. (2002). Predicting long-term treatment utilization among addicts entering detoxification: The contribution of help-seeking models. *Journal of Drug Issues, 32*(1), 209–230. https://doi.org/10.1177/002204260203200109

Laine, C., Hauck, W. W., Gourevitch, M. N., Rothman, J., Cohen, A., & Turner, B. J. (2001). Regular outpatient medical and drug abuse care and subsequent hospitalization of persons who use illicit drugs. *JAMA, 285*(18), 2355–2362. https://doi.org/10.1001/jama.285.18.2355

Lapham, G. T., Achtmeyer, C. E., Williams, E. C., Hawkins, E. J., Kivlahan, D. R., & Bradley, K. A. (2012). Increased documented brief alcohol interventions with a performance measure and electronic decision support. *Medical Care, 50*(2), 179–187. https://doi.org/10.1097/MLR.0b013e3181e35743

Larson, M. J., Saitz, R., Horton, N. J., Lloyd-Travaglini, C., & Samet, J. H. (2006). Emergency department and hospital utilization among alcohol and drug-dependent detoxification patients without primary medical care. *American Journal of Drug and Alcohol Abuse, 32*(3), 435–452. https://doi.org/10.1080/00952990600753958

Laudet, A. B., Stanick, V., & Sands, B. (2009). What could the program have done differently? A qualitative examination of reasons for leaving outpatient treatment. *Journal of Substance Abuse Treatment, 37*(2), 182–190. https://doi.org/10.1016/j.jsat.2009.01.001

Lee, E. B., An, W., Levin, M. E., & Twohig, M. P. (2015). An initial meta-analysis of Acceptance and Commitment Therapy for treating substance use disorders. *Drug and Alcohol Dependence, 155*, 1–7. https://doi.org/10.1016/j.drugalcdep.2015.08.004

Li, W., Howard, M. O., Garland, E. L., McGovern, P., & Lazar, M. (2017). Mindfulness treatment for substance misuse: A systematic review and meta-analysis. *Journal of Substance Abuse Treatment, 75*, 62–96. https://doi.org/10.1016/j.jsat.2017.01.008

Lipari, R. N., Park-Lee, E., & Van Horn, S. (2016, September 29). *America's need for and receipt of substance use treatment in 2015* (The CBHSQ Report). Rockville, MD: Substance Abuse and Mental Health Services Administration (SAMHSA). https://www.samhsa.gov/data/sites/default/files/report_2716/ShortReport-2716.html

Livingston, J. D., Milne, T., Fang, M. L., & Amari, E. (2012). The effectiveness of interventions for reducing stigma related to substance use disorders: A systematic review. *Addiction, 107*(1), 39–50. https://doi.org/10.1111/j.1360-0443.2011.03601.x

Lovi, R., & Barr, J. (2009). Stigma reported by nurses related to those experiencing drug and alcohol dependency: A phenomenological Giorgi study. *Contemporary Nurse, 33*(2), 166–178. https://doi.org/10.5172/conu.2009.33.2.166

Lubman, D. I., King, J. A., & Castle, D. J. (2010). Treating comorbid substance use disorders in schizophrenia. *International Review of Psychiatry, 22*(2), 191–201. https://doi.org/10.3109/09540261003689958

Lubman, D. I., & Sundram, S. (2003). Substance misuse in patients with schizophrenia: A primary care guide. *Medical Journal of Australia, 178*(Suppl), S71–S75. https://www.mja.com.au/journal/2003/178/9/substance-misuse-patients-schizophrenia-primary-care-guide

Lussier, J. P., Heil, S. H., Mongeon, J. A., Badger, G. J., & Higgins, S. T. (2006). A meta-analysis of voucher-based reinforcement therapy for substance use disorders. *Addiction, 101*(2), 192–203. https://doi.org/10.1111/j.1360-0443.2006.01311.x

Madras, B. K., Compton, W. M., Avula, D., Stegbauer, T., Stein, J. B., & Clark, H. W. (2009). Screening, brief interventions, referral to treatment (SBIRT) for illicit drug and alcohol use at multiple healthcare sites: comparison at intake and 6 months later. *Drug and Alcohol Dependence, 99*(1–3), 280–295. https://doi.org/10.1016/j.drugalcdep.2008.08.003

Masson, C. L., Shopshire, M. S., Sen, S., Hoffman, K. A., Hengl, N. S., Bartolome, J., … Iguchi, M. Y. (2013). Possible barriers to enrollment in substance abuse treatment among a diverse sample of Asian Americans and Pacific Islanders: Opinions of treatment clients. *Journal of Substance Abuse Treatment, 44*(3), 309–315. https://doi.org/10.1016/j.jsat.2012.08.005

McCarty, D., Gustafson, D., Capoccia, V. A., & Cotter, F. (2009). Improving care for the treatment of alcohol and drug disorders. *Journal of Behavioral Health Services and Research, 36*(1), 52–60. https://doi.org/10.1007/s11414-008-9108-4

McCrady, B. S., Epstein, E. E., Cook, S., Jensen, N. K., & Ladd, B. O. (2011). What do women want? Alcohol treatment choices, treatment entry and retention. *Psychology of Addictive Behaviors, 25*(3), 521–529. https://doi.org/10.1037/a0024037

McGovern, M. P., Lambert-Harris, C., Gotham, H. J., Claus, R. E., & Xie, H. (2014). Dual diagnosis capability in mental health and addiction treatment services: An assessment of programs across multiple state systems. *Administration and Policy in Mental Health, 41*(2), 205–214. https://doi.org/10.1007/s10488-012-0449-1

McKay, J. R. (2009). Continuing care research: What we have learned and where we are going. *Journal of Substance Abuse Treatment, 36*(2), 131–145. https://doi.org/10.1016/j.jsat.2008.10.004

McNeely, J., Strauss, S. M., Wright, S., Rotrosen, J., Khan, R., Lee, J. D., & Gourevitch, M. N. (2014). Test-retest reliability of a self-administered Alcohol, Smoking and Substance Involvement Screening Test (ASSIST) in primary care patients. *Journal of Substance Abuse Treatment, 47*(1), 93–101. https://doi.org/10.1016/j.jsat.2014.01.007

McQuade, W. H., Levy, S. M., Yanek, L. R., Davis, S. W., & Liepman, M. R. (2000). Detecting symptoms of alcohol abuse in primary care settings. *Archives of Family Medicine, 9*(9), 814–821. http://triggered.stanford.clockss.org/ServeContent?url=http%3A%2F%2Farchfami.ama-assn.org%2Fcgi%2Freprint%2F9%2F9%2F814

Meldrum, M. L. (2016). The ongoing opioid prescription epidemic: Historical context. *American Journal of Public Health, 106*(8), 1365–1366. https://doi.org/10.2105/ajph.2016.303297

Merikangas, K. R., & Kalaydjian, A. (2007). Magnitude and impact of comorbidity of mental disorders from epidemiologic surveys. *Current Opinion in Psychiatry, 20*(4), 353–358. https://doi.org/10.1097/YCO.0b013e3281c61dc5

Miller, W. R., & Rollnick, S. (2002). *Motivational interviewing: Preparing people for change.* New York, NY: Guilford Press.

Moos, R. H., & Moos, B. S. (2006). Participation in treatment and Alcoholics Anonymous: A 16-year follow-up of initially untreated individuals. *Journal of Clinical Psychology, 62*(6), 735–750. https://doi.org/10.1002/jclp.20259

Mowbray, O., Perron, B. E., Bohnert, A. S., Krentzman, A. R., & Vaughn, M. G. (2010). Service use and barriers to care among heroin users: Results from a national survey. *American Journal of Drug and Alcohol Abuse, 36*(6), 305–310. https://doi.org/10.3109/00952990.2010.503824

Mueser, K. T., & Gingerich, S. (2013). Treatment of co-occurring psychotic and substance use disorders. *Social Work in Public Health, 28*(3–4), 424–439. https://doi.org/10.1080/19371918.2013.774676

National Drug Intelligence Center. (2011). *The economic impact of illicit drug use on American society.* Johnstown, PA: U.S. Department of Justice, National Drug Intelligence Center.

Nowinski, J., Baker, S., Carroll, K., & National Institute on Alcohol Abuse and Alcoholism. (2007). *Twelve step facilitation therapy manual: A clinical research guide for therapists treating individuals with alcohol abuse and dependence.* Rockville, MD: U.S. Dept. of Health and

Human Services, Public Health Service, National Institutes of Health, National Institute on Alcohol Abuse and Alcoholism.

Office of the Surgeon General. (2016). *Facing addiction in America: The Surgeon General's report on alcohol, drugs, and health (Reports of the Surgeon General).* Washington, DC: US Department of Health and Human Services. https://addiction.surgeongeneral.gov/surgeon-generals-report.pdf

Oleski, J., Mota, N., Cox, B. J., & Sareen, J. (2010). Perceived need for care, help seeking, and perceived barriers to care for alcohol use disorders in a national sample. *Psychiatric Services, 61*(12), 1223–1231. https://doi.org/10.1176/ps.2010.61.12.1223

Oslin, D. W., Lynch, K. G., Maisto, S. A., Lantinga, L. J., McKay, J. R., Possemato, K., ... Wierzbicki, M. (2014). A randomized clinical trial of alcohol care management delivered in Department of Veterans Affairs primary care clinics versus specialty addiction treatment. *Journal of General Internal Medicine, 29*(1), 162–168. https://doi.org/10.1007/s11606-013-2625-8

Palmer, R. S., Murphy, M. K., Piselli, A., & Ball, S. A. (2009). Substance user treatment dropout from client and clinician perspectives: A pilot study. *Substance Use and Misuse, 44*(7), 1021–1038. https://doi.org/10.1080/10826080802495237

Perron, B. E., Mowbray, O. P., Glass, J. E., Delva, J., Vaughn, M. G., & Howard, M. O. (2009). Differences in service utilization and barriers among Blacks, Hispanics, and Whites with drug use disorders. *Substance Abuse Treatment, Prevention, and Policy, 4,* 3. https://doi.org/10.1186/1747-597x-4-3

Petry, N. M., Alessi, S. M., Olmstead, T. A., Rash, C. J., & Zajac, K. (2017). Contingency management treatment for substance use disorders: How far has it come, and where does it need to go? *Psychology of Addictive Behaviors, 31*(8), 897–906. https://doi.org/10.1037/adb0000287

Prendergast, M., Podus, D., Finney, J., Greenwell, L., & Roll, J. (2006). Contingency management for treatment of substance use disorders: A meta-analysis. *Addiction, 101*(11), 1546–1560. https://doi.org/10.1111/j.1360-0443.2006.01581.x

Pulford, J., Adams, P., & Sheridan, J. (2006). Unilateral treatment exit: A failure of retention or a failure of treatment fit? *Substance Use and Misuse, 41*(14), 1901–1920. https://doi.org/10.1080/10826080601025847

Rapp, R. C., Otto, A. L., Lane, D. T., Redko, C., McGatha, S., & Carlson, R. G. (2008). Improving linkage with substance abuse treatment using brief case management and motivational interviewing. *Drug and Alcohol Dependence, 94*(1–3), 172–182. https://doi.org/10.1016/j.drugalcdep.2007.11.012

Rash, C. J., Stitzer, M., & Weinstock, J. (2017). Contingency management: New directions and remaining challenges for an evidence-based intervention. *Journal of Substance Abuse Treatment, 72,* 10–18. https://doi.org/10.1016/j.jsat.2016.09.008

Riper, H., Andersson, G., Hunter, S. B., de Wit, J., Berking, M., & Cuijpers, P. (2014). Treatment of comorbid alcohol use disorders and depression with cognitive-behavioural therapy and motivational interviewing: A meta-analysis. *Addiction, 109*(3), 394–406. https://doi.org/10.1111/add.12441

Roberts, N. P., Roberts, P. A., Jones, N., & Bisson, J. I. (2016). Psychological therapies for post-traumatic stress disorder and comorbid substance use disorder. *Cochrane Database of Systematic Reviews, 4,* Cd010204. https://doi.org/10.1002/14651858.CD010204.pub2

Saitz, R., Horton, N. J., Larson, M. J., Winter, M., & Samet, J. H. (2005). Primary medical care and reductions in addiction severity: A prospective cohort study. *Addiction, 100*(1), 70–78. https://doi.org/10.1111/j.1360-0443.2005.00916.x

Saitz, R., Larson, M. J., Horton, N. J., Winter, M., & Samet, J. H. (2004). Linkage with primary medical care in a prospective cohort of adults with addictions in inpatient detoxification: Room for improvement. *Health Services Research, 39*(3), 587–606. https://doi.org/10.1111/j.1475-6773.2004.00246.x

Saitz, R., Palfai, T. P., Cheng, D. M., Alford, D. P., Bernstein, J. A., Lloyd-Travaglini, C. A., ... Samet, J. H. (2014). Screening and brief intervention for drug use in primary care: the ASPIRE randomized clinical trial. *JAMA, 312*(5), 502–513. https://doi.org/10.1001/jama.2014.7862

Samet, J. H., Friedmann, P., & Saitz, R. (2001). Benefits of linking primary medical care and substance abuse services: Patient, provider, and societal perspectives. *Archives of Internal Medicine, 161*(1), 85–91. https://doi.org/10.1001/archinte.161.1.85

Samet, J. H., Larson, M. J., Horton, N. J., Doyle, K., Winter, M., & Saitz, R. (2003). Linking alcohol- and drug-dependent adults to primary medical care: A randomized controlled trial of a multi-disciplinary health intervention in a detoxification unit. *Addiction, 98*(4), 509–516. https://doi.org/10.1046/j.1360-0443.2003.00328.x

Saxon, A. J., Malte, C. A., Sloan, K. L., Baer, J. S., Calsyn, D. A., Nichol, P., … Kivlahan, D. R. (2006). Randomized trial of onsite versus referral primary medical care for veterans in addictions treatment. *Medical Care, 44*(4), 334–342. https://doi.org/10.1097/01.mlr.0000204052.95507.5c

Sayegh, C. S., Huey, S. J., Zara, E. J., & Jhaveri, K. (2017). Follow-up treatment effects of contingency management and motivational interviewing on substance use: A meta-analysis. *Psychology of Addictive Behaviors, 31*(4), 403–414. https://doi.org/10.1037/adb0000277

Schierenberg, A., van Amsterdam, J., van den Brink, W., & Goudriaan, A. E. (2012). Efficacy of contingency management for cocaine dependence treatment: A review of the evidence. *Current Drug Abuse Reviews, 5*(4), 320–331. https://doi.org/10.2174/1874473711205040006

Schomerus, G., Lucht, M., Holzinger, A., Matschinger, H., Carta, M. G., & Angermeyer, M. C. (2011). The stigma of alcohol dependence compared with other mental disorders: A review of population studies. *Alcohol and Alcoholism, 46*(2), 105–112. https://doi.org/10.1093/alcalc/agq089

Skinner, N., Roche, A. M., Freeman, T., & Addy, D. (2005). Responding to alcohol and other drug issues: The effect of role adequacy and role legitimacy on motivation and satisfaction. *Drugs: Education, Prevention & Policy, 12*(6), 449–463. https://doi.org/10.1080/09687630500284281

Smith, P. C., Schmidt, S. M., Allensworth-Davies, D., & Saitz, R. (2009). Primary care validation of a single-question alcohol screening test. *Journal of General Internal Medicine, 24*(7), 783–788. https://doi.org/10.1007/s11606-009-0928-6

Smith, P. C., Schmidt, S. M., Allensworth-Davies, D., & Saitz, R. (2010). A single-question screening test for drug use in primary care. *Archives of Internal Medicine, 170*(13), 1155–1160. https://doi.org/10.1001/archinternmed.2010.140

Stevens, J., Kelleher, K. J., Gardner, W., Chisolm, D., McGeehan, J., Pajer, K., & Buchanan, L. (2008). Trial of computerized screening for adolescent behavioral concerns. *Pediatrics, 121*(6), 1099–1105. https://doi.org/10.1542/peds.2007-1878

Strathdee, S. A., Ricketts, E. P., Huettner, S., Cornelius, L., Bishai, D., Havens, J. R., … Latkin, C. A. (2006). Facilitating entry into drug treatment among injection drug users referred from a needle exchange program: Results from a community-based behavioral intervention trial. *Drug and Alcohol Dependence, 83*(3), 225–232. https://doi.org/10.1016/j.drugalcdep.2005.11.015

Sweeney, L. P., Samet, J. H., Larson, M. J., & Saitz, R. (2004). Establishment of a multidisciplinary Health Evaluation and Linkage to Primary care (HELP) clinic in a detoxification unit. *Journal of Addictive Diseases, 23*(2), 33–45. https://doi.org/10.1300/J069v23n02_03

Timko, C., & DeBenedetti, A. (2007). A randomized controlled trial of intensive referral to 12-step self-help groups: One-year outcomes. *Drug and Alcohol Dependence, 90*(2–3), 270–279. https://doi.org/10.1016/j.drugalcdep.2007.04.007

Timko, C., Kong, C., Vittorio, L., & Cucciare, M. A. (2016). Screening and brief intervention for unhealthy substance use in patients with chronic medical conditions: A systematic review. *Journal of Clinical Nursing, 25*(21–22), 3131–3143. https://doi.org/10.1111/jocn.13244

Timko, C., Sutkowi, A., Cronkite, R. C., Makin-Byrd, K., & Moos, R. H. (2011). Intensive referral to 12-step dual-focused mutual-help groups. *Drug and Alcohol Dependence, 118*(2–3), 194–201. https://doi.org/10.1016/j.drugalcdep.2011.03.019

Tofighi, B., Abrantes, A., & Stein, M. D. (2018). The role of technology-based interventions for substance use disorders in primary care: A review of the literature. *Medical Clinics of North America, 102*(4), 715–731. https://doi.org/10.1016/j.mcna.2018.02.011

Treloar, C., & Holt, M. (2006). Deficit models and divergent philosophies: Service providers' perspectives on barriers and incentives to drug treatment. *Drugs: Education, Prevention & Policy, 13*(4), 367–382. https://doi.org/10.1080/09687630600761444

U.S. Preventive Services Task Force. (2014). Screening and behavioral counseling interventions in primary care to reduce alcohol misuse: Recommendations statement. *American Family Physician, 89*(12), 970A–970D. https://www.aafp.org/afp/2014/0615/od1.html

Viggiano, T., Pincus, H. A., & Crystal, S. (2012). Care transition interventions in mental health. *Current Opinion in Psychiatry, 25*(6), 551–558. https://doi.org/10.1097/YCO.0b013e328358df75

Voluse, A. C., Gioia, C. J., Sobell, L. C., Dum, M., Sobell, M. B., & Simco, E. R. (2012). Psychometric properties of the Drug Use Disorders Identification Test (DUDIT) with substance abusers in outpatient and residential treatment. *Addictive Behaviors, 37*(1), 36–41. https://doi.org/10.1016/j.addbeh.2011.07.030

Wamsley, M., Satterfield, J. M., Curtis, A., Lundgren, L., & Satre, D. D. (2018). Alcohol and Drug Screening, Brief Intervention, and Referral to Treatment (SBIRT) training and implementation: Perspectives from 4 health professions. *Journal of Addiction Medicine, 12*(4), 262–272. https://doi.org/10.1097/adm.0000000000000410

Watkins, K. E., Ober, A. J., Lamp, K., Lind, M., Setodji, C., Osilla, K. C., … Pincus, H. A. (2017). Collaborative care for opioid and alcohol use disorders in primary care: The SUMMIT randomized clinical trial. *JAMA Internal Medicine, 177*(10), 1480–1488. https://doi.org/10.1001/jamainternmed.2017.3947

Weisner, C., Mertens, J., Parthasarathy, S., Moore, C., & Lu, Y. (2001). Integrating primary medical care with addiction treatment: A randomized controlled trial. *JAMA, 286*(14), 1715–1723. https://doi.org/10.1001/jama.286.14.1715

Weisner, C., Mertens, J., Tam, T., & Moore, C. (2001). Factors affecting the initiation of substance abuse treatment in managed care. *Addiction, 96*(5), 705–716. https://doi.org/10.1080/09652140020039071

Wendt, D. C., Hallgren, K. A., Daley, D. C., & Donovan, D. M. (2017). Predictors and outcomes of twelve-step sponsorship of stimulant users: Secondary analyses of a multisite randomized clinical trial. *Journal of Studies on Alcohol and Drugs, 78*(2), 287–295. https://doi.org/10.15288/jsad.2017.78.287

Westra, H. A., Aviram, A., & Doell, F. K. (2011). Extending motivational interviewing to the treatment of major mental health problems: Current directions and evidence. *Canadian Journal of Psychiatry. Revue Canadienne de Psychiatrie, 56*(11), 643–650. https://doi.org/10.1177/070674371105601102

Williams, E. C., Lapham, G. T., Hawkins, E. J., Rubinsky, A. D., Morales, L. S., Young, B. A., & Bradley, K. A. (2012). Variation in documented care for unhealthy alcohol consumption across race/ethnicity in the Department of Veterans Affairs Healthcare System. *Alcoholism, Clinical and Experimental Research, 36*(9), 1614–1622. https://doi.org/10.1111/j.1530-0277.2012.01761.x

Woodhead, E. L., Timko, C., Han, X., & Cucciare, M. A. (2018). *Stigma, treatment, and health among adult stimulant users: Life stage as a moderator.* San Jose, CA: San Jose State University.

World Health Organization. (2014). *Global status report on alcohol and health.* Geneva, Switzerland: Author (WHO). http://www.who.int/substance_abuse/publications/global_alcohol_report/msb_gsr_2014_1.pdf?ua=1

Yudko, E., Lozhkina, O., & Fouts, A. (2007). A comprehensive review of the psychometric properties of the Drug Abuse Screening Test. *Journal of Substance Abuse Treatment, 32*(2), 189–198. https://doi.org/10.1016/j.jsat.2006.08.002

Financing of Behavioral Health Services: Insurance, Managed Care, and Reimbursement

Samuel H. Zuvekas

Introduction

Behavioral health has evolved over time to largely insurance-based and insurance-financed systems of care, becoming much more like the rest of the health-care system. Up until the 1950s, most behavioral health services were provided in state and local long-term psychiatric hospitals and financed primarily through state and local general revenues. The Community Mental Health Centers Act of 1963 added federal funding for more community-based services through grants to the states. But it was the passage of the Medicare and Medicaid health insurance programs in the 1960s that fundamentally altered the way behavioral health services were financed in this country. Medicaid, in particular, created powerful incentives to provide services outside of state psychiatric facilities because only half the costs of treatment provided in the community were paid for by the states. In contrast, states were responsible for all of the costs of inpatient treatment in psychiatric and other long-term facilities under the Medicaid Institutions for Mental Disease (IMD) rule. The federal Social Security Disability Income (SSDI) program, passed in 1956, and later the Supplemental Security Income (SSI) program in the 1970s provided further impetus for community-based services by giving income support to those individuals disabled by mental disorders.

Private health insurance systems have also become central to the financing of behavioral health services. Most Americans under the age of 65 obtain health insurance coverage through employers and unions rather than through public insurance

---

The views expressed in this chapter are those of the author, and no official endorsement by the Agency for Healthcare Research and Quality, or the Department of Health and Human Services is intended or should be inferred.

S. H. Zuvekas (✉)
US Agency for Healthcare Research and Quality, Rockville, MD, USA
e-mail: Samuel.zuvekas@ahrq.hhs.gov

© Springer Nature Switzerland AG 2020
B. L. Levin, A. Hanson (eds.), *Foundations of Behavioral Health*,
https://doi.org/10.1007/978-3-030-18435-3_4

programs. The introduction of new classes of antidepressant in the 1980s and 1990s led millions more Americans into treatment, the majority with private health insurance coverage (Kessler et al., 2005; Zuvekas, 2001). Similarly, greater recognition and acceptance of medication-based treatment of ADHD, anxiety, and other behavioral disorders have led still more Americans into treatment. The availability of both public and private health insurance to finance medication-based and other treatments has considerably broadened the behavioral health systems beyond those with the most severe and persistent mental illnesses such as bipolar disorders and schizophrenia.

The movement to insurance-based behavioral health treatment systems also means tighter integration with the larger and constantly evolving health and social insurance systems. Thus, changes in the Medicaid and Medicare public insurance programs and private health plans largely drive how behavioral health services are organized, delivered, and financed. In particular, the expansions in insurance coverage under the 2010 Affordable Care Act (ACA) led to some 20 million Americans gaining insurance and, with coverage, a means of financing their behavioral health treatment (Uberoi, Finegold, & Gee, 2016). The ACA also extended the 2008 Mental Health Parity and Addiction Equity Act (MHPAEA) requiring equivalent coverage (or parity) between behavioral health and other health-care services and contained other important protections for behavioral health treatment (Barry, Goldman, & Huskamp, 2016; Beronio, Glied, & Frank, 2014).

The principal goals of this chapter are to (1) understand how insurance-based models of financing operate in theory and in practice and (2) understand the implications of increasing strains on private and public insurance systems, including the ACA insurance expansions and parity, for the future of behavioral health services.

Review of the Literature

Paying for Behavioral Health Treatment

Funding for behavioral health treatment comes from a complex array of public and private sources (SAMHSA, 2016), predominantly insurance-based. An estimated $220 billion was spent on behavioral health in 2014, accounting for 7.5% of all health-care spending in the United States (see Table 1). Public and private health plans together paid 64% of behavioral health care in 2014, up from 45% in 1986. In comparison, insurance financed 74% of all non-behavioral health spending in 2014 (Mark et al., 2016; SAMHSA, 2016). Private insurance coverage (26%) and Medicaid (24%) each accounted for about a quarter of all behavioral health spending in 2014, followed by Medicare (14%). Medicaid is a more important source of financing for behavioral health services compared to other health-care services, while Medicare and private insurance plans are less important.

Table 1 Distribution of spending by payment source, 1986, 2004, and 2014

| | Behavioral health care | | | | | | All health care | |
| | 1986 | | 2004 | | 2014 | | 2014 | |
	Billions ($)	Percent	Billions ($)	Percent	Billions ($)	Percent	Billions ($)	Percent
Private—total	18.5	44	50.8	39	86.3	39	1492.6	51
Out-of-pocket	6.9	17	14.6	11	22.3	10	343.8	12
Private insurance	9.5	23	32.4	25	58.1	26	1020.3	35
Other private	2.1	5	3.7	3	6.0	3	128.6	4
Public—total	23.1	56	79.4	61	133.6	61	1422.7	49
Medicare	2.4	6	8.5	7	30.3	14	616.8	21
Medicaid[a,b]	6.4	16	36.3	28	53.0	24	507.0	17
Other federal[b,c]	3.0	7	8.3	6	14.4	7	136.4	5
Other state and local[b]	11.2	27	26.3	20	35.9	16	162.5	6
Total	41.5	100	130.2	100	220.0	100	2915.3	100

Source: Adapted from Table A7, SAMHSA (2016)
[a]Includes state and local share of Medicaid
[b]State Children's Health Insurance Program (CHIP) spending is distributed across Medicaid, other federal, and other state and local categories, depending on whether the CHIP program was run through Medicaid or as a separate state CHIP program.
[c]SAMHSA block grants to "state and local" agencies are part of "other federal" government spending

It is important to note that the trend toward insurance-based financing of treatment over the last couple of decades extends mainly to mental health treatment services and not substance use disorders (Mark et al., 2016). The majority of funding for substance use disorders still comes from public sources other than Medicare and Medicaid and is unchanged over the last couple of decades (Mark et al., 2016; SAMHSA, 2016). Other sources of funding are still important for mental health treatment as well. State and local authorities still accounted for 16% of all behavioral health spending in 2014 apart from Medicaid (Table 1). Other federal sources, including Veterans Affairs, military health care, the Indian Health Services, and the $2.3 billion in SAMHSA block grants (SAMHSA, 2015) to state and local agencies, accounted for 7% of all behavioral health spending. Patients and their families financed 10% of all behavioral health care themselves out-of-pocket, while other private sources accounted for 3%.

Where Do Treatment Dollars Go?

Behavioral health treatment today is largely community-based. Only about one in four behavioral health treatment dollars was spent in specialty psychiatric and general hospitals in 2014, down from 43% in 1986 (Table 2). Because these aggregate

Table 2 Behavioral health services spending by type of service, 1986, 2004, and 2014

	1986		2004		2014	
	Billions ($)	Percent	Billions ($)	Percent	Billions ($)	Percent
Specialty sector	*27.2*	*65*	*67.3*	*52*	*108.9*	*50*
General hospitals. Specialty units[a]	5.6	14	13.8	11	25.3	12
Specialty hospitals	9.7	23	14.1	11	19.6	9
Psychiatrists	2.6	6	7.8	6	10.5	5
Other professionals[b]	2.2	5	7.4	6	14.5	7
Specialty mental health centers[c]	4.8	11	17.1	13	28.4	13
Specialty SUD centers[d]	2.3	6	7.2	6	10.5	5
General sector providers	*9.8*	*23*	*20.4*	*16*	*39.5*	*18*
General hospitals. Non-specialty units[a]	2.5	6	6.6	5	15.4	7
Nonpsychiatric physicians	2.0	5	6.0	6	11.3	5
Free-standing nursing homes	5.1	12	6.6	5	9.4	4
Free-standing home health	0.1	0	1.2	1	3.4	2
Retail prescription medications	*2.6*	*6*	*32.0*	*25*	*52.9*	*24*
Insurance administration	*2.0*	*5*	*10.5*	*8*	*18.7*	*9*
Total	*41.5*	*100*	*130.2*	*100*	*220.0*	*100*

Source: Adapted from Table A.4. (SAMHSA, 2016)
[a]All spending for psychiatric services in Department of Veterans Affairs hospitals is included in general hospital specialty unit providers.
[b]Includes psychologists, counselors, and social workers
[c]Includes residential treatment centers for children
[d]Includes other facilities for treating SUDs

figures for hospitals also include outpatient and partial day treatment, the amount spent on inpatient treatment is even less. Spending in psychiatric specialty hospitals now accounts for less than 1 of every 10 behavioral health-care dollars, down from 23% in 1986. Much of the drop was due to the rapid growth of specialty managed behavioral health-care organizations (MBHOs) during the 1980s and 1990s. MBHOs achieved cost savings primarily by promoting outpatient care in place of more expensive inpatient treatment (Ma & McGuire, 1998; National Advisory Mental Health Council, 2000; Sturm, 1997). However, administrative costs of insurance have increased as a by-product of increased management of behavioral health services. That is, over time proportionately fewer dollars are going to direct patient care.

Spending on psychiatrists has grown less rapidly than spending on other behavioral health professionals (Table 2). The nonpsychiatric physician share of total spending remains only about 5%. However, these aggregate estimates may understate the true amount spent on primary care physicians because behavioral health services and diagnoses are often not coded as such in the insurance claims data that form the basis for these estimates. In fact, the majority of people receiving behavioral health services get their care from nonspecialist providers, although they tend to have many fewer visits on average than people who receive services from specialists (Wang et al., 2005).

Prescription medications account for about a quarter of all behavioral health spending (Table 2). Spending on medications grew rapidly from the 1980s through the turn of the century with the introduction of expensive new classes of antidepressants, antipsychotics, and other behavioral health-related medications. These newer medications were many times more costly than older medications. Equally, if not more important, many more people were prescribed psychotropic medications. Spending on behavioral health medications has moderated over the last decade as generic versions of most of these medications became available and the growth in the number of Americans taking them flattened out.

Principles of Insurance

The main function of insurance is to protect people from financial risk when catastrophe strikes. In this sense, health insurance is much like automobile, homeowners, or life insurance. Instead of paying a fixed amount to your family if you die under a life insurance policy or paying to rebuild your house, health insurance helps pay medical bills when you are sick. When private health insurance plans first began in the 1940s and 1950s, they principally covered inpatient hospital stays. As other services grew in importance and expense, coverage expanded to include physician and other provider expenses and, more recently, prescription drugs. As late as the 1970s, many private plans did not offer prescription drug coverage—now it is almost universal. Likewise, Medicare did not offer the Part D prescription drug benefit until 2006—now approximately 86% of Medicare beneficiaries have drug coverage (Kaiser Family Foundation, 2018a). Health insurance, however, differs in crucial ways from other common types of insurance (Arrow, 1963).

Principles of Insurance: Moral Hazard

Health insurance contracts tend to be more open-ended than other types of insurance contracts because it is difficult to predict beforehand which of the many different types of illnesses you might get and how much health care you might need. That is, health insurance contracts are rarely written in such a way that if I get, say, leukemia, I will be paid a fixed $200,000, or if I get pneumonia, I will be paid $10,000. The open-ended nature of health insurance coverage leads to a situation that economists call *moral hazard*, where people overconsume health care. With health insurance coverage, out-of-pocket costs are generally less than the true cost of providing health care. At some point, the benefits of additional health-care services (e.g., extra tests) in terms of improving health are not worth their full costs, but because the insured only pay a fraction of the costs, they still want to use the services to get better.

Consumer cost-sharing evolved in response to this fundamental problem of moral hazard. By shifting at least some of the costs of health care to consumers, they become more sensitive to the true costs of health care. Current health-care reform discussions often refer to this idea as consumers having "skin in the game." Traditionally, health insurance plans imposed a *deductible*, where the health insurance plan only paid for services after consumers had paid a certain amount out of their own pockets (typically, $250 or $500). More recently, high-deductible health plans (HDHP), where health-care services, except for a limited set of preventive care services, are only covered after a deductible of $1350 or higher in 2018 is met (most often considerably higher), have become popular with employers (AHRQ, 2017; Claxton, Rae, Long, Damico, Foster, Whitmore, 2017).

Health plans also traditionally imposed cost-sharing in the form of *coinsurance*, where the consumer paid, typically, 20% of the cost of services (after the deductible had been met) and the plan 80%. As health insurance plans evolved, fixed *co-payments* for particular services, for example, $25 for an office visit or $35 for a brand-name prescription drug, have become common. While consumer cost-sharing can reduce excess use of health-care services, it can also reduce appropriate use of health-care services (Goldman, Dirani, Fastenau, & Conrad, 2014; Rice & Matsuoka, 2004). Thus, there is always a trade-off between the benefits of more generous insurance coverage and moral hazard. The goal with cost-sharing is to strike a balance in this trade-off (Besley, 1988; Zeckhauser, 1970).

The best-known evidence regarding moral hazard in health insurance coverage comes from the RAND Health Insurance Experiment (HIE), a large-scale, randomized control trial conducted from 1977 to 1982. This landmark study found that consumers' use of mental health services was twice as responsive to their out-of-pocket price as other medical services (Keeler, Manning, & Wells, 1988). The RAND HIE results became the main justification for providing less generous coverage for mental health services on economic efficiency grounds: moral hazard is greater where consumers are more sensitive to the price of services. However, several lines of evidence suggest that consumers are no longer as sensitive to the price of outpatient mental health services as they were four decades ago when treatment options were more limited (Goldman et al., 2006; Meyerhoefer & Zuvekas, 2010).

Principles of Insurance: Adverse and Favorable Risk Selection

Economists refer to moral hazard as a type of market failure because it leads to less than 100% insurance coverage. *Risk selection* can lead to even more serious market failure. Consumers with greater anticipated health needs are naturally more motivated to seek insurance coverage to cover the costs of services, and the more generous the coverage the better. This will drive up costs in plans that attract sicker-than-average patients (*adverse selection*). Insurers can respond by raising premiums, restricting coverage so as not to attract higher-risk consumers, and/or using other means to discourage higher-risk consumers. If insurers raise premiums, this can lead to a situation where the healthier consumers drop coverage (because it is no longer as good a deal). This causes premiums to go still higher, in turn, causing the next-healthiest consumers to drop coverage and so on (Rothschild & Stiglitz, 1976). In the extreme, this can lead to an insurance "death spiral," where the insurance market ceases to exist altogether, something that has been observed in the real world (Cutler & Reber, 1998; Cutler & Zeckhauser, 1998).

Adverse selection is thought to be especially acute in behavioral health (Frank, Glazer, & McGuire, 2000; Frank & McGuire, 2000; McGuire, 2016; Montz et al., 2016). Consumers with behavioral health disorders have much higher medical costs on average than other consumers and are thus unattractive risks from a health plan's perspective. For example, depression frequently co-occurs with diabetes and heart disease. The Federal Employees Health Benefits (FEHB) program during the 1960s and 1970s provides the classic illustration of adverse selection (Frank et al., 2000; Padgett, Patrick, Burns, Schlesinger, & Cohen, 1993). Federal employees have long had the choice of a number of health plans through the FEHBP. Several of the plans in the FEHBP began offering generous mental health coverage, others did not. Not surprisingly, consumers with behavioral health disorders migrated to the more generous plans, which raised costs. In response, the generous plans cut their behavioral health-care coverage so that coverage was low in all the plans by the late 1970s. Behavioral health coverage remained low in the federal health plans until 2001, when an executive order mandating parity coverage in all plans went into effect (Goldman et al., 2006).

Regulatory actions, such as parity mandates, are one potential solution to adverse selection. *Risk adjustment*, where payments vary according to the risk the plan faces in their population, is another standard approach to mitigating adverse selection. Risk adjustment is used, for example, in the payments made to Medicare and Medicaid managed care plans and in the ACA private insurance marketplaces. Much work has gone into devising better risk-adjustment methodologies over the last few decades, but they remain imperfect: predicting future medical expenditures is inherently difficult. With imperfect adjustments for risks, insurance plans have strong incentives to seek out better risks (favorable selection, often referred to as "cream skimming" or "cherry picking") and avoid sicker patients.

Mechanisms to induce pooling of consumers are another potential means for mitigating adverse selection. The dominance of employment-related health insurance arose partly by accident as employers used health insurance coverage as a means to attract and retain high-quality workers, much like retirement benefits. But public policy has also deliberately encouraged this development. Employer groups are seen as a convenient way to pool consumers independent of their health status. The value of health insurance benefits is not taxed, creating incentives for employers to provide, and employees to receive, compensation in the form of health insurance benefits, rather than higher wages, which are taxable. Some argue that this tax subsidy encourages too much insurance and overconsumption of medical care due to moral hazard. The ACA, for example, contains provisions to tax "Cadillac" plans above a certain threshold, although its implementation has been continually delayed. Other reform proposals would eliminate the tax subsidy altogether. Others argue that it is the glue that keeps the employment-related insurance system together and that the system might fall apart altogether due to adverse selection as the healthier workers opt out without the subsidy (Bernard & Selden, 2002; Monheit & Selden, 2000).

Principles of Insurance: Social Insurance

The Medicare and Medicaid programs that finance much of behavioral health services and the SSDI and SSI programs that provide many with severe and persistent mental illness with income support are examples of social insurance programs. Social insurance programs serve two primary purposes: (1) they are a means of overcoming market failure in private markets; and (2) they serve a redistributive function in providing safety net resources to vulnerable populations.

The Medicare program, enacted in 1965, serves both functions. Medicare Part A, which covers hospital services, was made compulsory explicitly to overcome adverse selection problems and is funded primarily out of payroll taxes. Nearly all people 65 and older are covered by Part A. Medicare, after a 2-year waiting period, also covers those under the age of 65 who have qualified for the SSDI program (those with a disability who paid into the Social Security System for 40 or more quarters).

The Medicare Part B program, which covers office-based and other services, while not compulsory, is funded 25% out of Medicare beneficiaries' own pockets and 75% out of general revenues.

The premiums for the optional Medicare Part D drug benefit are similarly heavily subsidized, encouraging high rates of participation, as well. Substantial penalties for late enrollment in Medicare Part B and Part D further encourage participation. The large subsidies combined with late enrollment penalties have also been effective in overcoming adverse selection: 86% of Medicare beneficiaries eligible for Part D prescription drug coverage have some form of drug coverage (Kaiser Family Foundation, 2018a).

The Medicaid program, unlike Medicare, was not designed to provide broad-based coverage for the population but as an insurer of last resort for vulnerable populations. It has long provided coverage to low-income children and their parents (many with Temporary Assistance to Needy Families), low-income pregnant women, low-income elderly, and people with disabilities. Eligibility varies widely by state. The 2010 ACA significantly expanded Medicaid coverage to childless adults and other low-income adult populations in states that chose to expand coverage.

Medicaid is an especially important source of coverage for people with mental disorders who qualify for SSI income support (many of whom do not have the 40 quarters of work needed to qualify for SSDI and, thus, Medicare). It also plays an important role in filling in gaps for Medicare, which requires significant cost-sharing and does not cover many behavioral health services.

Concerns regarding the potential loss of Medicaid and Medicare coverage create strong disincentives for people with disabilities to seek work and incentives to stay on social insurance programs and have led to a number of initiatives, such as the Ticket to Work program (Office of Disability Employment Policy, 2007).

Principles of Insurance: Managed Care

Managed care is ubiquitous in health care, no more so than in behavioral health treatment. But it also takes many different forms and is hard to categorize, especially with the extensive hybridization of models in recent years. Managed care evolved as another way to control the use of health-care services and restrain cost increases, which continued to rise rapidly in spite of the widespread use of consumer cost-sharing in health insurance plans.

Traditional staff/group model Health Maintenance Organizations (HMOs), such as Kaiser Permanente of Northern California and Group Health of Puget Sound, pioneered many of the basic managed care techniques. These staff/group model HMOs offered substantially reduced consumer cost-sharing compared to traditional fee-for-service (FFS) plans in return for (1) restrictive provider networks, with providers either salaried directly by the HMO or members of large groups contracted principally with the HMO; (2) physician gatekeeping, that is, requiring a referral from the patient's primary care provider to see specialists; (3) extensive utilization controls, such as prior authorization for services such as inpatient hospitals stays, physical therapy, and behavioral health services; and (4) drug formularies, where HMOs frequently offered market exclusivity to manufacturers in return for price breaks on specific drugs.

Traditional indemnity insurance has all but disappeared in private health insurance markets, supplanted by HMO plans, preferred provider organization (PPO) plans, and hybrid plans. PPOs consist of networks of providers, who provide services to plan members at a discounted price negotiated with the PPO. Consumer cost-sharing is much lower for network ("preferred") providers, but consumers have a choice of whether to use in-network providers or pay more for out-of-network providers. In contrast, in a closed HMO, consumers must use HMO providers or face denial of benefits (the HMO may either hire the provider directly as in a staff/group model HMO or contract with individual and groups of providers). PPOs also differ from closed HMOs in that they generally do not require referrals to access physician specialists. Some insurers offer both HMO and PPO products using the exact same network of providers, differing mainly in the use of physician gatekeeping and the ability to use of out-of-network providers.

Point-of-service (POS) plans contain elements of both HMO and PPO plans. For example, an "open-ended" HMO plan might allow consumers to see out-of-network providers (with higher cost-sharing) but still require referrals for specialists (gatekeeping).

HMOs enjoyed rapid growth into the late 1990s, doubling from 39.0 million enrollees in 1992 to a peak of 80.5 million in 1999 (Interstudy, 2002, 2003). A managed care "backlash" subsequently led to a decline in HMO enrollment to 71 million in 2006 (Interstudy, 2007). However, HMO enrollment has since risen to 92 million enrollees as of 2016 primarily due to increases among Medicare and Medicaid populations (Kaiser Family Foundation, 2018b). PPOs grew rapidly in the 1990s and 2000s and remain the most popular type of plan in the employer-sponsored insurance markets.

In contrast to private health insurance, Medicare remains largely a traditional fee-for-service program. Managed care plans were first introduced in the Medicare program in 1990. Enrollment in what are now called Medicare Advantage (Medicare Part C) plans has grown unevenly over time. However, it has accelerated recently with the introduction of new options reaching 34% of the Medicare population in 2018 (Centers for Medicare and Medicaid Services, 2018b).

State Medicaid programs continue to shift Medicaid recipients into managed care plans. In 1997, almost half (48%) of Medicaid recipients were enrolled in managed care plans, mostly in HMOs. By 2013, this had grown to 80% of all Medicaid recipients (Centers for Medicare and Medicaid Services, 2016).

Outside of the fee-for-service Medicare program, the majority of specialty behavioral health services for insured populations are organized and delivered through managed behavioral health organizations (MBHOs). Medicaid programs and private insurers alike contract with these specialty MBHOs, in what are termed behavioral health *carve-outs*. MBHOs generally develop their own networks of behavioral health specialists, usually reimbursed on a fee-for-service basis, along with extensive prior authorization and utilization review systems. Products marketed to both employers (direct carve-out) and health plans (indirect carve-out) range from employee assistance plans (EAP) to stand-alone utilization management products to comprehensive packages providing all specialty behavioral health services (network plus utilization management).

MBHOs spread rapidly during the 1980s and 1990s by successfully adapting many of the techniques originally pioneered by HMOs to the management of specialty behavioral health services. Industry sources show total enrollment in MBHO products increasing from 86 million in 1992 to an astounding 227 million in 2002 (Open Minds, 2002). MBHOs achieved impressive cost savings early on due primarily to dramatically reduced lengths of stays for inpatient hospitalizations (Ma & McGuire, 1998; National Advisory Mental Health Council, 1998, 2000; Sturm, 1997). This success led more and more plans and employers to contract with MBHOs. MBHOs also achieved cost savings partly through negotiated discounts from network providers and partly through what are termed "network" effects: the fear that a provider will be discontinued from the network if they provide too many services to patients (Ma & McGuire, 2004). Their growth, however, naturally reached a plateau as they came to dominate the market for specialty behavioral health services provided through insurance in the last couple of decades.

MBHOs' effects on access and quality of behavioral health services remain ambiguous. On balance, reducing lengthy inpatient stays and shifting resources to outpatient settings has likely been beneficial to patients. There is also evidence that MBHOs accelerated the diffusion of evidence-based practices (Ling Davina, Berndt, & Frank, 2007). But there are also concerns that MBHOs restrict access to specialty services, so that patients must seek treatment in primary care settings. MBHOs are also rarely at risk for the costs of psychotropic medications (management of prescription medications are generally contracted to yet another third party, see below). This creates incentives for psychotropic medication interventions, at the possible expense of evidence-based behavioral therapies (the cost for which they would be responsible). Evidence of cost shifting either to primary care settings or to prescription drugs, however, is mixed (Dickey, Normand, Norton, Rupp, & Azeni, 2001; Norton, Lindrooth, & Dickey, 1997; Zuvekas, Rupp, & Norquist, 2007).

Once a somewhat peripheral concern, prescription drug financing is now central to behavioral health treatment. Similar to specialty behavioral health services, management of prescription drugs in the private plans, including plans that serve Medicare and Medicaid populations, is now largely contracted out to third-party administrators called pharmacy benefit managers (PBMs). Also similar to MBHOs, PBMs contract directly with employers who have carved out their prescription benefits from the rest of their health coverage.

PBMs apply many of the basic tools of managed care to prescription medications. They develop and maintain networks of pharmacies with which they negotiate prices. They negotiate discounts and rebates from pharmaceutical manufacturers and wholesalers. Much like MBHOs, the PBM industry is highly concentrated, so PBMs are able to leverage their volume purchasing power with both pharmacies and manufacturers. Leverage with manufacturers is further increased through the use of drug formularies, essentially lists of approved drugs.

Multi-tiered formularies are the norm and, in private plans, are closely tied to consumer cost-sharing. In a standard three-tier plan, the first tier includes inexpensive generic medications with zero or low co-payment levels to encourage their use. The second tier includes a preferred medication(s) in a therapeutic class, with somewhat higher cost-sharing. The third tier includes non-preferred medications in a therapeutic class, with the highest cost-sharing.

Not all medications in a therapeutic class will necessarily appear in a formulary; formularies vary widely in their restrictiveness. Some particularly expensive medications, such as cancer drugs and atypical antipsychotics, may be listed but require prior authorization before use. PBMs, managed care plans that manage their own pharmacy benefits and Medicaid programs, use the leverage of tiers or preferred status of drugs, in return for discounts and rebates from manufacturers.

The treatment of psychotropic medications in drug formularies is an area of great controversy. Patients respond differently to the range of medications within therapeutic classes such as antidepressants and atypical antipsychotics. A restrictive formulary can thus create barriers to treatment for patients who do not respond to preferred drugs.

Consumer cost-sharing can also create barriers to treatment. Higher cost-sharing can lead to reduced use of medications (Goldman et al., 2004; Hodgkin, Parks Thomas, Simoni-Wastila, Ritter, & Lee, 2008; Huskamp et al., 2005; Landsman, Yu,

Liu, Teutsch, & Berger, 2005; Wang et al., 2008). In recognition of this potential problem, some employers and health plans have experimented with lower cost-sharing or eliminating it altogether for maintenance medications used to treat chronic conditions. For additional information on the topic of psychopharmacology, see chapter "Pharmacy Services in Behavioral Health" in this volume.

Principles of Reimbursement

Private health plans, public insurance programs, and state and local mental health authorities face difficult decisions in choosing how to organize and pay for health-care services provided to clients. A wide variety of reimbursement mechanisms has evolved over time. Each creates its own set of incentives, good and bad.

Closed systems, such as the Department of Veterans Affairs (VA), state and local psychiatric institutions, and the original staff/group HMOs typically own their own hospitals and clinics. That is, these closed systems combine insurance functions and health-care provision functions. They also typically hire providers directly, paying them a salary, or use other similar contractual methods to provide care. In principal, monitoring of provider behavior and patient outcomes is easier in a closed system, and providers can be made to more closely follow the dictates of the organization if their salary depends on it (either explicitly or implicitly). Success depends upon the strength of internal monitoring systems and organizational dynamics. In the public sector, political considerations also play a large role. Closed systems have other problems. The large investments needed to build, maintain, and staff closed systems, even in the private sector, reduce flexibility to shift resources as circumstances change. Many consumers also dislike the restricted choice of providers in closed systems.

The many variants of cost-based and fee-for-service reimbursement are administratively simpler alternatives to directly hiring providers. Cost-based reimbursement, where providers submit their actual costs, was once common for hospital services but is now the exception. Medicare, for example, paid hospitals on a strictly retrospective cost basis until 1982 (Hodgkin & McGuire, 1994). Under a fee-for-service system, providers receive a fixed amount for each service performed. This fee is administratively set in the traditional Medicare and Medicaid programs (although providers can indirectly influence fee setting through the political process). In private plans, the fees are usually set in negotiation with providers.

However, a significant percentage of behavioral health providers, especially in large metropolitan areas, have opted out of all insurance-based reimbursement, focusing on clients who pay up front out of their own pockets (with some patients filing claims with health plans and some declining to do so) at rates set by the providers (Bishop, Press, Keyhani, & Pincus, 2014; Cummings, 2015; Mitchell, 1991; O'Malley & Reschovsky, 2006; Wilk, West, Narrow, Rae, & Regier, 2005). Other providers opt out of specific plans, most commonly Medicaid plans, because of low reimbursement rates set by many states (Cunningham & Hadley, 2008; Mitchell,

1991; Zuckerman, McFeeters, Cunningham, & Nichols, 2004). The declining number of providers willing to treat patients with Medicaid raises concerns that access to care for individuals with low incomes and disabilities has diminished (Atherly & Mortensen, 2014; Cohen & Cunningham, 1995; Cunningham & Hadley, 2008; Decker, 2012; Sharma et al., 2018).

Cost-based and fee-for-service reimbursement also create incentives to over-provide services, as providers earn more revenue the more services they perform as long as the actual reimbursement amount covers their costs. For example, there is substantial evidence that paying hospitals fixed per diem rates creates incentives for longer lengths of stay (Berenson, Upadhyay, Delbanco, & Murray, 2016, April; Hodgkin & McGuire, 1994). Actual costs tend to be front-loaded, so patients become increasingly profitable the longer they stay. Perversely, cost-based and fee-for-service reimbursement can even create incentives for poor quality care, since there are often no real consequences for bad outcomes and providers can earn still more revenue correcting their mistakes.

Fee-for-service systems have the additional disadvantage of distorting treatment decisions, as some types of services are more profitable than others. For example, primary care providers are rarely separately reimbursed for screening for depression, addiction, and other behavioral health disorders, while they are routinely reimbursed for laboratory tests, a significant barrier to wide-scale behavioral health screening.

Capitation and other prospective payment systems were developed in response to the poor incentives created under fee-for-service or cost-based reimbursement systems. The basic idea is to shift some or all of the financial risk of additional services to providers, creating incentives to be as efficient as possible in providing services. Capitation to health plans and capitation to providers are commonly confused. Under provider capitation, providers receive a fixed amount per month for each patient in that provider's panel (or at least those covered by the plan), regardless of the amount of services they use or whether a particular patient uses services at all. Under plan capitation, the health plan receives a fixed amount for each patient to cover all the health-care services for all the providers in the plan, essentially an insurance premium. Plan capitation is far more common than provider capitation. Even in capitated managed care plans, including carve-outs to MBHOs, the predominant form of reimbursement to providers is fee-for-service or salary (Strunk & Reschovsky, 2002; Zuvekas & Cohen, 2016). This is primarily due to the administrative complexity of determining capitation formulas and unwillingness of providers, especially in small or solo practices, to assume risk (Berenson & Rich, 2010; Frakt & Mayes, 2012; Goldsmith, 2010; Mechanic & Altman, 2009).

Medicare's Prospective Payment System, where hospitals receive a fixed payment for all patients within a Diagnosis Related Group (DRGs) regardless of the services they use (with provisions for outliers), works in similar fashion to capitation. Lengths of inpatient hospital stays fell dramatically after Medicare switched to this system in 1983. Many state Medicaid programs and even private health insurance plans have adopted similar prospective payment systems.

While there is some evidence that capitation and prospective payment increase efficiency of care, they also create incentives to under-provide care (in contrast to the over-provision of care in fee-for service systems). This is especially true where outcomes are difficult to monitor. Capitation and prospective payment reimbursement also create strong incentives for the same types of risk selection behavior (cream skimming or cherry picking) evident in health insurance markets. Healthier patients will obviously be more profitable than sicker patients. As a result, the same types of risk-adjustment methods are also commonly applied to capitated and prospective payments systems, again imperfectly.

There is increasing recognition that both fee-for-service and capitation are imperfect reimbursement methods if they are not linked explicitly to outcomes and/ or quality. The term "pay for performance" has become ubiquitous in recent years to describe various attempts to create better incentives in payment systems. The Centers for Medicare and Medicaid Services (CMS) prefers the terms "alternative payment models." Results to date are mixed, but the CMS and private payers continue to experiment with wide variety of payment models (Hussey, Ridgely, & Rosenthal, 2011; Rosenthal, Landon, Narmond, et al., 2007; Rosenthal, Frank, Li, & Epstein, 2005; Rosenthal, Landon, Howitt, Song, & Epstein, 2007; Rosenthal, Landrum, Robbins, & Schneider, 2016; Sinaiko et al., 2017). Among the models being tested are various forms of bundled payment linked to clinical outcomes for episodes of treatment (e.g., knee replacement) encompassing most or all components of treatment (hospital, physician, laboratory, rehab) rather than paying individual providers separately.

Closely related are Accountable Care Organizations (ACOs), which combine hospitals, physicians, and other providers to accept bundled payments or to participate in other alternative payment models, as well as patient-centered medical homes (PCMHs) (Centers for Medicare and Medicaid Services, 2018a). These new payment models may have accelerated a growing trend of consolidation and integration of health-care providers (e.g., hospitals buying up physician practices). Adoption of these new payment models has been much slower in behavioral health, partly because of concerns about adverse selection and partly because of concerns about measuring behavioral health outcomes.

Presentation of Critical Issues

As we have seen, the financing of behavioral health services is closely and increasingly tied to the health insurance coverage Americans hold (Mark et al., 2016). Loss of health insurance reduces use of behavioral health services, while extending health insurance coverage tends to improves access (Beronio et al., 2014; Frank & McGuire, 1986; Garfield, Zuvekas, Lave, & Donohue, 2011; Zuvekas, 1999). Thus, changes in the health insurance system have immediate consequences for behavioral health services. We consider here the impact of long-run structural changes in the health insurance system along with two major health reform initiatives of the last decade or so: the 2010 Affordable Care Act (ACA) and the 2008 Mental Health Parity and Addiction Equity Act (MHPAEA).

Long-Run Trends in Health Insurance Coverage

The mixed public and private nature of US health-care systems extends to health insurance coverage. Only those aged 65 and above have near universal coverage through the federally funded Medicare health insurance program. In contrast, working-age Americans and their children still depend primarily on private insurance obtained through employers or unions to pay for their health care. However, not all Americans have access to employment-related insurance. Some employers do not offer health insurance coverage or offer coverage only to certain types of employees (e.g., full-time but not part-time workers). Some employees decline their employer's offer of insurance either because they are covered by other insurance or cannot or do not wish to pay the employee out-of-pocket share of the insurance premium.

Prior to the ACA, the percentage of non-elderly Americans who were uninsured remained stable for decades. Approximately 17% of the non-elderly US population was uninsured in both 1997 and 2013 with little variation in between (Fig. 1). This stability masks enormous changes. In 1997, 71% of the non-elderly population was covered by private health insurance. By 2013, this had declined a full 10 percentage

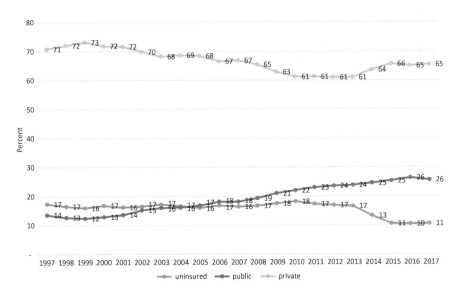

Fig. 1 Trends In insurance coverage, under 65, 1997–2017. Note: Percentages add to more than 100 because a small percentage of people report both public and private coverage. Source: Adapted from Tables 1.1b, 1.2a, 1.2b. Clarke, Schiller, and Norris (2017)

points to 61%. Rising insurance premiums are thought to be a major factor in the decline. For example, the average total cost of an employer-sponsored family plan rose from $4954 in 1996 to $16,029 in 2013 and to $17,710 in 2016 (Fig. 2). Economists generally believe that employees absorb most of these increased insurance costs in the form of lower wage increases. For example, unions have been willing to make wage concessions in return for continuing guarantees of health insurance coverage in collective bargaining agreements.

However, as total premiums continue to rise, so too do the amounts employees are required to pay out of pocket for their coverage by employers. The average out-of-pocket share for a single plan was $1325 and $4956 for a family plan in 2016 (Agency for Healthcare Research and Quality, 2017, September). This is a likely reason why Americans are increasingly declining employer offers of insurance coverage (Agency for Healthcare Research and Quality, 2017, September; Cooper & Schone, 1997; Cooper & Vistnes, 2003). It is this declining "take-up rate" that is largely responsible for the decline in private health insurance coverage prior to the ACA.

Several successive federal and state expansions of Medicaid coverage beginning in the 1990s and the State Children's Health Insurance Program (SCHIP), enacted in 1996 for lower-income uninsured children, have compensated for the loss of private health insurance. The percentage of non-elderly Americans covered by public programs rose substantially from 14% in 1997 to 24% in 2013, fully offsetting the 10-percentage point decline in private insurance coverage over that same period (Fig. 1).

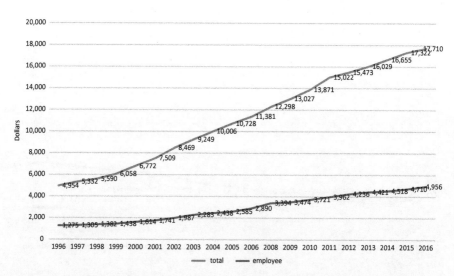

Fig. 2 Total family premium per enrolled employee, private sector establishments, 1996–2016. Source: AHRQ (2017)

Recent Trends Under the Affordable Care Act

The 2010 Affordable Care Act (ACA) legislated substantial changes in the structure of health insurance coverage in the United States and led to a decline in the number of uninsured Americans. The most widely known of the ACA's many provisions were three expansions of insurance coverage: (1) dependent coverage to age 25 in private plans, (2) ACA marketplace coverage, and (3) Medicaid expansions.

The first expansion implemented allowed parents to cover any of their children through the age of 25 through their employer's family plan beginning in 2010. This popular provision is especially important for young adults with behavioral health needs. The vast majority of uninsured young adults are healthy. Yet they are also vulnerable as they transition from their parents' homes to school (for some) and into the workforce (for others). The onset of many mental disorders, such as schizophrenia and bipolar disorder, tends to occur at precisely this time. Previously, only students up to the age of 22 (or less commonly, age 25) were generally covered, and if the student was forced to drop out of school because of behavioral health issues, they might lose that coverage. The expansion significantly increased coverage in young adults by 5–8 percentage points (Barbaresco, Courtemanche, & Qi, 2015; McClellan, 2017).

Correspondingly, use of mental health but not substance use disorder treatment increased (McClellan, 2017; Saloner & Le Cook, 2014), and out-of-pocket treatment costs decreased (Ali, Chen, Mutter, Novak, & Mortensen, 2016). However, it is important to note that many young adults do not have access to this type of coverage because their parents do not have private employer-sponsored coverage themselves.

A second expansion under the ACA established state-based private insurance marketplaces (operated by states alone or in partnership with the federal government) providing new options for individually purchased and small employer plans beginning in 2014. Premiums paid by eligible individuals and families in the marketplace are subsidized for those with family incomes between 100 and 400% of the federal poverty line, with larger subsidies for those with lower incomes. These subsidies are tied to a cap on the percentage of income that a person has to pay for the second lowest cost "silver" (benchmark) plan offered in the area.

Silver plans are required to cover a minimum of 70%, on average, of medical costs (bronze plans (60%), gold (80%), platinum (90%)) with the rest paid out-of-pocket by individuals. Individuals and families under 250% of poverty are also eligible for "cost-sharing reduction" silver plans, where in addition to premium subsidies they also have more generous coverage with fewer out-of-pocket costs. These subsidies were coupled with a mandate that individuals must be covered by insurance or face a "shared responsibility" tax penalty.

This "carrot and stick approach" of combining subsidies on the one hand with mandates and tax penalties on the other hand was intended to minimize the amount of adverse selection faced by insurers and reduce premium increases. The ACA also contained a number of other provisions to both encourage private insurers and consumers alike to participate in the marketplaces and to limit adverse selection. Particularly relevant for behavioral health, the ACA mandates that all plans offered in the marketplaces (as well as non-grandfathered individual and small group market plans offered outside of marketplaces) must contain coverage for ten essential health benefits (EHBs). Included among these EHBs are mental health and substance use disorder services.

The third expansion under the ACA gave states generous subsidies to provide Medicaid coverage to individuals with family income up to 138% of the federal poverty level beginning in 2014. Initially, the federal government covered 100% of the cost of newly eligible enrollees falling to 95% in 2017 and 90% in 2020 and beyond (Kaiser Family Foundation, 2018c, January 16). The Supreme Court ruled in 2012 that this Medicaid expansion was effectively optional for states, rather than mandatory for continued participation in the overall Medicaid program as originally enacted in the ACA. Subsequently, not all states adopted this expansion (18 in all as of January 2018) including large states such as Texas and Florida.

The ACA led an estimated 20 million previously uninsured Americans to gain coverage (Uberoi et al., 2016). This reduced the share of the uninsured to 11% of the non-elderly population in 2017, down from approximately 17% before the ACA was enacted (Fig. 1). Notably, after declining for many years, the share of Americans covered by private insurance coverage stabilized and then increased from 61% in 2010 to 65% of the non-elderly in 2017 (Fig. 1). This represents the combined effect of the dependent coverage expansions, individual mandates and Marketplace coverage, along with other new mandates and subsidies to employers to provide coverage. Public coverage too continued to increase in importance through the ACA Medicaid expansions (Fig. 2).

Parity

For decades, coverage for behavioral health services in private health insurance plans lagged behind other services with much higher co-pays and coinsurance (e.g., 50% vs 20%) and strict limits on the number of days, visits, or dollars covered in most plans (Barry et al., 2016; Beronio et al., 2014). The main argument advanced in favor of this discriminatory coverage was on economic efficiency grounds, because of the potential for moral hazard the RAND HIE study found. More likely, adverse selection was the driving force with insurers seeking to deter more expensive consumers with behavioral health problems from enrolling in their plans (Barry et al., 2016).

Proponents of parity in coverage advanced two main arguments. First, it is discriminatory to provide less generous coverage to those with behavioral health disorders, regardless of economic efficiency arguments. Second, parity was affordable in the context of managed care, as a number of studies strongly supported (Barry et al., 2016; Goldman et al., 2006; National Advisory Mental Health Council, 1998, 2000).

Mental health advocates successfully pushed almost every state to enact at least some legislation designed to strengthen mental health coverage in private health plans. However, most of these state mandates fell well short of parity. Even in states with fairly strong parity laws, parity failed to cover most people (Buchmueller, Cooper, Jacobson, & Zuvekas, 2007). Under the provisions of the 1974 Employment Retirement and Income Security Act (ERISA), firms that self-insure are exempt from state health insurance regulations including parity mandates. Consequently, strong parity laws covered only 20% of working Americans with health coverage (Buchmueller et al., 2007). In addition, most of these strong laws covered only severe or "biologically based" disorders and typically did not apply to drug and alcohol services.

The federal 2008 Mental Health Parity and Addiction Equity Act (MHPAEA) went far beyond these state parity mandates and the earlier 1996 federal law in at least four important ways. First, the MHPAEA eliminated differential co-payments and coinsurance, deductibles, and limits on number of visits and days of treatment for firms that offer behavioral health coverage beginning in 2010–2011.

Second, unlike the state mandates, it applies to all employers with 50 or more employees that offer behavioral health coverage. The subsequent 2010 ACA legislation further extended parity to all non-grandfathered small group and individual market plans by requiring both that behavioral health services be covered as an EHB and requiring these plans to also meet MHPAEA requirements.

Third, the MHPAEA is applied not only to services related to mental health conditions but also drug and alcohol disorders. Fourth, the federal administrative regulations implementing MHPAEA interpreted parity to apply not only to quantitative plan features like deductibles and out-of-pocket maximums but also to "nonquantitative treatment limits" (NQTLs) such as medical necessity requirements and prior authorization. For example, if a plan had no prior authorization requirements for office-based visits for a physical condition, the plan could not impose prior authorization requirements for behavioral health visits.

Congress also extended parity to the Medicare program. HR 6331 gradually reduced cost-sharing for mental health services from 50% to 20% between 2010 and 2014.

Parity does not seem to cost insurers much (Barry et al., 2016; Goldman et al., 2006), but what does it mean for consumers? The available evidence suggests that parity does indeed reduce the out-of-pocket burden of behavioral health services, albeit modestly (Barry et al., 2016; Ettner et al., 2016; Goldman et al., 2006). Parity's effects on access to behavioral health services are less certain with modest improvements at best (Barry & Busch, 2008; Barry et al., 2016; Busch et al., 2006; Ettner et al., 2016; Goldman et al., 2006; Pacula & Sturm, 2000). The majority of Americans receiving behavioral health services (especially for mental disorders such as depression, anxiety, and ADHD) get the bulk of them through their primary care doctors and/or pharmacies. For all intents and purposes, these services were already largely covered at parity before the MHPAEA and state parity mandates.

However, in theory all else being equal, parity should have increased access to those needing more intensive, specialty-based behavioral health services. But all else is not equal. Parity creates incentives to tighten other aspects of the management of behavioral health services to offset cost increases in several ways (Barry et al., 2016; National Advisory Mental Health Council, 1998, 2000; Ridgely, Burnam, Barry, Goldman, & Hennessy, 2006).

First, NQTLs are by their nature more difficult to monitor and enforce than quantitative limits such as deductible, co-pays, and other cost-sharing features that are written down in policy booklets. Second, plans might use restrictive provider networks to limit access to behavioral health providers. Third, plans can use low reimbursement rates to providers to discourage participation in their plans.

Significance for Behavioral Health

Closer integration with the constantly changing and evolving insurance-based and insurance-financed systems of health care in the United States has profound implications for the way behavioral health-care services are financed, organized, and delivered. The costs of providing health care continue to rise increasing pressure for further reforms in health-care systems. The direction these reforms take will have significant impacts on Americans with behavioral health-care needs.

Less than a decade old, the ACA faces an uncertain future. Providing insurance coverage for millions of American, it significantly reduced the ranks of the uninsured, many with behavioral health needs (Garfield et al., 2011; Mark, Wier, Malone, Penne, & Cowell, 2015). Adults with behavioral health conditions tend to have lower incomes on average and less access to employer-sponsored coverage than other Americans (Garfield et al., 2011). Thus, the ACA Medicaid expansions and substantial premium and cost-sharing reduction subsidies in the marketplaces for lower-income Americans are especially important for them. However, many of the specific provisions of the ACA are unpopular (although some also enjoy fairly widespread support, such as the dependent coverage expansion) leading to calls for either further reform to ACA provisions at the federal level or outright appeal.

Short of full repeal, the future of the ACA Medicaid expansions is dependent mainly on the decisions of individual states. As of January 2018, 33 states (including the District of Columbia) have opted to expand Medicaid, with several adopting after the initial 2014 start year (Kaiser Family Foundation, 2018, January 16).

Debate continues in many of the remaining 18 states so more may opt to eventually expand. However, there have also been discussions in states that have already expanded about whether to drop the program. Some, like Kentucky, have also sought waivers from the federal government to reduce the scope of the expansion programs offered either in terms of populations served or services offered, including behavioral health services. The Centers for Medicare and Medicaid Services has signaled to states that they are interested in giving states more flexibility in the program.

Changes in how the ACA marketplaces operate may also have disproportionate effects on Americans with behavioral health needs. For example, the 2017 Tax

Reform eliminated the unpopular individual mandate for insurance coverage and shared responsibility tax penalties after 2019. It remains to be seen whether this actually leads to adverse selection, the main conceptual argument for why the mandate is necessary, and significantly higher premiums in the marketplaces. It is possible that, in practice, this "stick" side of the equation is less important than subsidies to consumers and insurers in maintaining a stable marketplace.

Other proposed changes to the marketplaces, besides outright repeal, include eliminating the EHB requirements altogether and thus allowing insurers to sell plans without coverage for behavioral health or other EHB services. These reduced coverage plans would likely be unattractive to consumers with behavioral needs but might be attractive to healthier individuals, potentially leading to adverse selection and higher costs in plans that meet behavioral health needs.

The Centers for Medicare and Medicaid Services (2018c) is already giving states more flexibility in selecting essential health benefit benchmark plans beginning in 2020. This might reduce behavioral health coverage and increase the potential for adverse selection if states select less generous plans as their benchmarks for coverage.

Even without further legislative action, concerns remain that provider networks are more limited and NQTLs greater for behavioral health services in marketplace plans compared to other private coverage (Stewart et al., 2018). In addition, there is concern that the flexibility given to states has led to uneven implementation of parity requirements in the marketplaces and considerable variation in the scope of mental health and especially addiction treatment services covered (Berry, Huskamp, Goldman, & Barry, 2015; Tran Smith et al., 2017).

Proposed reforms to public insurance and other health programs extend well beyond further ACA reform or outright repeal. As health-care costs continue to rise and the population ages, the Medicare program share of the federal budget continues to grow. Many argue this growth is unsustainable in the long run. The ACA itself contained a number of provisions to limit the growth of spending in Medicare, but many of these are unpopular especially with providers and insurers.

Market-based proposals include turning Medicare into a voucher system. Instead of providing a defined set of benefits universally to all Medicare beneficiaries, individuals would receive a fixed dollar amount to purchase private plans. Plans would compete against each other to most efficiently provide coverage to consumers (in many respects, like the ACA marketplace). Instead of an open-ended commitment on the government's part, federal contributions under many of these proposals would be limited to an inflation-indexed voucher value, regardless of how much health-care costs rise. If competition between plans drives substantial innovation leading to better coverage, greater health outcomes, and reduced costs, then consumers clearly gain. If not, Medicare beneficiaries may see their premiums increase and/or the value of their insurance coverage erode over time. Moreover, there are concerns about how higher-risk consumers, including those with behavioral health needs, would fare in markets where insurers might find them unattractive risks.

The share of the federal budget devoted to Medicaid also continues to rise. Reform proposals range from giving states more flexibility within the current program (e.g., changing eligibility requirements, cutting benefits, and/or increasing enrollee cost-sharing) to converting Medicaid to a block grant program. Currently, Medicaid is jointly financed by the federal government and individual states with the federal government matching state outlays a minimum of 50% but often higher for traditional Medicaid programs and 95% for the Medicaid expansion populations (falling to 90% by 2020).

Under some block grant proposals, states would receive a fixed per capita allocation with constrained growth over time and allowed flexibility to run the Medicaid program as they wish. A per capita allocation would significantly shift resources away from higher spending states, many of whom provide extensive recovery and support services (sometimes termed "wrap around services") to those with behavioral health needs in addition to paying for health-care treatment. These potential reforms in turn are likely to place increasing pressure on public mental health systems at a time when those systems are already experiencing financial pressures.

Calls for reform extend as well to the Veterans Health Administration (VHA) health-care system, a significant provider of behavioral health treatment for millions of veterans (Tsai & Rosenheck, 2016). Proposals range from giving veterans more treatment options outside VA owned and operated facilities to converting the program from a wholly government owned and operated closed system to entirely a private insurance-based system, such as the TRICARE program for spouses and dependents of active duty military personnel.

Rising health-care costs and premiums continue to threaten the employment-based private health insurance system that provides health insurance coverage to most Americans under the age 65. In spite of its recent stabilization, many predict the employer-based insurance system will continue to slowly erode, increasing the pressure on the ACA marketplaces, state Medicaid budgets, and public mental health and addiction systems.

Market-based reform efforts to shore up the private health insurance system also have implications for the coverage of behavioral health services. The 2003 Medicare Modernization Act contained provisions to encourage the creation of *Health Savings Accounts (HSAs)*. HSAs allow individuals to pay for health-care services and save for future health expenses tax-free. However, these accounts can only be used by consumers who purchase high-deductible health plans (for individuals, a deductible of at least $1350 and families $2700 in 2018). This requirement means that individuals and families pay more for health care including behavioral health services directly out of their own pockets. Legislation has also encouraged employers to offer similar types of savings accounts in combination with high-deductible health plan coverage.

Not all of these high-deductible plans provide behavioral health benefits (Wildsmith, 2009, October). High-deductible plans grew slowly at first but have accelerated in recent years. In 2016, 85% of all employer provided coverage contained a deductible with an average individual deductible of $1696 and an average family deductible of $3069 (Agency for Healthcare Research and Quality, 2017, September).

Other proposed market-based reforms would supplant the employment-based system altogether with vouchers or tax credits for the purchase of individual health insurance plans. Lacking the pooling mechanism of a large employer, there are concerns that adverse selection would lead to problems accessing affordable and adequate insurance coverage for those with behavioral health needs if these individual markets are not well-designed.

Implications for Behavioral Health

The share of the nation's resources devoted to behavioral services, as measured by gross domestic product (GDP), has remained largely level since the 1970s (Frank & Glied, 2006; Substance Abuse and Mental Health Services Administration, 2016). This stands in marked contrast with the health-care system as a whole, which has grown from 7% to 18% of GDP since 1970 (Centers for Medicare and Medicaid Services, 2018, January 8). In one sense, this represents a phenomenal success (Druss, 2006; Frank & Glied, 2006). The continued movement away from hospitals to community settings has allowed millions more Americans to be drawn into behavioral health treatment, without increasing the share of the country's resources needed to finance these services.

However, the shift to insurance-financed treatment systems has also led to a relative shift in resources away from individuals with severe and persistent mental illness and addiction toward those with other mental disorders such as anxiety, depression, and attention-deficit/hyperactivity disorder (ADHD). Treatment has undoubtedly improved for most people with serious and persistent mental illness (SPMI), but the still fragmentary nature of financing creates substantial gaps, especially for addiction treatment (Druss, 2006; Frank & Glied, 2006; Mechanic, 2007). Plugging these gaps within ever changing and increasingly costly insurance-based systems of financing remains a challenge.

References

Agency for Healthcare Research and Quality. (2017, September). *Medical Expenditure Panel Survey insurance component 2016 chartbook* (AHRQ Publication No. 17-0034-EF)). Rockville, MD: Agency for Healthcare Research and Quality. https://meps.ahrq.gov/mepsweb/data_files/publications/cb21/cb21.pdf

Ali, M. M., Chen, J., Mutter, R., Novak, P., & Mortensen, K. (2016). The ACA's dependent coverage expansion and out-of-pocket spending by young adults with behavioral health conditions. *Psychiatric Services, 67*(9), 977–982. https://doi.org/10.1176/appi.ps.201500346

Arrow, K. J. (1963). Uncertainty and the welfare economics of medical care. *The American Economic Review, 53*(5), 941–973. https://www.jstor.org/stable/1812044

Atherly, A., & Mortensen, K. (2014). Medicaid primary care physician fees and the use of preventive services among Medicaid enrollees. *Health Services Research, 49*(4), 1306–1328. https://doi.org/10.1111/1475-6773.12169

Barbaresco, S., Courtemanche, C. J., & Qi, Y. (2015). Impacts of the Affordable Care Act dependent coverage provision on health-related outcomes of young adults. *Journal of Health Economics, 40,* 54–68. https://doi.org/10.1016/j.jhealeco.2014.12.004

Barry, C. L., & Busch, S. H. (2008). Caring for children with mental disorders: Do state parity laws increase access to treatment? *The Journal of Mental Health Policy and Economics, 11*(2), 57–66.

Barry, C. L., Goldman, H. H., & Huskamp, H. A. (2016). Federal parity in the evolving mental health and addiction care landscape. *Health Affairs, 35*(6), 1009–1016. https://doi.org/10.1377/hlthaff.2015.1653

Berenson, R. A., & Rich, E. C. (2010). US approaches to physician payment: The deconstruction of primary care. *Journal of General Internal Medicine, 25*(6), 613–618. https://doi.org/10.1007/s11606-010-1295-z

Berenson, R. A., Upadhyay, D. K., Delbanco, S. F., & Murray, R. (2016, April). *Per diem payments to hospitals for inpatient stays* (Research report: Payment methods and benefit designs: How they work and how they work together to improve health care). Washington, DC: Urban Institute. https://www.urban.org/sites/default/files/03_per_diem_payment_to_hospitals_for_inpatient_stays.pdf

Bernard, D., & Selden, T. M. (2002). Employer offers, private coverage, and the tax subsidy for health insurance: 1987 and 1996. *International Journal of Health Care Finance and Economics, 2*(4), 297–318. https://doi.org/10.1023/A:1022360202017

Beronio, K., Glied, S., & Frank, R. (2014). How the Affordable Care Act and Mental Health Parity and Addiction Equity Act greatly expand coverage of behavioral health care. *The Journal of Behavioral Health Services & Research, 41*(4), 410–428. https://doi.org/10.1007/s11414-014-9412-0

Berry, K. N., Huskamp, H. A., Goldman, H. H., & Barry, C. L. (2015). A tale of two states: Do consumers see mental health insurance parity when shopping on state exchanges? *Psychiatric Services, 66*(6), 565–567. https://doi.org/10.1176/appi.ps.201400582

Besley, T. J. (1988). Optimal reimbursement health insurance and the theory of Ramsey taxation. *Journal of Health Economics, 7*(4), 321–336. https://doi.org/10.1016/0167-6296(88)90019-7

Bishop, T. F., Press, M. J., Keyhani, S., & Pincus, H. A. (2014). Acceptance of insurance by psychiatrists and the implications for access to mental health care. *JAMA Psychiatry, 71*(2), 176–181. https://doi.org/10.1001/jamapsychiatry.2013.2862

Buchmueller, T. C., Cooper, P. F., Jacobson, M., & Zuvekas, S. H. (2007). Parity for whom? Exemptions and the extent of state mental health parity legislation. *Health Affairs, 26*(4), w483–w487. https://doi.org/10.1377/hlthaff.26.4.w483

Busch, A. B., Huskamp, H. A., Normand, S. L., Young, A. S., Goldman, H., & Frank, R. G. (2006). The impact of parity on major depression treatment quality in the Federal Employees' Health Benefits Program after parity implementation. *Medical Care, 44*(6), 506–512. https://doi.org/10.1097/01.mlr.0000215890.30756.b2

Centers for Medicare and Medicaid Services. (2016). *Medicaid managed care enrollment and program characteristics, 2015.* Baltimore, MD: Centers for Medicare and Medicaid Services. https://www.medicaid.gov/medicaid/managed-care/downloads/enrollment/2015-medicaid-managed-care-enrollment-report.pdf

Centers for Medicare and Medicaid Services. (2018a). *Innovation models* [Web page]. Baltimore, MD: Centers for Medicare and Medicaid Services. https://innovation.cms.gov/initiatives/index.html#views=models

Centers for Medicare and Medicaid Services. (2018b). *Medicare enrollment dashboard.* Baltimore, MD: Centers for Medicare and Medicaid Services. https://www.cms.gov/Research-Statistics-Data-and-Systems/Statistics-Trends-and-Reports/Dashboard/Medicare-Enrollment/Enrollment%20Dashboard.html

Centers for Medicare and Medicaid Services. (2018c, January 8). *National Health Expenditures by type of service and source of funds, CY 1960-2016.* Baltimore, MD: Centers for Medicare and Medicaid Services. https://www.cms.gov/Research-Statistics-Data-and-Systems/Statistics-Trends-and-Reports/NationalHealthExpendData/NationalHealthAccountsHistorical.html

Clarke, T. C., Schiller, J. S., & Norris, T. (2017). *Early release of selected estimates based on data from the January–June 2017 National Health Interview Survey*, from https://www.cdc.gov/nchs/data/nhis/earlyrelease/earlyrelease201712.pdf

Claxton, G., Rae, M., Long, M., Damico, A., Foster, G., & Whitmore, H. (2017). 2017 employer health benefits survey. Menlo Park, CA, US; Chicago, IL, US: Kaiser Family Foundation; Health Research & Educational Trust. https://files.kff.org/attachment/Report-Employer-Health-Benefits-Annual-Survey-2017

Cohen, J. W., & Cunningham, P. J. (1995). Medicaid physician fee levels and children's access to care. *Health Affairs, 14*(1), 255–262. https://doi.org/10.1377/hlthaff.14.1.255

Cooper, P. F., & Schone, B. S. (1997). More offers, fewer takers for employment-based health insurance: 1987 and 1996. *Health Affairs, 16*(6), 142–149. https://doi.org/10.1377/hlthaff.16.6.142

Cooper, P. F., & Vistnes, J. (2003). Workers' decisions to take-up offered health insurance coverage: Assessing the importance of out-of-pocket premium costs. *Medical Care, 41*(7 Suppl), III35–III43. https://doi.org/10.1097/01.Mlr.0000076050.73075.51

Cummings, J. R. (2015). Rates of psychiatrists' participation in health insurance networks. *JAMA, 313*(2), 190–191. https://doi.org/10.1001/jama.2014.12472

Cunningham, P. J., & Hadley, J. (2008). Effects of changes in incomes and practice circumstances on physicians' decisions to treat charity and Medicaid patients. *The Milbank Quarterly, 86*(1), 91–123. https://doi.org/10.1111/j.1468-0009.2007.00514.x

Cutler, D. M., & Reber, S. J. (1998). Paying for health insurance: The trade-off between competition and adverse selection. *The Quarterly Journal of Economics, 113*(2), 433–466. https://doi.org/10.1162/003355398555649

Cutler, D. M., & Zeckhauser, R. J. (1998). Adverse selection in health insurance. In A. M. Garber & D. M. Cutler (Eds.), *Frontiers in health policy research* (Vol. 1). Cambridge, MA: National Bureau of Economic Research.

Decker, S. L. (2012). In 2011 nearly one-third of physicians said they would not accept new Medicaid patients, but rising fees may help. *Health Affairs, 31*(8), 1673–1679. https://doi.org/10.1377/hlthaff.2012.0294

Dickey, B., Normand, S. L., Norton, E. C., Rupp, A., & Azeni, H. (2001). Managed care and children's behavioral health services in Massachusetts. *Psychiatric Services, 52*(2), 183–188. https://doi.org/10.1176/appi.ps.52.2.183

Druss, B. G. (2006). Rising mental health costs: What are we getting for our money? *Health Affairs, 25*(3), 614–622. https://doi.org/10.1377/hlthaff.25.3.614

Ettner, S. L., Harwood, J. M., Thalmayer, A., Ong, M. K., Xu, H., Bresolin, M. J., … Azocar, F. (2016). The Mental Health Parity and Addiction Equity Act evaluation study: Impact on specialty behavioral health utilization and expenditures among "carve-out" enrollees. *Journal of Health Economics, 50*, 131–143. https://doi.org/10.1016/j.jhealeco.2016.09.009

Frakt, A. B., & Mayes, R. (2012). Beyond capitation: How new payment experiments seek to find the 'sweet spot' in amount of risk providers and payers bear. *Health Affairs, 31*(9), 1951–1958. https://doi.org/10.1377/hlthaff.2012.0344

Frank, R. G., Glazer, J., & McGuire, T. G. (2000). Measuring adverse selection in managed health care. *Journal of Health Economics, 19*(6), 829–854. https://doi.org/10.1016/S0167-6296(00)00059-X

Frank, R. G., & Glied, S. (2006). Changes in mental health financing since 1971: Implications for policymakers and patients. *Health Affairs, 25*(3), 601–613. https://doi.org/10.1377/hlthaff.25.3.601

Frank, R. G., & McGuire, T. G. (1986). A review of studies of the impact of insurance on the demand and utilization of specialty mental health services. *Health Services Research, 21*(2 Pt 2), 241–265. https://www.ncbi.nlm.nih.gov/pmc/articles/PMC1068951/, https://www.ncbi.nlm.nih.gov/pmc/articles/PMC1068951/pdf/hsresearch00502-0009.pdf

Frank, R. G., & McGuire, T. G. (2000). Economics and mental health. In A. J. Culyer & J. P. Newhouse (Eds.), *Handbook of health economics* (Vol. 1B). New York, NY: Elsevier.

Garfield, R. L., Zuvekas, S. H., Lave, J. R., & Donohue, J. M. (2011). The impact of national health care reform on adults with severe mental disorders. *The American Journal of Psychiatry, 168*(5), 486–494. https://doi.org/10.1176/appi.ajp.2010.10060792

Goldman, D. P., Dirani, R., Fastenau, J., & Conrad, R. M. (2014). Do strict formularies replicate failure for patients with schizophrenia? *American Journal of Managed Care, 20*(3), 219–228. http://www.ajmc.com/journals/issue/2014/2014-vol20-n3/do-strict-formularies-replicate-failure-for-patients-with-schizophrenia?p=2

Goldman, D. P., Joyce, G. F., Escarce, J. J., Pace, J. E., Solomon, M. D., Laouri, M., ... Teutsch, S. M. (2004). Pharmacy benefits and the use of drugs by the chronically ill. *JAMA, 291*(19), 2344–2350. https://doi.org/10.1001/jama.291.19.2344

Goldman, H. H., Frank, R. G., Burnam, M. A., Huskamp, H. A., Ridgely, M. S., Normand, S. L., ... Blasinsky, M. (2006). Behavioral health insurance parity for federal employees. *The New England Journal of Medicine, 354*(13), 1378–1386. https://doi.org/10.1056/NEJMsa053737

Goldsmith, J. (2010). Analyzing shifts in economic risks to providers in proposed payment and delivery system reforms. *Health Affairs, 29*(7), 1299–1304. https://doi.org/10.1377/hlthaff.2010.0423

Hodgkin, D., & McGuire, T. G. (1994). Payment levels and hospital response to prospective payment. *Journal of Health Economics, 13*(1), 1–29. https://doi.org/10.1016/0167-6296(94)90002-7

Hodgkin, D., Parks Thomas, C., Simoni-Wastila, L., Ritter, G. A., & Lee, S. (2008). The effect of a three-tier formulary on antidepressant utilization and expenditures. *The Journal of Mental Health Policy and Economics, 11*(2), 67–77.

Huskamp, H. A., Deverka, P. A., Epstein, A. M., Epstein, R. S., McGuigan, K. A., Muriel, A. C., & Frank, R. G. (2005). Impact of 3-tier formularies on drug treatment of attention-deficit/hyperactivity disorder in children. *Archives of General Psychiatry, 62*(4), 435–441. https://doi.org/10.1001/archpsyc.62.4.435

Hussey, P. S., Ridgely, M. S., & Rosenthal, M. B. (2011). The PROMETHEUS bundled payment experiment: Slow start shows problems in implementing new payment models. *Health Affairs, 30*(11), 2116–2124. https://doi.org/10.1377/hlthaff.2011.0784

Interstudy. (2002). *The interstudy competitive edge 13.1: Part II, HMO industry report*. St. Paul, MN: Interstudy.

Interstudy. (2003). *The interstudy competitive edge 13.1: Part II, HMO industry report*. St. Paul, MN: Interstudy.

Interstudy. (2007). *The Interstudy Competitive Edge 17.1: Part II, HMO industry report*. St. Paul, MN: Interstudy.

Kaiser Family Foundation. (2018a). *Medicare prescription drug plans: Number of medicare beneficiaries with creditable prescription drug coverage, by type: Timeframe: March 2014*. Washington, DC: Kaiser Family Foundation. https://www.kff.org/medicare/state-indicator/medicare-rx-drug-coverage/

Kaiser Family Foundation. (2018b). *Total HMO enrollment [Timeframe: Jan 2016]*. [Web page]. Washington, DC: Kaiser Family Foundation. https://www.kff.org/other/state-indicator/total-hmo-enrollment

Kaiser Family Foundation. (2018c, January 16). *Status of state action on the Medicaid Expansion decision, as of January 16, 2018*. [Web page]. Washington, DC: Kaiser Family Foundation. https://www.kff.org/health-reform/state-indicator/state-activity-around-expanding-medicaid-under-the-affordable-care-act/

Keeler, E. B., Manning, W. G., & Wells, K. B. (1988). The demand for episodes of mental health services. *Journal of Health Economics, 7*(4), 369–392. https://doi.org/10.1016/0167-6296(88)90021-5

Kessler, R. C., Demler, O., Frank, R. G., Olfson, M., Pincus, H. A., Walters, E. E., ... Zaslavsky, A. M. (2005). Prevalence and treatment of mental disorders, 1990 to 2003. *The New England Journal of Medicine, 352*(24), 2515–2523. https://doi.org/10.1056/NEJMsa043266

Landsman, P. B., Yu, W., Liu, X., Teutsch, S. M., & Berger, M. L. (2005). Impact of 3-tier pharmacy benefit design and increased consumer cost-sharing on drug utilization. *The American Journal of Managed Care, 11*(10), 621–628.

Ling Davina, C., Berndt, E. R., & Frank, R. G. (2007). Economic incentives and contracts: The use of psychotropic medications. *Contemporary Economic Policy, 26*(1), 49–72. https://doi.org/10.1111/j.1465-7287.2007.00063.x

Ma, A., & McGuire, T., G. (2004). Network incentives in managed health care. *Journal of Economics & Management Strategy, 11*(1), 1-35. doi:https://doi.org/10.1111/j.1430-9134.2002.00001.x

Ma, A., & McGuire, T. G. (1998). Costs and incentives in a behavioral health carve-out. *Health Affairs, 17*(2), 53–69. https://doi.org/10.1377/hlthaff.17.2.53

Mark, T. L., Wier, L. M., Malone, K., Penne, M., & Cowell, A. J. (2015). National estimates of behavioral health conditions and their treatment among adults newly insured under the ACA. *Psychiatric Services, 66*(4), 426–429. https://doi.org/10.1176/appi.ps.201400078

Mark, T. L., Yee, T., Levit, K. R., Camacho-Cook, J., Cutler, E., & Carroll, C. D. (2016). Insurance financing increased for mental health conditions but not for substance use disorders, 1986-2014. *Health Affairs, 35*(6), 958–965. https://doi.org/10.1377/hlthaff.2016.0002

McClellan, C. B. (2017). The Affordable Care Act's dependent care coverage expansion and behavioral health care. *Journal of Mental Health Policy and Economics, 20*(3), 111–130.

McGuire, T. G. (2016). Achieving mental health care parity might require changes in payments and competition. *Health Affairs, 35*(6), 1029–1035. https://doi.org/10.1377/hlthaff.2016.0012

Mechanic, D. (2007). Mental health services then and now. *Health Affairs, 26*(6), 1548–1550. https://doi.org/10.1377/hlthaff.26.6.1548

Mechanic, R. E., & Altman, S. H. (2009). Payment reform options: Episode payment is a good place to start. *Health Affairs, 28*(2), w262–w271. https://doi.org/10.1377/hlthaff.28.2.w262

Meyerhoefer, C. D., & Zuvekas, S. H. (2010). New estimates of the demand for physical and mental health treatment. *Health Economics, 19*(3), 297–315. https://doi.org/10.1002/hec.1476

Mitchell, J. B. (1991). Physician participation in Medicaid revisited. *Medical Care, 29*(7), 645–653.

Monheit, A. C., & Selden, T. M. (2000). Cross-subsidization in the market for employment-related health insurance. *Health Economics, 9*(8), 699–714.

Montz, E., Layton, T., Busch, A. B., Ellis, R. P., Rose, S., & McGuire, T. G. (2016). Risk-adjustment simulation: Plans may have incentives to distort mental health and substance use coverage. *Health Affairs, 35*(6), 1022–1028. https://doi.org/10.1377/hlthaff.2015.1668

National Advisory Mental Health Council. (1998). *Parity in financing mental health services: Managed care effects on cost, access, and quality; an interim report to Congress.* Rockville, MD: Department of Health and Human Services, National Institutes of Health, National Institute of Mental Health. https://www.nimh.nih.gov/about/advisory-boards-and-groups/namhc/reports/nimh-parity-report_42572_42572.pdf

National Advisory Mental Health Council. (2000). *Insurance parity for mental health: Cost, access, and quality; final report to Congress* (NIH Publication No. 00-4787). Bethesda, MD: Department of Health and Human Services, National Institutes of Health, National Institute of Mental Health. https://www.nimh.nih.gov/about/advisory-boards-and-groups/namhc/reports/insurance-parity-for-mental-health-cost-access-and-quality-final-report-to-congress-by-the-national-advisory-mental-health-council.shtml

Norton, E. C., Lindrooth, R. C., & Dickey, B. (1997). Cost shifting in a mental health carve-out for the AFDC population. *Health Care Financing Review, 18*(3), 95–108. https://www.ncbi.nlm.nih.gov/pmc/articles/PMC4194497/

O'Malley, A. S., & Reschovsky, J. D. (2006). No exodus: physicians and managed care networks. *Tracking report*(14), 1–4. http://www.hschange.org/CONTENT/838/?PRINT=1

Office of Disability Employment Policy. (2007). *Increasing options: The Ticket to Work and Self Sufficiency Program. [Fact sheet].* Washington, DC: U. S. Department of Labor. https://www.dol.gov/odep/pubs/fact/options.htm

Open Minds. (2002). *Open Minds yearbook of managed behavioral health & employee assistance program market share in the United States, 2002–2003*. Gettysburg, PA: Behavioral Health Industry News.

Pacula, R. L., & Sturm, R. (2000). Mental health parity legislation: Much ado about nothing? *Health Services Research, 35*(1 Pt 2), 263–275. https://www.ncbi.nlm.nih.gov/pmc/articles/PMC1089100/

Padgett, D. K., Patrick, C., Burns, B. J., Schlesinger, H. J., & Cohen, J. (1993). The effect of insurance benefit changes on use of child and adolescent outpatient mental health services. *Medical Care, 31*(2), 96–110. https://doi.org/10.1097/00005650-199302000-00002

Rice, T., & Matsuoka, K. Y. (2004). The impact of cost-sharing on appropriate utilization and health status: a review of the literature on seniors. *Medical Care Research & Review, 61*(4), 415–452. https://doi.org/10.1177/1077558704269498

Ridgely, M. S., Burnam, M. A., Barry, C. L., Goldman, H. H., & Hennessy, K. D. (2006). Health plans respond to parity: Managing behavioral health care in the Federal Employees Health Benefits Program. *The Milbank Quarterly, 84*(1), 201–218. https://doi.org/10.1111/j.1468-0009.2006.00443.x

Rosenthal, M. B., Frank, R. G., Li, Z., & Epstein, A. M. (2005). Early experience with pay-for-performance: From concept to practice. *JAMA, 294*(14), 1788-1793. doi:https://doi.org/10.1001/jama.294.14.1788

Rosenthal, M. B., Landon, B. E., Howitt, K., Song, H. R., & Epstein, A. M. (2007). Climbing up the pay-for-performance learning curve: Where are the early adopters now? *Health Affairs, 26*(6), 1674–1682. https://doi.org/10.1377/hlthaff.26.6.1674

Rosenthal, M. B., Landon, B. E., Normand, S. L., Frank, R. G., Ahmad, T. S., & Epstein, A. M. (2007). Employers' use of value-based purchasing strategies. *JAMA, 298*(19), 2281–2288. https://doi.org/10.1001/jama.298.19.2281

Rosenthal, M. B., Landrum, M. B., Robbins, J. A., & Schneider, E. C. (2016). Pay for performance in Medicaid: Evidence from three natural experiments. *Health Services Research, 51*(4), 1444–1466. https://doi.org/10.1111/1475-6773.12426

Rothschild, M., & Stiglitz, J. (1976). Equilibrium in competitive insurance markets: An essay on the economics of imperfect information. *Quaterly Journal of Economics, 90*(4), 629–649. https://doi.org/10.1007/978-94-015-7957-5_18

Saloner, B., & Le Cook, B. (2014). An ACA provision increased treatment for young adults with possible mental illnesses relative to comparison group. *Health Affairs, 33*(8), 1425–1434. https://doi.org/10.1377/hlthaff.2014.0214

Sharma, R., Tinkler, S., Mitra, A., Pal, S., Susu-Mago, R., & Stano, M. (2018). State Medicaid fees and access to primary care physicians. *Health Economics, 27*(3), 629–636. https://doi.org/10.1002/hec.3591

Sinaiko, A. D., Landrum, M. B., Meyers, D. J., Alidina, S., Maeng, D. D., Friedberg, M. W., … Rosenthal, M. B. (2017). Synthesis of research on patient-centered medical homes brings systematic differences into relief. *Health Affairs, 36*(3), 500–508. https://doi.org/10.1377/hlthaff.2016.1235

Stewart, M. T., Horgan, C. M., Hodgkin, D., Creedon, T. B., Quinn, A., Garito, L., … Garnick, D. W. (2018). Behavioral health coverage under the Affordable Care Act: What can we learn from marketplace products? *Psychiatric Services, 69*(3), 315–321. https://doi.org/10.1176/appi.ps.201700098

Strunk, B. C., & Reschovsky, J. D. (2002). Kinder and gentler: Physicians and managed care, 1997-2001. *Tracking report*(5), 1–4. http://www.hschange.org/CONTENT/486/?PRINT=1

Sturm, R. (1997). How expensive is unlimited mental health care coverage under managed care? *JAMA, 278*(18), 1533–1537. https://doi.org/10.1007/BF02287491

Substance Abuse and Mental Health Services Administration. (2015, February 15). *HHS FY2016 budget in brief: Substance Abuse and Mental Health Services Administration (SAMHSA)*. Washington, DC: U. S. Department of Health and Human Services. https://www.hhs.gov/about/budget/budget-in-brief/samhsa/index.html

Substance Abuse and Mental Health Services Administration. (2016). *Behavioral health spending and use accounts, 1986–2014* (HHS Publication No. SMA-16-4975). Rockville, MD: Substance Abuse and Mental Health Services Administration. https://store.samhsa.gov/shin/content/SMA16-4975/SMA16-4975.pdf

Tran Smith, B., Seaton, K., Andrews, C., Grogan, C. M., Abraham, A., Pollack, H., ... Humphreys, K. (2017). Benefit requirements for substance use disorder treatment in state health insurance exchanges. *The American Journal of Drug and Alcohol Abuse, 1–5.* https://doi.org/10.1080/00952990.2017.1411934

Tsai, J., & Rosenheck, R. A. (2016). US veterans' use of VA mental health services and disability compensation increased from 2001 to 2010. *Health Affairs, 35*(6), 966–973. https://doi.org/10.1377/hlthaff.2015.1555

Uberoi, N., Finegold, K., & Gee, E. (2016). Health insurance coverage and the Affordable Care Act, 2010-2016. *ASPE Issue Brief* (March 3, 2016), 1–14. https://aspe.hhs.gov/system/files/pdf/187551/ACA2010-2016.pdf

Wang, P. S., Lane, M., Olfson, M., Pincus, H. A., Wells, K. B., & Kessler, R. C. (2005). Twelve-month use of mental health services in the United States: Results from the National Comorbidity Survey Replication. *Archives of General Psychiatry, 62*(6), 629–640. https://doi.org/10.1001/archpsyc.62.6.629

Wang, P. S., Patrick, A. R., Dormuth, C. R., Avorn, J., Maclure, M., Canning, C. F., & Schneeweiss, S. (2008). The impact of cost sharing on antidepressant use among older adults in British Columbia. *Psychiatric Services, 59*(4), 377–383. https://doi.org/10.1176/ps.2008.59.4.377

Wildsmith, T. F. (2009, October). *Individual health insurance 2009: A comprehensive survey of affordability, access, and benefits.* Washington, DC: America's Health Insurance Plan. https://kaiserhealthnews.files.wordpress.com/2013/02/2009individualmarketsurveyfinalreport.pdf

Wilk, J. E., West, J. C., Narrow, W. E., Rae, D. S., & Regier, D. A. (2005). Access to psychiatrists in the public sector and in managed health plans. *Psychiatric Services, 56*(4), 408–410. https://doi.org/10.1176/appi.ps.56.4.408

Zeckhauser, R. (1970). Medical insurance: A case study of the tradeoff between risk spreading and appropriate incentives. *Journal of Economic Theory, 2*(1), 10–26. https://doi.org/10.1016/0022-0531(70)90010-4

Zuckerman, S., McFeeters, J., Cunningham, P., & Nichols, L. (2004). Changes in Medicaid physician fees, 1998-2003: Implications for physician participation. *Health Affairs, Supplement Web Exclusives,* W4-374–384. https://doi.org/10.1377/hlthaff.w4.374

Zuvekas, S. H. (1999). Health insurance, health reform, and outpatient mental health treatment: Who benefits? *Inquiry, 36*(2), 127–146.

Zuvekas, S. H. (2001). Trends in mental health services use and spending, 1987–1996. *Health Affairs, 20*(2), 214–224. https://doi.org/10.1377/hlthaff.20.2.214

Zuvekas, S. H., & Cohen, J. W. (2016). Fee-for-service, while much maligned, remains the dominant payment method for physician visits. *Health Affairs, 35*(3), 411–414. https://doi.org/10.1377/hlthaff.2015.1291

Zuvekas, S. H., Rupp, A., & Norquist, G. (2007). Cost shifting under managed behavioral health care. *Psychiatric Services, 58*(1), 100–108. https://doi.org/10.1176/ps.2007.58.1.100

The Role of Implementation Science in Behavioral Health

Oliver T. Massey and Enya B. Vroom

Introduction

Health and behavioral health professionals recognize a critical *research-to-practice gap* in the provision of community-based services. This gap lies between what is known about effective services developed through careful research and what is typically provided in community-based behavioral health services. Effective services, practices, and programs, defined as *evidence-based programs* (EBPs), have demonstrated evidence of their effectiveness under controlled research settings. EBPs were developed with the expectations that professionals would readily adopt services of proven efficacy to improve the quality of outcomes for service recipients. It was believed good programs would easily find a home in service agencies that are genuinely interested in using the best interventions for their clients.

Unfortunately, it is now recognized that programs are not adopted readily and there are significant gaps in the translation of EBPs into working programs in the field (Proctor et al., 2009; Urban & Trochim, 2009). Simply providing an effective new program is not sufficient to ensure that it is implemented in the real world.

This inability to translate effective programs into practices in the field has led to an emphasis on implementation science (IS). IS attempts to bridge the gap between research and practice by identifying and accounting for the barriers that prevent effective programs from being easily identified, accepted, and utilized in clinical practice. Known as tracing blue highways, a two-way adaptation, research-practice integration, and research translation (Fixsen, Naoom, Blase, Friedman, & Wallace, 2005; Hoagwood & Johnson, 2003; Urban & Trochim, 2009; Wandersman et al., 2008; Westfall, Mold, & Fagnan, 2007), IS deals with the capacity to move what is known about effective treatment into services (Proctor et al., 2009).

O. T. Massey (✉) · E. B. Vroom
Department of Child and Family Studies, College of Behavioral and Community Sciences,
University of South Florida, Tampa, FL, USA
e-mail: massey@usf.edu

© Springer Nature Switzerland AG 2020
B. L. Levin, A. Hanson (eds.), *Foundations of Behavioral Health*,
https://doi.org/10.1007/978-3-030-18435-3_5

IS encompasses the investigation of methods, variables, interventions, and strategies to promote appropriate adoption, support, and sustainability of EBPs (Titler, Everett, & Adams, 2007). This perspective recognizes the complex problem of ensuring that an effective intervention is adapted and integrated into practice where community acceptability, applicability, organizational and political demands, resources, and cultural differences may compromise program effectiveness and consumer outcomes.

This chapter reviews and discusses research and practice in the fields of behavioral health and public health from the perspective of IS, with an emphasis on critical questions researchers and practice professionals must address as they attempt to improve services in the community. While a complete discussion of the research-to-practice gap might include the early stages involved with converting basic science findings into human applications and interventions (often labeled translational science), this chapter concentrates on latter stages concerned with moving programs that have been conceptualized and tested under controlled conditions into clinical practices. We are concerned with the issues that help in moving programs of proven efficacy into programs of ongoing effectiveness in the field. We pay particular attention to the process of implementation, issues in program fidelity, fit, and adaptation and conclude with a discussion of integration and sustainability.

Evidence-Based Programs

As we are concerned with the implementation of evidence-based programs and practices (EBPs), it may be helpful to clarify how we define EBPs. The term "evidence-based practice" has a number of definitions. One definition revolves around evidence-based treatments, practices, and interventions and those related sets of programs or policies that have empirical proof of their effectiveness. Empirical proof, by definition, is based in a demonstration of therapeutic change, an outcome that is different from a no-treatment or treatment as usual condition (Kazdin, 2008), and focuses on approaches shown to be effective through research rather than through professional experience or opinion (Guevara & Solomon, 2009).

A second definition of EBPs addresses the practice of clinical service that is based on an evidence-informed philosophy in which services for consumers should emerge from careful consideration of the professional's clinical expertise and accumulated experience, available research evidence, and the wishes, needs, and preferences of the patient. An EBP then becomes one that integrates these perspectives in the process of making decisions about patient care. Research evidence is just one source of information that helps support an effective patient care process. This broader term is often used by health disciplines including medicine, public health, and psychology (APA Presidential Task Force on Evidence-Based Practice, 2006; Hoagwood & Johnson, 2003; Sackett, Rosenberg, Gray, Haynes, & Richardson, 1996) and is a source of confusion among professionals and laypersons alike. Our use of the term EBP aligns with the first definition, as in those practices, programs, or interventions shown to be empirically efficacious under controlled research situations.

The emphasis on the use of EBPs has significantly increased in the last three decades. In 1999, the US Surgeon General reported that despite the widespread availability of EBPs, persons with mental illnesses were not actually receiving them (Office of the Surgeon General, 1999).

Of the many programs and services that were in use, only a relatively small number had evidence of their effectiveness (Kazdin, 2000). This led to the President's New Freedom Commission on Mental Health (2003), which suggested all clinical practice should have a foundation in evidence in order to increase the effectiveness of mental health services. From this emphasis, IS emerged as a key component in the improvement of clinical services.

Barriers to the Use of EBPs

As EBPs are widely available, any discussion of IS must begin with why programs of proven efficacy are not used. The difficulty inherent in the translation of programs into the community does not lie with the lack of effectiveness studies or sufficient evidence to convince skeptics of a program's utility or value. A large number of evidence-based programs and interventions are available for many behavioral health concerns. Rather, the difficulties rest with the EBP and its fit with a range of issues germane to the service organization and professionals providing services. These include staffing, clientele, political climate, funding limitations, and cultural expectations at both the organizational and community levels (Aarons, 2004, 2006; Green, 2008; Lehman, Greener, & Simpson, 2002).

A number of implementation models suggest six sets of factors are relevant for program implementation success (Chaudoir, Dugan, & Barr, 2013; Damschroder et al., 2009; Durlak & DuPre, 2008; Nilsen, 2015). These factors include (1) characteristics of the EBP itself, (2) characteristics of the professionals providing services, (3) consumer/patient and stakeholder variables, (4) the context and culture of the organization providing services, (5) the community, and (6) the strategies used to facilitate or implement the EBP (see Table 1).

Characteristics of the EBP relevant for successful implementation may include the source of the intervention the strength of the evidence supporting its use, the advantage of its use, and issues of cost, complexity, adaptability, and "trialability" (Damschroder et al., 2009). A program or practice that can be used on a trial basis, adapted to fit the needs or qualifications of current staff, and costs little to implement is more likely to be adopted than one that does not. The presence of a standard "manualized" approach is also an important characteristic of the EBP (Stichter, Herzog, Owens, & Malugen, 2016).

Characteristics of the professionals providing services also play a critical role in the successful adoption of new or different services. A fundamental concern for staff is if they have the qualifications and skills to provide the new service and, if

Table 1 Factors relevant for program implementation success

Factors	Relevant variables
EBP characteristics	Evidence of effectiveness, relative advantage (ROI), cost, complexity, trialability, adaptability (Damschroder et al., 2009)
Professional characteristics	Qualifications, relevant skills, readiness for change, training, trust in leadership (Aarons, 2004; Durlak & DuPre, 2008; Fixsen et al., 2005)
Client characteristics	Trust in the organization, perceived relevance, perceived value, culture, faith, individual differences (Dovidio et al., 2008; Feldstein & Glasgow, 2008)
Organization characteristics	Leadership, resources, procedural supports, billing systems, referral systems, funding strategies (Aarons & Sommerfeld, 2012; Aarons, Sommerfeld, & Walrath-Greene, 2009; Durlak & DuPre, 2008)
Community characteristics	Acceptance, awareness, political support, community support (Chaudoir et al., 2013; Durlak & DuPre, 2008; Isett et al., 2007)
The implementation process	Training, coaching, preparation efforts, consensus building, clarity of manualization, implementation planning (Blase, Kiser, and Van Dyke, 2013; Damschroder et al., 2009)

not, is training available and readily obtained. The National Implementation Research Network (NIRN) model of implementation suggests the selection, training, and coaching of professional staff are critical drivers of successful implementation (Fixsen et al., 2005). Even with the requisite skills, staff readiness for change and willingness to try a new program may determine if it is implemented successfully (Aarons, 2004). Finally, staff attitudes toward the new effort, their faith in its value, and their trust that the program will be supported all bear on eventual implementation success (Durlak & DuPre, 2008).

Characteristics of the clientele receiving services include considerations of those who will eventually receive the service or program. Even the most effective program will not succeed if it confronts the culture, faith, or beliefs of the consumers for whom it is intended (Feldstein & Glasgow, 2008). Patient values and preferences will determine if they are willing to participate in interventions proposed on their behalf. Culture may trump evidence in the ultimate test of successful implementation. Those belonging to cultures who have suffered historic disparities may not trust the program or its purveyors and may refuse to engage in services they did not have a say in developing (Dovidio et al., 2008).

Characteristics of the organization providing services such as organizational type, leadership styles, organizational climate, and the management processes that support the program or practice all contribute to implementation success (Aarons & Sommerfeld, 2012; Aarons, Sommerfeld, & Walrath-Greene, 2009; Durlak & DuPre, 2008). An adaptive leadership style has been proposed as increasing successful program implementation and having appropriate decision support systems, middle management support, and administrative supports (Fixsen et al., 2005; Tabrizi, 2014).

Another major consideration is the importance of change agents or program champions who may be engaged in the implementation process (Greenhalgh, Robert, Macfarlane, Bate, & Kyriakidou, 2004; Rogers, 2003). These individuals believe in the purpose and mission of the EBP that their organization is implementing and can assist in creating the organizational culture and climate conducive to accepting innovation. Finally, adequate staffing patterns and supervision may also impact the successful implementation of new services (Walker et al., 2003), as can larger issues of organizational structure such as identifying lines of authority and accountability (Massey, Armstrong, Boroughs, Henson, & McCash, 2005).

Organizations are embedded in broader communities that influence the implementation of new programs and practices. Thus, *characteristics of the community* also influence successful implementation. Public policies; local, state, and federal laws and regulations; political climate; and realities of funding may all contribute to the utilization of new programs and services (Chaudoir et al., 2013; Durlak & DuPre, 2008). Legal, political, and human capital are often required to ensure successful implementation, and each EBP brings its own set of political, regulatory, and leadership issues (Isett et al., 2007). Damschroder et al. (2009) include communication and social network channels and the resulting community culture that encourages or discourages adoption of new programs and policies.

Lastly, characteristics of *the implementation process* itself may influence the eventual success of a new program or practice. Damschroder et al. (2009) suggest at least four considerations in how programs are implemented including the process of planning, engaging, executing, and evaluating programs as they are implemented. Blase, Kiser, and Van Dyke (2013) suggest successful implementation requires consideration of resources, capacity, readiness, and fit as part of the planning and engaging process. As will be discussed later, implementation occurs in stages, with different considerations emerging over time. Much research remains regarding how to move programs optimally into practice. Crucial questions also remain regarding how much each of these domains weighs in the implementation of new programs and where scarce resources should be placed to maximally encourage successful program innovation.

Fidelity and Adaptation of EBPs

Given the many barriers to successful implementation, an overarching concern is what must be done to address these challenges to ensure that programs are implemented successfully. Successful program implementation demands a balance between maintaining the fidelity of the program and allowing program adaptations that are required to overcome any barriers to its successful use. The challenge is to resolve the tension between fidelity and fit. This tension deals with the match between programs as developed and the needs, interests, and concerns of populations in the community and may include the degree to which efforts account for cultural, community, and family standards and expectations (Lieberman et al., 2011).

Fidelity has been variously labeled as integrity, implementation fidelity, and treatment fidelity (Allen, Shelton, Emmons, & Linnan, 2018; Carroll et al., 2007;

Dane & Schneider, 1998) and defined as the extent to which a program or innovation is implemented as it was originally designed or intended (Allen et al., 2018; Carroll et al., 2007; Durlak & DuPre, 2008). It involves attention to measuring and maintaining the elements of a program or practice that are critical for programmatic impact as the program is brought into the community setting (Bond, Evans, Salyers, Williams, & Kim, 2000; Bruns, 2008; Center for Substance Abuse Treatment, 2007).

The conceptualization and operationalization of fidelity has evolved to include five core elements: (1) adherence, (2) dose or exposure, (3) quality of delivery, (4) participant responsiveness, and (5) program differentiation (Allen et al., 2018; Durlak & DuPre, 2008) (see Table 2).

Adherence refers to the degree to which a program or practice was implemented consistent with the structure, components, and procedures under which it was designed (Carroll et al., 2007). For example, if a substance abuse prevention program delivered in a classroom setting required the teacher to implement the curriculum based on a weekly schedule utilizing an adult learning model, utilizing a biweekly schedule without the adult learning model would reflect poor program adherence.

Dose or *exposure* refers to the degree to which the amount of a program participants receive matches the program model as designed (Durlak & DuPre, 2008). While dose in medical terminology is readily defined, in behavioral health settings, dose may correspond to appropriate exposure to program elements, the duration of the program as it was originally prescribed, or even the number of therapeutic sessions attended (Baldwin, Johnson, & Benally, 2009). In an evaluation of a school-based intervention program, Yampolskaya, Massey, and Greenbaum (2006) measured dose as time spent in hours in academic and behavioral programming.

Quality of delivery is the manner in which the implementer (e.g., teacher, clinician, or staff) delivers a program or practice (Allen et al., 2018). This can include how well an implementer answers questions or addresses concerns and how knowledgeable they are of the program model and curriculum. Often, observation and a trained rater or observer measure this element based on components included in a

Table 2 Core elements of fidelity

Elements	Definition
Adherence	The degree to which a program or practice was implemented as it was originally designed by the developer (Durlak & DuPre, 2008)
Dose or exposure	The amount, frequency, and/or duration of a program or practice an individual receives (Allen et al., 2018)
Quality of delivery	How well the components of a program or practice are delivered (e.g., clarity and knowledge of topic) (Carroll et al., 2007)
Participant responsiveness	The degree to which a program or practice engages, stimulates, and is accepted by the target population (Allen et al., 2018; Durlak & DuPre, 2008)
Program differentiation	A program's theoretical roots and practices that exert influence and are unique from other programs (Allen et al., 2018; Durlak & DuPre, 2008)

fidelity measure or checklist. For example, raters observing a classroom-based substance abuse prevention program may be interested in observing and rating a teacher's clarity of instruction on how to complete a marijuana myth-busting assignment.

Participant responsiveness refers to how engaged and responsive a participant is to a program or practice as well as their level of understanding of program materials or the importance of a practice (e.g., deep breathing or adherence to medication) (Allen et al., 2018; Durlak & DuPre, 2008). Although much emphasis has been put on the examination of adherence and dosage, achieving high levels of adherence can be influenced by other elements like participant responsiveness (Carroll et al., 2007) and may not always be the most significant predictor of participant outcomes.

Program differentiation refers to components that have been identified as unique to a program, without which, programmatic success would be impossible (Allen et al., 2018). The identification of the critical common elements of a program or intervention constitutes and defines the program (Chorpita, Daleiden, & Weisz, 2005). Program differentiation may also be important for evaluations of new interventions in order to identify components of the program that are essential for positive outcomes (Carroll et al., 2007). While some researchers suggest that all core elements of fidelity are equally important, others argue those implementing need to prioritize the elements based on the intervention, its purpose, and the resources and personnel that are available (Allen et al., 2018; Harn, Parisi, & Stoolmiller, 2013).

Fidelity and Outcomes

There is significant evidence supporting the relationship between fidelity and participant outcomes (c.f. Carroll et al., 2007; Durlak & DuPre, 2008), and a thorough evaluation of fidelity is integral to understanding why an intervention succeeds or fails. If fidelity is not monitored and evaluated, it may not be possible to determine if the failure of an intervention is related to poor implementation, the shortcomings of the intervention itself (labeled as a "type III error"), or other ancillary variables (Allen et al., 2018; Carroll et al., 2007; Harn et al., 2013). The emphasis in fidelity has resulted in numerous attempts to identify critical elements and standards of programs and to conduct fidelity assessments to measure the degree to which programs maintain these standards (c.f. Deschênes, Clark, & Herrygers, 2008; Hernandez, Worthington, & Davis, 2005). For example, Pullmann, Bruns, and Sather (2013) developed a fidelity index that assessed the degree to which providers followed the essential principles of wraparound in their service delivery. The index assesses the degree to which critical components of wraparound such as family participation, strength-based approaches, and cultural competence are present in therapeutic encounters. Thus, fidelity has become the cornerstone of effective implementation (Lendrum, Humphrey, & Greenberg, 2016).

Balanced against the concern for program fidelity is the need for EBPs to fit the communities where they are implemented. This contrasting perspective may be characterized as the relevance of the program for the community and the realities of not only resources and capacity but also characterized by culture, family and community preferences, and acceptance by professionals who recognize the unique characteristics and needs of their consumers. Not all EBPs are necessarily developed for members of specific communities or all proven interventions appropriate for all communities in need of services. In efforts to ensure the internal validity of research studies, interventions are developed and tested on narrowly defined, homogeneous populations.

The emphasis on internal validity, a critical concern for the development of evidence-based research, comes at the expense of external validity and the effectiveness of interventions across populations (Green, 2008; Green & Glasgow, 2006; Hoagwood, Burns, Kiser, Ringeisen, & Schoenwald, 2001). Thus, one difficulty rests with establishing a match between the program developed for a narrow, specifically defined clientele and the diverse clientele residing in the community. A second difficulty rests with the match between the EBPs' programmatic requirements and the needs, capacity, and constraints operating in community service agencies. Community organizations may simply not have the resources to provide an EBP under the same conditions or at the same level of intensity as the program was developed. Adaptations are then necessary in order to provide an intervention that is effective at the local level (Castro, Barrera Jr, & Martinez Jr, 2004; Harn et al., 2013).

Adaptations can be defined as modifications or changes made to an EBP in order to serve the needs of a particular setting or to increase the fit of a program to a target population. Adaptations typically take place during the adaption and implementation of the intervention. They improve a program's fit and compatibility with a new setting and the needs of the individual(s) and population(s) of interest (Carvalho et al., 2013; Rabin & Brownson, 2018; Stirman, Miller, Toder, & Calloway, 2013). Client and provider attributes (e.g., language, cultural norms, understanding of the EBP) may also be taken into consideration to enhance the fit between the EBP and consumers (Cabassa & Baumann, 2013).

For example, a study in Zambia looked to adapt adult trauma-focused cognitive behavioral therapy (TF-CBT) for use with children and adolescents. Murray et al. (2013) discovered it was critical to work collaboratively with local stakeholders and counselors in order to create culturally responsive and high-fidelity adaptations to increase "fit" and acceptability of the intervention. The collaborative process by which TF-CBT was selected and adapted assisted in creating strong buy-in from the local community, including the support and recommendation of the Ministry of Health in Zambia (Murray et al., 2013).

Tension exists in the research community over the competing ideas of fidelity versus adaptation (Castro et al., 2004; Morrison et al., 2009). While some argue adaptations are essential in order to meet the needs of a particular setting, others argue a program that has been adapted will be significantly less effective when compared to the original program (Carvalho et al., 2013; Castro et al., 2004; Chambers & Norton, 2016). This distinction rests with the emphasis on ensuring the effectiveness of an intervention under clearly specified conditions versus the emphasis on generalizability and effectiveness in less consistent, real-world settings. While adaptations may threaten internal validity, the intent is to improve external validity and thus enhance outcomes for program participants in the real world (Baumann, Cabassa, & Stirman, 2018).

To address the issues associated with adaptations and fidelity, it is important for consumers (e.g., schools, clinicians, mental health organizations) to identify the core components or "active ingredients" (Chorpita et al., 2005; Harn et al., 2013) of a program or practice in order to preserve them during the adaptation process. Once these core components are defined, frameworks, such as the Interactive Systems Framework (Wandersman et al., 2008), the Modification Framework (Stirman et al., 2013), or the Adaptome data platform (Chambers & Norton, 2016), can assist in monitoring adaptations to ensure critical components are left unchanged. If significant program modification does occur, then it is incumbent on implementers to conduct rigorous outcome evaluations in order to assess the possible impact the changes may have on intended outcomes (Carvalho et al., 2013) (for a more comprehensive discussion of managing adaptations and fidelity, c.f. Cabassa & Baumann, 2013; Castro et al., 2004; Chambers & Norton, 2016; Lee, Altschul, & Mowbray, 2008; Stirman et al., 2013; Wandersman et al., 2008).

The question remains as to whether a program reaching optimal fidelity would be sufficient to obtain significant outcomes (Chambers & Norton, 2016). More research is needed to identify the appropriate balance between fidelity and adaptation.

Stages of Implementation

Given the tension between program fidelity and community fit, a natural question is how the implementation process might work. In human service settings, practitioners usually serve to enable a new intervention. As a result, innovations have to be built into thousands of practitioners in multiple organizations that operate under different regulations (e.g., state and federal) and contexts (Fixsen, Blase, Naoom, & Wallace, 2009). It has been suggested the ultimate success of a program and its sustainability (described below) will be largely dependent on laying an appropriate foundation for change (Adelman & Taylor, 2003).

To assist in building innovations into community settings, researchers have proposed several models of implementation that emphasize the implementation process as occurring in stages (Aarons, Hurlburt, & Horwitz, 2011; Fixsen et al., 2005, 2009). The EPIS (exploration, adoption/preparation, implementation, sustainment) is an example of a four-stage model which has different stages that span outer (e.g., sociopolitical) and inner (e.g., organization characteristics) contexts (Aarons et al., 2011). To provide a concrete example of implementation stages, we review another four-stage model, the National Implementation Research Network's (NIRN) model, that includes exploration, installation, initial implementation, and full implementation (Fixsen et al., 2005; National Implementation Research Network, 2015).

The National Implementation Research Network (NIRN) Model

The first stage in the NIRN model is *exploration*. Exploration begins when an organization, community, or an individual within an organization/community decides to make use of a new program or practice. The purpose of this stage is to explore the potential fit between the community and the EBP, the needs of the community, the needs of the EBP, and the amount of community resources needed and available in order to implement the new program. The stage helps determine whether the organization should proceed with the innovation or not. A critical question in this stage is the degree of an organization's readiness for implementation. Research has shown that taking time for exploration and planning saves time and money and can increase the likelihood of success (Fixsen et al., 2005; National Implementation Research Network, 2015; Saldana, Chamberlain, Wang, & Hendricks Brown, 2012).

The second stage of implementation in the NIRN model is *installation*. During installation, the resources and structural supports needed to assist the implementation of an EBP are procured. Resources can include selecting staff, finding sources for training and coaching and providing the initial training for staff, ensuring location/space (e.g., classroom or office space) and access to materials or equipment (e.g., computer or projector), finding or developing fidelity tools, and identifying funding streams and human resource strategies. This is the stage where a community or organization prepares their staff for the new innovation During (Fixsen et al., 2005; National Implementation Research Network 2015).

The third stage is *initial implementation*. This stage involves using the new EBP for the first time. Often referred to as the "initial awkward stage" of implementation, this is where practitioners become familiar with the new program or practice (Fixsen et al., 2005). It also happens to be the most delicate stage of implementation, because organizations and practitioners are changing their normal, comfortable routines and have to fight the urge of reverting to old routines. In order to sustain these changes in a practitioner's routine, it is essential to establish external supports (e.g., coaches, implementation teams, or leadership) on the practice, organization, and system levels (National Implementation Research Network 2015).

The final stage in the NIRN model is *full implementation*. Full implementation is achieved when the new ways of providing services have become standard practice with practitioners, staff, and organizational leaders. Concomitant changes in policies and procedures also are standardized. At this point, the anticipated benefits of an EBP are realized, with staff and practitioners skilled in the procedures of their new routine. Achieving and sustaining full implementation is an arduous process and may be enabled by the success of the preceding stages (National Implementation Research Network 2015). However, research has shown that success in early stages of implementation may not always guarantee full implementation (Abdinnour-Helm, Lengnick-Hall, & Lengnick-Hall, 2003).

One of the main benefits from adhering to a theoretical model or conceptual framework is it allows consumers and researchers to plan for potential barriers and recognize the facilitators of implementation before resources and time are depleted.

More examples and information on other models of implementation are found elsewhere (c.f. Aarons et al., 2011; Damschroder et al., 2009; Rogers, 2003; Saldana, 2014; Saldana et al., 2012).

Sustainability of EBPs

Once a program is in place, the question becomes how to sustain it. Sustainability is involved with the continuity and maintenance of programs after implementation and must be a major consideration of IS. Sustainability may be broadly defined to encompass several aspects of the continuity of an EBP, including maintenance of the procedural processes, commitments, financing (Fixsen et al., 2005), obtaining resources, gaining visibility, status and organizational place (Massey et al., 2005), and supporting the continued benefits and positive outcomes of the program effort (Moore, Mascarenhas, Bain, & Straus, 2017). Sustainability may be best thought of as a continuation of the implementation process, where the emphasis shifts from putting a program into place to maintaining the program through ongoing adaptation and continuous quality improvement efforts (Chambers, Glasgow, & Stange, 2013).

While there have been major advances in understanding the adoption, integration, and implementation of EBPs, program sustainability is not always adequately considered (Shelton, Cooper, & Stirman, 2018). This lack of attention can not only lead to economic and resource losses from wasted effort but also limits the likelihood of successful improvements. EBPs that are discontinued or deserted can result in lower levels of buy-in when a new EBP is proposed for an organization/community and limit the trust that individuals place in research and organizations that conduct research (Shelton et al., 2018).

A number of challenges exist to the sustainability of even well-implemented programs. For example, a systematic review examining the sustainability of health interventions implemented in sub-Saharan Africa found that weak health systems, lack of financial leadership, lack of a consistent workforce, and social and political climates limited an organization's ability to build capacity and sustain interventions (Iwelunmor et al., 2016).

Those who implement EBPs frequently fail to consider the ongoing changes that happen within communities and organizations (Chambers et al., 2013). Prevention programs implemented within a community or organization evolve over time due to changes and level of understanding of staff (i.e., buy-in), feedback from the community or organization, and improvement in the quality of delivery (Shelton et al., 2018). Consistent with the implementation process, research suggests, among other factors, successful sustainability requires modifiable programs, internal champions, readily perceived benefits, and adequate funding and infrastructure support (Hunter, Han, Slaughter, Godley, & Garner, 2017; Scheirer, 2005). It is also critical to ensure all the important stakeholders are included in the sustainability planning. For example, failing to include the individuals who deliver the practice or program (e.g., clinicians or teachers) may lead to issues with long-term buy-in (Cooper, Bumbarger, & Moore, 2015).

Planning for sustainability should be an ongoing discussion that takes place from the initial exploration stage. This allots time dedicated to planning for long-term financing, commitment and organizational support, training and coaching for the workforce, and procedural evaluation and monitoring (Chambers et al., 2013).

Implications for Behavioral Health

IS has clearly defined the difficulties of bringing programs of proven efficacy into the community where they may serve the public interest. For the researcher, it is clear that simply developing a program with the expectation that it will be adopted readily into the field is naïve. While preliminary studies may narrowly focus on exemplary conditions to demonstrate an intervention is effective, it behooves the researcher to move into the community to assess effectiveness as well.

For the practitioner in the field, there is an opportunity to work collaboratively to identify the critical components of interventions and work to match those demands to the needs and characteristics of the organization, the community, and the clientele for whom the program is intended. This bi-directional effort that links the practitioner to the researcher strengthens not only the development of programs and their relevance for the community but also helps identify and build the conditions under which new programs may be maximally effective.

A collaborative process can be established by which consumers, families, practicing clinicians, communities, and cultures develop common agendas for the improvement of service outcomes and actively participate through all stages of program development and implementation (Baumbusch et al., 2008; Gonzales, Ringeisen, & Chambers, 2002; Green, 2008; Hoagwood et al., 2001; McDonald & Viehbeck, 2007). Models for this approach include community-based participatory research (CBPR), which strays from traditional applied research paradigms and strives to incorporate community partnership and action-oriented approaches to behavioral health research (Minkler & Wallerstein, 2013).

In addition, IS training efforts that prepare researchers for program development and implementation may also benefit from expanded opportunities to work in community settings. For example, service-learning opportunities that place researchers in the settings where programs are implemented offers training opportunities for expanding the implementation process and strengthening the cooperation between program implementers and program users (Burton, Levin, Massey, Baldwin, & Williamson, 2016).

The push for policy and regulations requiring EBPs in multiple health services, lack of buy-in from health practitioners, and poor dissemination methods for evidence remain critical in the research-to-practice gap. Estimates suggest it can take up to 17 years for EBPs to make their way from research to practice (Green, Ottoson, Garcia, & Hiatt, 2009). IS addresses this gap by assisting researchers and communities with the translation of research to real-world practice by identifying the implementation factors that are essential for consistent, sufficient, and effective use of EBPs. IS is an essential driver for ensuring effective and efficacious programs and practices and will lead to significant health benefits for the diverse populations and communities requiring behavioral health services.

References

Aarons, G. A. (2004). Mental health provider attitudes toward adoption of evidence-based practice: The Evidence-Based Practice Attitude Scale (EBPAS). *Mental Health Services Research, 6*(2), 61–74. https://doi.org/10.1023/B:MHSR.0000024351.12294.65

Aarons, G. A. (2006). Transformational and transactional leadership: Association with attitudes toward evidence-based practice. *Psychiatric Services, 57*(8), 1162–1169. https://doi.org/10.1176/ps.2006.57.8.1162

Aarons, G. A., Hurlburt, M., & Horwitz, S. M. (2011). Advancing a conceptual model of evidence-based practice implementation in public service sectors. *Administration and Policy in Mental Health, 38*(1), 4–23. https://doi.org/10.1007/s10488-010-0327-7

Aarons, G. A., & Sommerfeld, D. H. (2012). Leadership, innovation climate, and attitudes toward evidence-based practice during a statewide implementation. *Journal of the American Academy of Child and Adolescent Psychiatry, 51*(4), 423–431. https://doi.org/10.1016/j.jaac.2012.01.018

Aarons, G. A., Sommerfeld, D. H., & Walrath-Greene, C. M. (2009). Evidence-based practice implementation: The impact of public versus private sector organization type on organizational support, provider attitudes, and adoption of evidence-based practice. *Implementation Science, 4*, 83. https://doi.org/10.1186/1748-5908-4-83

Abdinnour-Helm, S., Lengnick-Hall, M. L., & Lengnick-Hall, C. A. (2003). Pre-implementation attitudes and organizational readiness for implementing an Enterprise Resource Planning system. *European Journal of Operational Research, 146*(2), 258–273. https://doi.org/10.1016/S0377-2217(02)00548-9

Adelman, H. S., & Taylor, L. (2003). On sustainability of project innovations as systemic change. *Journal of Educational and Psychological Consultation, 14*(1), 1–25. https://doi.org/10.1207/S1532768XJEPC1401_01

Allen, J. D., Shelton, R. C., Emmons, K. M., & Linnan, L. A. (2018). Fidelity and its relationship to implementation, effectiveness, adaptation, and dissemination. In R. C. Brownson, G. A. Colditz, & E. K. Proctor (Eds.), *Dissemination and implementation research in health: Translating science to practice* (2nd ed., pp. 267–284). New York, NY: Oxford University Press.

APA Presidential Task Force on Evidence-Based Practice. (2006). Evidence-based practice in psychology. *American Psychologist, 61*(4), 271–285. https://doi.org/10.1037/0003-066x.61.4.271

Baldwin, J. A., Johnson, J. L., & Benally, C. C. (2009). Building partnerships between indigenous communities and universities: Lessons learned in HIV/AIDS and substance abuse prevention research. *American Journal of Public Health, 99*(Suppl 1), S77–S82. https://doi.org/10.2105/ajph.2008.134585

Baumann, A. A., Cabassa, L. J., & Stirman, S. W. (2018). Adaptation in dissemination and implementation science. In R. C. Brownson, G. A. Colditz, & E. K. Proctor (Eds.), *Dissemination and implementation research in health: Translating science to practice* (2nd ed., pp. 285–300). New York, NY: Oxford University Press.

Baumbusch, J. L., Kirkham, S. R., Khan, K. B., McDonald, H., Semeniuk, P., Tan, E., & Anderson, J. M. (2008). Pursuing common agendas: A collaborative model for knowledge translation between research and practice in clinical settings. *Research in Nursing and Health, 31*(2), 130–140. https://doi.org/10.1002/nur.20242

Blase, K., Kiser, L., & Van Dyke, M. (2013). *The Hexagon Tool: Exploring context*. Chapel Hill, NC: National Implementation Research Network, FPG Child Development Institute, University of North Carolina at Chapel Hill. https://www.pbis.org/Common/Cms/files/pbisresources/NIRN-Education-TheHexagonTool.pdf

Bond, G. R., Evans, L., Salyers, M. P., Williams, J., & Kim, H. W. (2000). Measurement of fidelity in psychiatric rehabilitation. *Mental Health Services Research, 2*(2), 75–87. https://doi.org/10.1023/A:1010153020697

Bruns, E. (2008). *Measuring wraparound fidelity. The resource guide to wraparound*. Portland, OR: Portland State University, National Wraparound Initiative, Research and Training Center on Family Support and Children's Mental Health. http://depts.washington.edu/wrapeval/sites/default/files/Bruns-5e.1-%28measuring-fidelity%29.pdf

Burton, D. L., Levin, B. L., Massey, T., Baldwin, J., & Williamson, H. (2016). Innovative graduate research education for advancement of implementation science in adolescent behavioral health. *Journal of Behavioral Health Services and Research, 43*(2), 172–186. https://doi.org/10.1007/s11414-015-9494-3

Cabassa, L. J., & Baumann, A. A. (2013). A two-way street: Bridging implementation science and cultural adaptations of mental health treatments. *Implementation Science, 8*, 90. https://doi.org/10.1186/1748-5908-8-90

Carroll, C., Patterson, M., Wood, S., Booth, A., Rick, J., & Balain, S. (2007). A conceptual framework for implementation fidelity. *Implementation Science, 2*, 40. https://doi.org/10.1186/1748-5908-2-40

Carvalho, M. L., Honeycutt, S., Escoffery, C., Glanz, K., Sabbs, D., & Kegler, M. C. (2013). Balancing fidelity and adaptation: Implementing evidence-based chronic disease prevention programs. *Journal of Public Health Management and Practice, 19*(4), 348–356. https://doi.org/10.1097/PHH.0b013e31826d80eb

Castro, F. G., Barrera, M., Jr., & Martinez, C. R., Jr. (2004). The cultural adaptation of prevention interventions: Resolving tensions between fidelity and fit. *Prevention Science, 5*(1), 41–45. https://doi.org/10.1023/B:PREV.0000013980.12412.cd

Center for Substance Abuse Treatment. (2007). *Understanding evidence-based practices for co-occurring disorders: Overview paper 5* (DHHS Publication No. (SMA) 07–4278). Rockville, MD: Substance Abuse and Mental Health Services Administration, Center for Mental Health Services, Center for Substance Abuse Treatment. http://purl.access.gpo.gov/GPO/LPS84453

Chambers, D. A., Glasgow, R. E., & Stange, K. C. (2013). The dynamic sustainability framework: Addressing the paradox of sustainment amid ongoing change. *Implementation Science, 8*, 117. https://doi.org/10.1186/1748-5908-8-117

Chambers, D. A., & Norton, W. E. (2016). The adaptome: Advancing the science of intervention adaptation. *American Journal of Preventive Medicine, 51*(4 Suppl 2), S124–S131. https://doi.org/10.1016/j.amepre.2016.05.011

Chaudoir, S. R., Dugan, A. G., & Barr, C. H. (2013). Measuring factors affecting implementation of health innovations: A systematic review of structural, organizational, provider, patient, and innovation level measures. *Implementation Science, 8*, 22. https://doi.org/10.1186/1748-5908-8-22

Chorpita, B. F., Daleiden, E. L., & Weisz, J. R. (2005). Identifying and selecting the common elements of evidence based interventions: A distillation and matching model. *Mental Health Services Research, 7*(1), 5–20. https://doi.org/10.1007/s11020-005-1962-6

Cooper, B. R., Bumbarger, B. K., & Moore, J. E. (2015). Sustaining evidence-based prevention programs: Correlates in a large-scale dissemination initiative. *Prevention Science, 16*(1), 145–157. https://doi.org/10.1007/s11121-013-0427-1

Damschroder, L. J., Aron, D. C., Keith, R. E., Kirsh, S. R., Alexander, J. A., & Lowery, J. C. (2009). Fostering implementation of health services research findings into practice: A consolidated framework for advancing implementation science. *Implementation Science, 4*, 50. https://doi.org/10.1186/1748-5908-4-50

Dane, A. V., & Schneider, B. H. (1998). Program integrity in primary and early secondary prevention: Are implementation effects out of control? *Clinical Psychology Review, 18*(1), 23–45. https://doi.org/10.1016/S0272-7358(97)00043-3

Deschênes, N., Clark, H. B., & Herrygers, J. (2008). The development of fidelity measures for youth transition programs. In C. Newman, C. Liberton, K. Kutash, & R. M. Friedman (Eds.), *The 20th annual research conference proceedings: A system of care for children's mental health: Expanding the research base* (pp. 333–338). Tampa, FL: University of South Florida, Louis de la Parte Florida Mental Health Institute, Research and Training Center for Children's Mental Health. http://rtckids.fmhi.usf.edu/rtcconference/proceedings/20thproceedings/20thChapter10.pdf

Dovidio, J. F., Penner, L. A., Albrecht, T. L., Norton, W. E., Gaertner, S. L., & Shelton, J. N. (2008). Disparities and distrust: The implications of psychological processes for understanding racial disparities in health and health care. *Social Science and Medicine, 67*(3), 478–486. https://doi.org/10.1016/j.socscimed.2008.03.019

Durlak, J. A., & DuPre, E. P. (2008). Implementation matters: A review of research on the influence of implementation on program outcomes and the factors affecting implementation. *American Journal of Community Psychology, 41*(3–4), 327–350. https://doi.org/10.1007/s10464-008-9165-0

Feldstein, A. C., & Glasgow, R. E. (2008). A practical, robust implementation and sustainability model (PRISM) for integrating research findings into practice. *Joint Commission Journal on Quality and Patient Safety, 34*(4), 228–243. https://doi.org/10.1016/S1553-7250(08)34030-6

Fixsen, D. L., Blase, K. A., Naoom, S. F., & Wallace, F. (2009). Core implementation components. *Research on Social Work Practice, 19*(5), 531–540. https://doi.org/10.1177/1049731509335549

Fixsen, D. L., Naoom, S. F., Blase, K. A., Friedman, R. M., & Wallace, F. (2005). *Implementation research: A synthesis of the literature* (FMHI Publication No. 231). Tampa, FL: University of South Florida, Louis de la Parte Florida Mental Health Institute, National Implementation Research Network. https://nirn.fpg.unc.edu/sites/nirn.fpg.unc.edu/files/resources/NIRN-MonographFull-01-2005.pdf

Gonzales, J. J., Ringeisen, H. L., & Chambers, D. A. (2002). The tangled and thorny path of science to practice: Tensions in interpreting and applying "evidence". *Clinical Psychology: Science and Practice, 9*(2), 204–209. https://doi.org/10.1093/clipsy/9.2.204

Green, L. W. (2008). Making research relevant: If it is an evidence-based practice, where's the practice-based evidence? *Family Practice, 25*(Suppl 1), i20–i24. https://doi.org/10.1093/fampra/cmn055

Green, L. W., & Glasgow, R. E. (2006). Evaluating the relevance, generalization, and applicability of research: Issues in external validation and translation methodology. *Evaluation and the Health Professions, 29*(1), 126–153. https://doi.org/10.1177/0163278705284445

Green, L. W., Ottoson, J. M., Garcia, C., & Hiatt, R. A. (2009). Diffusion theory and knowledge dissemination, utilization, and integration in public health. *Annual Review of Public Health, 30*, 151–174. https://doi.org/10.1146/annurev.publhealth.031308.100049

Greenhalgh, T., Robert, G., Macfarlane, F., Bate, P., & Kyriakidou, O. (2004). Diffusion of innovations in service organizations: Systematic review and recommendations. *Milbank Quarterly, 82*(4), 581–629. https://doi.org/10.1111/j.0887-378X.2004.00325.x

Guevara, M., & Solomon, E. (2009). *Implementing evidence-based policy and practice in community corrections*. Washington, DC: U.S. Department of Justice, National Corrections Institute. https://s3.amazonaws.com/static.nicic.gov/Library/024107.pdf

Harn, B., Parisi, D., & Stoolmiller, M. (2013). Balancing fidelity with flexibility and fit: What do we really know about fidelity of implementation in schools? *Exceptional Children, 79*(3), 181–193. https://doi.org/10.1177/001440291307900204

Hernandez, M., Worthington, J., & Davis, C. S. (2005). *Measuring the fidelity of service planning and delivery to system of care principles: The system of care practice review (SOCPR)* (Making children's mental health services successful series; FMHI Publication #223-1). Tampa, FL. http://rtckids.fmhi.usf.edu/rtcpubs/SOCPR/SOCPR-Monograph.pdf

Hoagwood, K., Burns, B. J., Kiser, L., Ringeisen, H., & Schoenwald, S. K. (2001). Evidence-based practice in child and adolescent mental health services. *Psychiatric Services, 52*(9), 1179–1189. https://doi.org/10.1176/appi.ps.52.9.1179

Hoagwood, K., & Johnson, J. (2003). School psychology: A public health framework I. From evidence-based practices to evidence-based policies. *Journal of School Psychology, 41*(1), 3–21. https://doi.org/10.1016/s0022-4405(02)00141-3

Hunter, S. B., Han, B., Slaughter, M. E., Godley, S. H., & Garner, B. R. (2017). Predicting evidence-based treatment sustainment: Results from a longitudinal study of the Adolescent-Community Reinforcement Approach. *Implementation Science, 12*(1), 75. https://doi.org/10.1186/s13012-017-0606-8

Isett, K. R., Burnam, M. A., Coleman-Beattie, B., Hyde, P. S., Morrissey, J. P., Magnabosco, J., … Goldman, H. H. (2007). The state policy context of implementation issues for evidence-based practices in mental health. *Psychiatric Services, 58*(7), 914–921. https://doi.org/10.1176/ps.2007.58.7.914

Iwelunmor, J., Blackstone, S., Veira, D., Nwaozuru, U., Airhihenbuwa, C., Munodawafa, D., … Ogedegebe, G. (2016). Toward the sustainability of health interventions implemented in sub-Saharan Africa: A systematic review and conceptual framework. *Implementation Science, 11*, 43. https://doi.org/10.1186/s13012-016-0392-8

Kazdin, A. E. (2000). *Psychotherapy for children and adolescents: Directions for research and practice*. New York, NY: Oxford University Press.

Kazdin, A. E. (2008). Evidence-based treatment and practice: New opportunities to bridge clinical research and practice, enhance the knowledge base, and improve patient care. *American Psychologist, 63*(3), 146–159. https://doi.org/10.1037/0003-066x.63.3.146

Lee, S. J., Altschul, I., & Mowbray, C. T. (2008). Using planned adaptation to implement evidence-based programs with new populations. *American Journal of Community Psychology, 41*(3–4), 290–303. https://doi.org/10.1007/s10464-008-9160-5

Lehman, W. E., Greener, J. M., & Simpson, D. D. (2002). Assessing organizational readiness for change. *Journal of Substance Abuse Treatment, 22*(4), 197–209. https://doi.org/10.1016/S0740-5472(02)00233-7

Lendrum, A., Humphrey, N., & Greenberg, M. (2016). Implementing for success in school-based mental health promotion: The role of quality in resolving the tension between fidelity and adaptation. In R. H. Shute & P. T. Slee (Eds.), *Mental health and wellbeing through schools: The way forward* (pp. 53–63). London: Routledge.

Lieberman, R., Zubritsky, C., Martínez, K., Massey, O. T., Fisher, S., Kramer, T., … Obrochta, C. (2011, February). *Issue brief: Using practice-based evidence to complement evidence-based practice in children's behavioral health*. Atlanta, GA: ICF Macro, Outcomes Roundtable for Children and Families. http://cfs.cbcs.usf.edu/_docs/publications/OutcomesRoundtableBrief.pdf

Massey, O. T., Armstrong, K., Boroughs, M., Henson, K., & McCash, L. (2005). Mental health services in schools: A qualitative analysis of challenges to implementation, operation, and sustainability. *Psychology in the Schools, 42*(4), 361–372. https://doi.org/10.1002/pits.20063

McDonald, P. W., & Viehbeck, S. (2007). From evidence-based practice making to practice-based evidence making: Creating communities of (research) and practice. *Health Promotion Practice, 8*(2), 140–144. https://doi.org/10.1177/1524839906298494

Minkler, M., & Wallerstein, N. (2013). Introduction to community-based participatory research: New issues and emphases. In M. Minkler & N. Wallerstein (Eds.), *Community-based participatory research for health: From process to outcomes* (5th ed., pp. 5–24). San Francisco, CA: Jossey-Bass. http://rbdigital.oneclickdigital.com

Moore, J. E., Mascarenhas, A., Bain, J., & Straus, S. E. (2017). Developing a comprehensive definition of sustainability. *Implementation Science, 12*(1), 110. https://doi.org/10.1186/s13012-017-0637-1

Morrison, D. M., Hoppe, M. J., Gillmore, M. R., Kluver, C., Higa, D., & Wells, E. A. (2009). Replicating an intervention: The tension between fidelity and adaptation. *AIDS Education and Prevention, 21*(2), 128–140. https://doi.org/10.1521/aeap.2009.21.2.128

Murray, L. K., Dorsey, S., Skavenski, S., Kasoma, M., Imasiku, M., Bolton, P., … Cohen, J. A. (2013). Identification, modification, and implementation of an evidence-based psychotherapy for children in a low-income country: The use of TF-CBT in Zambia. *International Journal of Mental Health Systems, 7*(1), 24. https://doi.org/10.1186/1752-4458-7-24

National Implementation Research Network. (2015). *Implementation stages*. [Web page]. Chapel Hill, NC: University of North Carolina, Chapel Hill, FPG Child Development Institute, The National Implementation Research Network. https://nirn.fpg.unc.edu/learn-implementation/implementation-stages

Nilsen, P. (2015). Making sense of implementation theories, models and frameworks. *Implementation Science, 10*, 53. https://doi.org/10.1186/s13012-015-0242-0

Office of the Surgeon General. (1999). *Mental health: A report of the Surgeon General*. Rockville, MD: U. S. Department of Health and Human Services, U.S. Public Health Service. https://profiles.nlm.nih.gov/ps/retrieve/ResourceMetadata/NNBBHS

President's New Freedom Commission on Mental Health. (2003). *Achieving the promise: Transforming mental health care in America: Final report* (DHHS publication no.). Rockville, MD: U. S. Department of Health and Human Services. http://www.eric.ed.gov/PDFS/ED479836.pdf

Proctor, E. K., Landsverk, J., Aarons, G., Chambers, D., Glisson, C., & Mittman, B. (2009). Implementation research in mental health services: An emerging science with conceptual, methodological, and training challenges. *Administration and Policy in Mental Health, 36*(1), 24–34. https://doi.org/10.1007/s10488-008-0197-4

Pullmann, M. D., Bruns, E. J., & Sather, A. K. (2013). Evaluating fidelity to the wraparound service model for youth: Application of item response theory to the Wraparound Fidelity Index. *Psychological Assessment, 25*(2), 583–598. https://doi.org/10.1037/a0031864

Rabin, B. A., & Brownson, R. C. (2018). Terminology for dissemination and implementation research. In R. C. Brownson, G. A. Colditz, & E. K. Proctor (Eds.), *Dissemination and implementation research in health: Translating science to practice* (2nd ed., pp. 19–45). New York, NY: Oxford University Press.

Rogers, E. M. (2003). *Diffusion of innovations*. New York, NY: Free Press.

Sackett, D. L., Rosenberg, W. M., Gray, J. A., Haynes, R. B., & Richardson, W. S. (1996). Evidence based medicine: What it is and what it isn't. *BMJ, 312*(7023), 71–72. https://doi.org/10.1136/bmj.312.7023.71

Saldana, L. (2014). The stages of implementation completion for evidence-based practice: Protocol for a mixed methods study. *Implementation Science, 9*(1), 43. https://doi.org/10.1186/1748-5908-9-43

Saldana, L., Chamberlain, P., Wang, W., & Hendricks Brown, C. (2012). Predicting program start-up using the stages of implementation measure. *Administration and Policy in Mental Health, 39*(6), 419–425. https://doi.org/10.1007/s10488-011-0363-y

Scheirer, M. A. (2005). Is sustainability possible? A review and commentary on empirical studies of program sustainability. *American Journal of Evaluation, 26*(3), 320–347. https://doi.org/10.1177/1098214005278752

Shelton, R. C., Cooper, B. R., & Stirman, S. W. (2018). The sustainability of evidence-based interventions and practices in public health and health care. *Annual Review of Public Health, 39*, 55–76. https://doi.org/10.1146/annurev-publhealth-040617-014731

Stichter, J. P., Herzog, M. J., Owens, S. A., & Malugen, E. (2016). Manualization, feasibility, and effectiveness of the School-Based Social Competence Intervention for Adolescents (SCI-A). *Psychology in the Schools, 53*(6), 583–600. https://doi.org/10.1002/pits.21928

Stirman, S. W., Miller, C. J., Toder, K., & Calloway, A. (2013). Development of a framework and coding system for modifications and adaptations of evidence-based interventions. *Implementation Science, 8*, 65. https://doi.org/10.1186/1748-5908-8-65

Tabrizi, B. (2014, October). The key to change is middle management. *Harvard Business Review*. [Web page]. https://hbr.org/2014/10/the-key-to-change-is-middle-management

Titler, M. G., Everett, L. Q., & Adams, S. (2007). Implications for implementation science. *Nursing Research, 56*(4 Suppl), S53–S59. https://doi.org/10.1097/01.NNR.0000280636.78901.7f

Urban, J. B., & Trochim, W. (2009). The role of evaluation in research – Practice integration working toward the "golden spike". *American Journal of Evaluation, 30*(4), 538–553. https://doi.org/10.1177/1098214009348327

Walker, J. S., Koroloff, N. M., Schutte, K., & Portland State University. Research and Training Center on Family Support and Children's Mental Health. (2003). *Implementing high-quality collaborative individualized service/support planning: Necessary conditions.* Portland, OR: Research and Training Center on Family Support and Children's Mental Health, Portland State University. https://nwi.pdx.edu/NWI-book/Chapters/App-6f-Individualized-Service-And-Support%20Planning.pdf

Wandersman, A., Duffy, J., Flaspohler, P., Noonan, R., Lubell, K., Stillman, L., … Saul, J. (2008). Bridging the gap between prevention research and practice: The interactive systems framework for dissemination and implementation. *American Journal of Community Psychology, 41*(3–4), 171–181. https://doi.org/10.1007/s10464-008-9174-z

Westfall, J. M., Mold, J., & Fagnan, L. (2007). Practice-based research – "Blue Highways" on the NIH roadmap. *JAMA, 297*(4), 403–406. https://doi.org/10.1001/jama.297.4.403

Yampolskaya, S., Massey, O. T., & Greenbaum, P. E. (2006). At-risk high school students in the "Gaining Early Awareness and Readiness" Program (GEAR UP): Academic and behavioral outcomes. *Journal of Primary Prevention, 27*(5), 457–475. https://doi.org/10.1007/s10935-006-0050-z

Challenges with Behavioral Health Services Research Data

Ardis Hanson and Bruce Lubotsky Levin

Introduction

Behavioral health services research is a multidisciplinary area of study that evolved during the 1980s. Those who participate in behavioral health services research examine the organization, financing, and delivery of behavioral health systems and services and the implications for cost, quality, access, and outcomes. While the broad field of behavioral health services research has continued to rapidly evolve over the past 30 years, there has been an accompanying exponential growth in the amount and type of data.

This chapter examines the complexity of data being generated by a multitude of individuals and organizations within the various areas of behavioral health (alcohol, drug abuse, and mental health) services research. It will also examine the role of technology in the complexity of services research and in accessing research databases. In addition, this chapter will identify some of the major databases in behavioral health services research and illustrate the complexity of collecting, organizing, and accessing information from a vast array of data collection sources.

A. Hanson (✉)
Research and Education Unit, Shimberg Health Sciences Library,
University of South Florida, Tampa, FL, USA
e-mail: hanson@health.usf.edu

B. L. Levin
Department of Child and Family Studies, College of Behavioral and Community Sciences,
University of South Florida, Tampa, FL, USA

Behavioral Health Concentration, College of Public Health, University of South Florida,
Tampa, FL, USA

© Springer Nature Switzerland AG 2020   119
B. L. Levin, A. Hanson (eds.), *Foundations of Behavioral Health*,
https://doi.org/10.1007/978-3-030-18435-3_6

Behavioral Health System Challenges

The "de facto" behavioral health systems are very complex. They have numerous distinct sectors, organizational settings, financing streams, and differences in the type and duration of care. These systems are comprised of public sector services, private sector services, and increasingly hybridized services crossing over both public and private sectors (Hanson & Levin, 2013). The existing delivery systems provide acute and long-term care in homes, communities, and institutional settings. In addition, these systems provide services across the specialty behavioral health sector, the general primary care sector, and the voluntary care sector. In the United States, various other sectors that provide behavioral health services include the military, the Veterans Administration (VA), long-term care facilities, and the criminal justice systems (e.g., juvenile facilities, jails, and prisons) (Hanson, 2014).

Furthermore, there are multiple stakeholders involved in these systems, from providers to clients. There are numerous federal, state, local, and tribal agencies, professional licensing and accreditation organizations, managed care provider organizations, advocacy and regulatory agencies, and healthcare policy-making entities involved with impacting policy and services delivery. Stakeholders also include service users of all ages, their families, and their caregivers (including family members, advocates, guardians ad litem, and ombudsmen). Providers include clinicians, such as psychologists, psychiatrists, psychiatric nurses, social workers, mental health counselors, pastoral counselors, primary care providers, pharmacists, supportive services personnel, vocational and rehabilitation staff, administrative and clerical staff, and peer and lay workers, among many others who work in the prevention, intervention, and treatment of individuals with behavioral health problems. The number and variety of interested stakeholders, in turn, contribute to the complexity of collecting, maintaining, and accessing data in behavioral health service delivery systems.

Collecting data and the use of technology to develop information systems in behavioral health service systems are not new initiatives. Rosen and Weil (1997) described the use of electronic office management and psychological assessment software in clinical practice. Sujansky (1998) wrote the need for decision support tools and bibliographic retrieval systems, such as PubMed, to be embedded in the then-emerging electronic health record (EHR). Others have written the use of the Internet and national administrative data to collect behavioral health data, to address changes to existing services systems, and to establish mental health promotion campaigns (Andrade et al., 2014; Berry, Lobban, Emsley, & Bucci, 2016; Rhodes, Bowie, & Hergenrather, 2003).

Today, numerous types of networked informatics programs and applications handle in-house administrative tasks, such as billing and scheduling, as well as many functions within the managed care environment, such as certifications, authorizations, treatment plans, medication evaluation forms, treatment summary forms, and outcome assessments, and reporting requirements at the state and national level. Transportability issues surrounding innovations (such as treatment effectiveness and treatment context), standardization of terminology to reduce ambiguity, quality of care issues, and building improved behavioral health information and practice infrastructures continue to be addressed at the federal, tribal, and state levels.

As discussed throughout this volume, the often fragmented and rapidly changing policy and practice landscape exacerbates the lag between development and ultimate implementation of innovative, empirically tested practices which may take between 15 and 20 years for actual implementation (President's New Freedom Commission on Mental Health, 2003).

Further, the rapid change in behavioral health technology over the past decade has brought even more volatility to research and practice settings. For example, not only are "soft" behavioral health service technologies particularly vulnerable to problems of fidelity in implementation (Allen, Shelton, Emmons, & Linnan, 2018); there also are significant challenges to implementing and sustaining comprehensive behavioral health service programs at consumer, provider, program administrator, and developer levels (Aarons et al., 2012; Chaudoir, Dugan, & Barr, 2013; Gotham, 2004; Williams, Ehrhart, Aarons, Marcus, & Beidas, 2018).

Since challenges come from and across service, interorganizational, and consumer/advocacy sectors, intraorganizational and individual levels, and system/environment fit, specific data needed to address these challenges may become difficult to tease out, define, collect, or synthesize. These are universal challenges for nations, regardless of socioeconomic status of countries or levels of technologies easily available to their citizens. Today's multiple systems for the delivery of behavioral health services represent an increasingly diversified, interrelated, and complex information framework where data are collected, information is synthesized, and treatment, law, and policy decisions are made based upon the available data.

Behavioral Health Services Research Data

There are three main types of data in behavioral health services research: (1) primary data, (2) secondary data, and (3) tertiary data. Primary data are original, often "raw" data that can be in any format (e.g., numeric, spatial, textual, or interview data). Secondary data are analyses run on primary data that interpret, review, or synthesize original research. One example would be a report that repurposes a county infrastructure and services data for a neighborhood assessment of benefits and deficits. Another example is a summary report generated from the Centers for Disease Control and Prevention's (CDC) Web-Based Injury Statistics Query and Reporting System (WISQARS™) mortality and morbidity database. Tertiary data are the synthesis of data and secondary reports that place repurposed and/or collected data within a specific context within behavioral health services research. An example would be an agency report that included a series of articles from a peer-reviewed journal on formulary management with cost data from a report from Massachusetts on its public formulary.

However, behavioral health services research is complex. Often a research project or research data may address only a very specific portion of a larger issue. There are bits and pieces of data from multiple publishers/carriers/vendors across different time frames and in different formats. Further, not only are there numerous disciplines that work within behavioral health services research; there are different weights given to different types or elements of data and how these data may be used within those disciplines and professional practices. Numeric data, for example, in the form of actual datasets or predefined tables of variables, may be available for public use through the National Institutes of Health (NIH) federal data management requirements for research conducted under receipt of a federal grant (NIH, 2003, February 26) or through the Open Government Directive, a presidential memorandum signed by former President Barack Obama (2009).

While there are a significant variety of data sets in behavioral health at the federal level, they do not always exist in formats immediately usable for all individuals accessing these databases. For example, data are collected for a variety of federal data sets and organized into very different information formats (e.g., numeric, spatial, and textual) and contexts (e.g., clinical, statistical, and services delivery). The data are collected based upon specific objectives established for data collection and are based upon the specific plans for the utilization of that data set. Two examples are QuickFacts and FastStats.

QuickFacts, by the US Census Bureau, is a very thin slice of data that estimates selected characteristics of a population of a specific place at a specific point in time, as well as selected business and geographical data. However, data from a QuickFacts page comes from 12 different Census Bureau datasets: (1) Population Estimates, (2) American Community Survey, (3) Census of Population and Housing, (4) Current Population Survey, (5) Small Area Health Insurance Estimates, (6) Small Area Income and Poverty Estimates, (7) State and County Housing Unit Estimates, (8) County Business Patterns, (9) Non-employer Statistics, (10) Economic Census, (11) Survey of Business Owners, and (12) Building Permits.

A second example is the Mental Health FastStats from the National Center for Health Statistics. It offers four central data points: (1) morbidity, (2) physician office visits, (3) emergency room visits, and (4) mortality, with links to other reports that may also be of interest as well as other related agency data or sites. And while users can also look for FastStats on depression, there are no corresponding pages for schizophrenia, bipolar, or anxiety disorders. These examples reinforce some of the problems with publically accessible datasets and predefined tables, such as the granularity of data one may be seeking is not available through these resources; the combination of variables one is seeking may not be available; and the age of the data may make them unusable in a more current context. These problems plague many of the publicly available federal, state, and academic data.

Data also may be repurposed from primary data into secondary data analyses or tertiary data sources, such as reports and white papers. Information on how data are collected or characteristics of state behavioral health agency data systems for federal systems should always be reviewed to ensure the relevance and accuracy of the data for researchers and practitioners. Reports, such as *Characteristics of State*

Mental Health Agency Data Systems (Lutterman, Phelan, Berhane, Shaw, & Rana, 2008) or the most recent Mental Health Client-Level Data/Mental Health Treatment Episode Data Set (MH-CLD/MH-TEDS) for services provided through state mental health agencies, provide information on what researchers and practitioners may or may not find in agency data systems.

A basic EHR system, for example, may contain patient history and demographics, a patient problem list, physician clinical notes, a comprehensive list of patient's medications and allergies, computerized orders for prescriptions, and laboratory and imaging results. However, other documentation, such as the reports mentioned above, often include crosswalk tables, reporting methods, data dictionaries of included variables, federal definitions used in the reports, and behavioral health diagnosis codes. Federal legislation, such as the 45 CFR 170 (2011), addresses standards, implementation specifications, and certification criteria that apply to the EHR and EHR modules.

Public Domain and Public Sector Data

Federal and state governments are moving to digital-only data and documents available on the Internet. Public domain data and public sector data are not interchangeable (Abresch, Hanson, & Reehling, 2008). Public domain is a legal status, that is, items in the public domain are copyright-free. Public domain material may be modified, giving the person who did the modification both intellectual property rights and copyrights for the *modification*, not the *original* product.

Public sector data, however, are data produced by a public sector body. These data may either be in the public domain or be protected data. Governmental and institutional policies determine access, which potentially vary. Since constitutional, federal, or state law may govern access to public sector information, changes in access to government information, particularly after passage of the Homeland Security Act, potentially affect content and access (Abresch et al., 2008).

There are licensing and distribution issues associated with the use of primary and secondary data sets, such as data size, format complexity, and potential use restrictions. These restrictions may be due to copyright, access, or license agreements created by either public or private data producers. There are also intellectual property rights, liability issues, distribution methods, and data management practices to address in the acquisition, use, repurposing, and publishing of data and its results. There may be significant legal risks related to numeric and spatial data and analysis tools, including models, methodologies, and services, based upon the data and tools. Defective data used in decision-making may have consequences at a planning or population-based level of policy or practice. Since behavioral health services research often uses personal data obtained with informed consent, there may be restrictions and authorizations required for its use, with de-identified, aggregated data used in the final product.

Definitional Data

The first question in collecting data on behavioral disorders starts with definition and contextualization. In the United States, the authoritative guide to the diagnosis of behavioral disorders is the DSM-5 (American Psychiatric Association, 2013); the international standard for behavioral health diagnosis is the ICD-11 (International Classification of Diseases and Related Health Problems) in concert with the ICF (International Classification of Functioning, Disability and Health) to determine burden of disease (World Health Organization, 2017, 2018b).

While the ICD is used for reporting diseases, health conditions, and baseline statistics, the ICF is used to classify the functional components of health conditions. Also, there is language in the ICD-11 that suggests a relationship between the clinical effects of mental, behavioral, and neurodevelopmental disorders and the ability of individuals to function effectively across interpersonal, family, social, educational, occupational, and other levels of functioning. The ICF extends the context of disability (level of functioning) to environmental factors. This is an important consideration, as there is a continued global focus on the social determinants of health and how these determinants and their effects can be collected (Atkinson, Page, Wells, Milat, & Wilson, 2015; Hosseini Shokouh et al., 2017; Thomsen et al., 2013; Vest, Grannis, Haut, Halverson, & Menachemi, 2017; World Health Organization, 2016).

Behavioral Health System Data

Data can focus on an individual, an at-risk population, a facility, or a system. In the United States, behavioral health system data spans private and public providers (including both individual and organizational providers) of care, treatment and delivery, financing of care, law, and policy. It also spans medicine, social services, and rehabilitation. Behavioral healthcare data may address acute (or crisis) or long-term (maintenance) care. Although behavioral healthcare takes place in hospitals, providers' offices, community mental health centers, peer-run centers, religious organizations (pastoral care), academic health centers, jails and prisons, state or local government facilities, and private facilities, not all of these facilities are required to collect or report to or across local, state, regional, or national entities (see Fig. 1).

Common measures include behavioral health service history, severity and level of functioning, and quality assessment. Behavioral health service history is the patient's treatment history, defined as whether he/she had ever received behavioral health treatment prior to the current episode of care and, if so, where.

Severity and level of functioning measures an individual's level of everyday functioning and comparison with premorbid (before onset of diseases) functioning. Relevant aspects of daily living include daily living skills, social and recreational

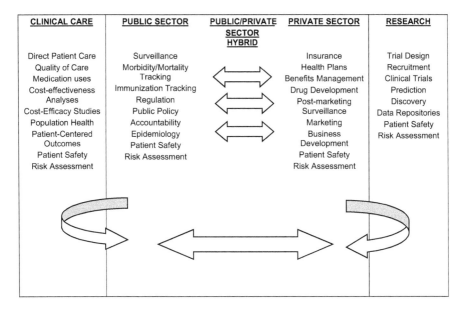

CLINICAL CARE	PUBLIC SECTOR	PUBLIC/PRIVATE SECTOR HYBRID	PRIVATE SECTOR	RESEARCH
Direct Patient Care	Surveillance		Insurance	Trial Design
Quality of Care	Morbidity/Mortality		Health Plans	Recruitment
Medication uses	Tracking		Benefits Management	Clinical Trials
Cost-effectiveness	Immunization Tracking		Drug Development	Prediction
Analyses	Regulation		Post-marketing	Discovery
Cost-Efficacy Studies	Public Policy		Surveillance	Data Repositories
Population Health	Accountability		Marketing	Patient Safety
Patient-Centered	Epidemiology		Business	Risk Assessment
Outcomes	Patient Safety		Development	
Patient Safety	Risk Assessment		Patient Safety	
Risk Assessment			Risk Assessment	

Fig. 1 Uses of behavioral health data across sectors

skills, and financial, vocational, interpersonal, and parental skills. The point of measuring level of functioning is to assess how much the illness has affected the person. This information is then used to design appropriate levels of psychosocial treatment and relevant social supports.

Quality assessment tools include individual treatment and system performance indicators, report cards, and consumer outcome measures, all of which use guideline fidelity measures (standards).

Data and assessment tools are comprised of domains that are issues, categories, or topics of interest. Indicators are discrete measurable activities, events, characteristics, or items that represent a domain. Measures are the instruments used to assess, evaluate, and measure an indicator.

In addition, behavioral health data is collected and used in a number of ways, such as client information systems and decision support functions. Such systems and functions would need to contain enough data to provide clinical consultations, update disease profiles, and create semantic relationships to map algorithms for diagnoses and etiologies. To achieve requires production rules, hierarchical classification trees, heuristic questions, and diagnostic criteria. Production rules would require probabilities to ensure findings are related accurately to diagnoses. Hierarchical classification tree(s) would represent disease categories and allow mapping to preferred, narrower, and current terminology. In addition, heuristic questions and evidence-based diagnostic criteria would be necessary to narrow the diagnostic hypotheses and conclude the clinical query. However, these and other elements are critical to ensure precision and relevance in discovery.

All types of data (computational, spatial, social, and environmental) increasingly are used in behavioral health services research. Integration of research into practice, the development of "best practices," fidelity in implementation, and the issues surrounding translational research require more and more data and use many different lenses and tools to view the data. Data mining large quantitative datasets, modeling real-life phenomena, and prediction or forecasting of long-term behaviors and activity are common activities in data collection and analysis.

Behavioral Health Clinical Data

Behavioral health clinical data exists in many forms. There is the raw data (i.e., patient-level fact data), knowledge data (best practices), aggregate patient data at the facility or system level, and surveillance data; any or all may be reported in varying degrees across local, state, national, regional, and global reporting levels. Data comes from medical records, administrative data, incidence data, patient satisfaction surveys, and more (see Table 1).

Linking client data from different health and behavioral healthcare sectors and agencies is necessary to assure the continuity of care, evaluation, and planning of behavioral health services. Integrating client, human resources, financial, services, and organizational databases create a foundation for both clinical and administrative data-based decision support and for programmatic and outcomes evaluation, program planning, and research. Reuse of behavioral health clinical data is found across numerous settings, from clinical, research, governmental, and business, and is often dependent on the source of data and the models used in the studies (Hutter, Rodriguez-Ibeas, & Antonanzas, 2014).

Three common models address cost-effectiveness, cost utility, or quality of life. Cost-effectiveness analysis (CEA) of treatment in healthcare facilities examines health outcomes more one-dimensionally, as in the number of psychotic events prevented or number of life years a patient gained. Cost-utility analysis (CUA) moves to two-dimensional measures, such as measures of change in patient survival *and* changes in the quality of a patient life. Health-related quality of life (HRQoL) measures often are multiplied by number of life years gained, which then generates the number quality-adjusted life years (QALYs) gained by the patient. These analyses also use patient survey data and cost data in a hospital or network. Table 2 shows a common CEA data collection and analysis process.

Data collection in healthcare facilities falls under process management (i.e., task/procedure processes, standardization, coordination, reorganization, using a cross-functional viewpoint examining strategy, operations, techniques, and people). This is particularly key as healthcare facilities, systems, and provider networks continue to automate their administrative processes to derive outcomes, quality improvement, and assessment data on patient care and business operations. However, three major challenges to the effective analysis, use, and decision-making with data are incomplete data and undefined management processes (Monto et al., 2016), as well as knowing what to count.

Table 1 Data and program types

| Data | Community-based programs | | | |
	Supported services	Evaluation	Treatment	Research
Admissions Patient history Caregiver/ clinician reports Medical/lab tests Genomic profiles Treatment Emergency/crisis Medical records Patient satisfaction Surveys Accreditation Administrative Programmatic outcomes Patient report cards	Supported employment/education/ housing Mobile care team Case management Hotline/crisis service	Consultation Client liaison Referral to service/ treatment	Integrated care Specialty care Rehabilitation (vocational, physical) Emergency/crisis services	Day program Peer-run program Ambulatory care Case management

Table 2 CEA data collection process

	Patient	Facility	CEA analysis
First visit	First HRQoL survey	Patient data: personal, demographic, medical, etc. Data entry and storage	Calculation of scores
3 months posttreatment	Second HRQoL survey	Data entry and storage	Calculation of patient scores
			Calculation of difference between scores
			Calculation of QALYS
			Cost of treatment data
			Cost-effectiveness analysis

Knowing What to Count in Behavioral Health

One of the most challenging factors in collecting data on behavioral disorders is what data elements are collected. This ranges from setting, status as a primary or secondary diagnosis, levels of functioning, family, and societal burden. In 2001a, the World Health Organization's (WHO) *World Health Report* acknowledged the burden of mental, neurological, and substance use (MNS) disorders. Almost a decade later, the 2010 Global Burden of Disease Study confirmed that nearly one quarter of all years lived with a disability (DALYS) can be attributed to behavioral disorders (Murray et al., 2012; Vos et al., 2012; Whiteford et al., 2013). As part of the larger group of noncommunicable diseases (NCDs), MNS disorders account for more than 60% of deaths worldwide and frequently occur as comorbid disorders with both NCD and infectious diseases (Bahorik, Satre, Kline-Simon, Weisner, & Campbell, 2017; Charlson et al., 2016; Goodell, Druss, Walker, & Mat, 2011; Prince et al., 2007).

However, without addressing the relatedness of comorbid NCDs, infectious disease, and MNS, a paradox is created. MNS disorders are often less acknowledged in a global integrated health context, but often play a major part in a patient's quality of life, level of functioning, burden of disease, wellness, and years lived with a disability. Hence, achieving desired outcomes for global and national health programs becomes more problematic, especially when looking at the issues involved in gathering accurate data to answer the questions asked and yet to be asked.

How the ICD and ICF Are Used

The ICD is used extensively for the diagnostic classification of routine collection of population-based health information (morbidity and mortality) and for the mandatory statistical reporting required of WHO member countries. Depending upon the level of information required, the ICD ranges from a set of 100 codes to 10,000 codes which can be related to diagnosis-related groups (DRGs) and other case-mix systems. Categories include "diseases, disorders, syndromes, signs, symptoms, findings, injuries, external causes of morbidity and mortality, factors influencing health status, reasons for encounter of the health system, and traditional medicine," complemented by additional data on "anatomy, substances, infectious agents, or place of injury" (World Health Organization, 2018a). From a classification perspective, each ICD entity has a unique identifier (URI) and is grouped within and across hierarchies of groups, categories, and narrower terms. For a more detailed discussion on the elements of the ICD-11, see the WHO ICD-11 Reference Guide.

The ICD is increasingly used in the public health sector as a frame for (1) accessible services that address epidemiology, natural course of a disease, and disease burden of these disorders and (2) health promotion efforts to destigmatize mental illnesses (International Advisory Group, 2011). More recent discussions on the ICD suggest its importance in research, including formative, case-controlled, and clinical utility field studies, national diagnostic quality studies, and administrative data reviews (Gologorsky, Knightly, Lu, Chi, & Groff, 2014; Keeley et al., 2016; Nesvag et al., 2017). More importantly, the recent revision of the ICD (ICD-11) includes a "functioning properties" component that integrates the ICF activities and participation domains specific to disorders along with body functions and contextual factors (Escorpizo et al., 2013). The intent of the ICD-ICF cross-coding is to improve operationalization of an integrated disease-functioning model across health systems in all countries, from low resource to high resource.

Over the past 30 years, the ICD has been steadily integrated into national health policy and clinical care by the governments of WHO Member States (countries) through a number of stakeholder groups. These diverse groups include clinical care providers, healthcare coverage and reimbursement agencies, social and community support services, disability benefits agencies, payers of healthcare services, consumer and family advocacy groups, government agencies, criminal justice systems, educational systems, and judicial systems (International Advisory Group for the Revision of ICD-10 Mental and Behavioural Disorders, 2011). However, not all WHO Member States gather data from all of these trajectories of care.

Underreporting Prevalence

A major challenge in behavioral health data is underreporting. This means accurate and representative data on the prevalence of disorders is difficult to define. A number of resources are used to define prevalence, from medical and national records and epidemiologic and survey data to meta-regression modeling. However, raw data for countries that lack adequate collection and reporting infrastructure require comparisons that are created running sophisticated statistical models on epidemiologic data from neighboring countries. This affects studies, such as the Global Burden of Disease (GBD) studies, which rely upon epidemiological studies for its global and national estimates. These studies may not match data across age groups, countries, disorders, and epidemiologic parameters (Whiteford, Ferrari, & Degenhardt, 2016). To compensate, the GBD researchers use a specific statistical tool, Bayesian meta-regression, which (1) pools the epidemiological data available for a given disorder into a weighted average and (2) adjusts for known sources of variability in reported study estimates (Whiteford et al., 2016).

Since disorders and prevalence are not defined the same across researchers or nations, it can be confounding to compare data. For example, the GBD prevalence data on depression varies from the prevalence data used by the WHO, which varies from the US Centers for Disease Control and Prevention (CDC) prevalence of depression. Unlike the GBD and the WHO definitions of depression, the CDC includes anxiety as a subset of depression in its examination of the prevalence of depression (Whiteford et al., 2016).

Underreporting Population Subgroups

There is a relative lack of standards for collecting data on population subgroups. Numerous policy documents, such as the Sustainable Development Goals or Healthy People 2020, promote the elimination of health disparities[1] (US) or health inequities (WHO) as an overarching goal for the next decade. However, attaining this elusive

---

[1] Health disparities include but are not limited to language; culture; socioeconomic status; gender; age; mental health; cognitive, sensory, or physical disability; sexual orientation or gender identity; geographic location (e.g., rural vs. urban); or other characteristics historically linked to discrimination or exclusion, such as race or ethnicity.

goal has been challenging. The lack of standardized data relevant to the many factors that identify vulnerable and at-risk populations makes it difficult to identify and implement effective actions to reduce specific health disparities. Health disparities/inequities are closely linked with the social and physical determinants of health (e.g., social, economic, and/or environmental factors) that affect health, level of functioning, and quality of life outcomes. A social determinants approach can help reframe the way policy-makers, public and private sectors, and the general public think about achieving and sustaining behavioral health.

Addressing Pathology and Etiology

Since their respective inceptions DSM (American Psychiatric Association, 1952); ICD (International Statistical Institute, 1893); ICF (World Health Organization, 2001b), these diagnostic standards have been the benchmarks for how behavioral disorders are diagnosed and "accounted" in incidence, prevalence, and treatment data. In addition, the ICD and DSM are used heavily in public health, clinical diagnosis, service provision, and specific research applications. However, their categorical and dimensional models fail to address the pathology and etiology of these disorders. The National Institute of Mental Health's Research Domain Criteria (RDoC) provides a different framework for understanding MNS disorders, including etiology, categories and dimensions, disorder thresholds, and comorbidity (Clark, Cuthbert, Lewis-Fernandez, Narrow, & Reed, 2017).

In the RDoC, etiology examines mental disorders from a multi-causality frame, in that these disorders develop from multiple influences (e.g., physiological, environmental, and societal). This parallels the SDH and social and behavioral determinants of health (SBD) frames. Mental disorders are complex, dimensional disorders, and different categories of disorders often have common, overlapping characteristics. Hence, categorizing mental disorders and their dimensions is problematic. Disorder thresholds are central in clinical decision-making; however, thresholds may vary greatly based on which component is under review (e.g., emotional, behavioral, cognitive, or physical) and can have negative or positive consequences (e.g., stigma or eligibility). Comorbidity denotes the simultaneous co-occurrence of two distinct disorders; however, Clark et al. (2017) suggest that co-existence of mental disorders may be a better way of framing the complexity and interrelatedness of mental disorders.

Data and Standards

An EHR documents (1) each episode (evaluation and treatment) of a patient's illness, (2) the plan for patient care and recovery, and (3) communication between all patient care staff. From an administrative perspective, the EHR is used for fiscal review and evaluation of the care and services, as it is a record of all events over time and locations. Since the EHR holds identifiable patient data, it is subject to legislative, regulatory, and confidentiality requirements at the staff, facility, provider, state, and national levels.

Accordingly, there are standards for the collection, coding, classification, and exchange of clinical and administrative data for behavioral health. Terminology, data interchange, and knowledge representation schema are the most common standards. Much like a controlled vocabulary, there are specific terms and concepts used to describe, classify, and code healthcare data, as well as to create relationships among the terms and concepts. Data interchanges encode healthcare data elements for exchange among facilities, providers, and networks. Knowledge representation schema codify how healthcare literature, clinical guidelines, and other information are used for clinical decision-making within the EHR or how other clinical or administrative documents link to or use information from the EHR.

The global emphasis on the social determinants of health and the Sustainable Development Goals (SDGs) has effects on the acquisition of a number of health indicators, especially to show national achievements of the SDGs. However, the success of a global health initiative depends on the development of a series of standards for national health infrastructures. A health record is but one tiny part of a national health infrastructure, which also must address interorganizational and cross-system communication, such as storage, processing, and transmission hardware and physical facilities, software applications, and network standards.

National and international standards for programming languages, operating systems, data formats, communications protocols, applications interfaces, services delivery, and record formats ensure compatibility and interoperability between systems and compatibility of data for comparative statistical or analytical purposes. Standards also establish a common ontology and ensure conformity assessment and usability.

Standards may also limit data collection, especially in remote or rural areas. National definitions of what constitutes a village, town, city, or metropolitan area vary significantly. Many national statistical systems provide data at the province or state level, with national definitions of what constitutes an urban area, a city, a town, an unincorporated area, or a village. If everything outside the "urban" class is designated as rural or the level of administrative oversight stops several steps above the village area, as may be the case in low- or lower-middle-income countries, then population data may be under- or overestimated. How a nation or locale defines a geographic area or its level of administrative oversight affects how it classes populations, settings, and workforce in its data collection and in final analyses of such. These "definitional caveats," which may or may not be stated in health or accompanying statistical reports, may affect our understanding of a national or locale.

Standards also play an important part in the development and use of monitoring and evaluation frameworks. National health information systems rely upon a range of population-based and health facility-based data sources, such as census data, household surveys, vital registration systems, public health surveillance, administrative data, health services data, and health system monitoring data, derived from local, state, regional, and national sources. With the development of the SDGs, a common monitoring and evaluation framework to strengthen health systems is essential (World Health Organization, 2010).

Health systems and research on these systems are often framed around financing, organization, payment, services delivery, and regulation (Hoffman et al., 2012, February 29). However, not all instances of the same theoretical framework are equivalent; hence, it is important to determine if there has been any divergence or convergence from or to a given standard framework or definition. Consider the case of universal health coverage (UHC). Although many countries rely on disaggregated survey data coupled with facility data, the survey data does not occur frequently enough to be a reliable indicator of current health sector performance. A focus on levels of health services coverage and equitable financial protection can provide indicators on how well a system is moving toward achieving UHC (Boerma et al., 2014).

From both global and national perspectives, syntheses of health data sources should focus on monitoring performance, harmonizing indicators and measurement strategies, and reconciliation of system disparities and discrepancies within and across systems. Harmonizing national indicators to a global measurement strategy may be problematic. To partner with WHO's monitoring and evaluation framework for health systems performance assessment and the SDG goals, US health data may need to be crosswalked to WHO, United Nations, and World Bank frameworks, among others. Since global indicators are used in comparative analyses, data quality assurance is critical across the breadth of diverse healthcare systems and policies. Data quality frameworks that can be used across national and global levels add complexity to the data collection, management, sharing, and conduct of analyses. Hence, it is critical to ensure for each metric or framework used there is consistency in the standards adopted to ensure objectivity and comparability over time and across localities, states, regions, and countries.

Implications for Behavioral Health

We talk about the importance of numbers in behavioral health services delivery, research, practice, and policy. Numbers are rhetorical devices, support implementation, drive policy, determine need, and determine success of treatment. Numbers are important. If you cannot be counted, you simply do not exist. A state (as in a country) has no obligation to you.

Examining the discussion on data presented above, we can articulate, with certainty, the following conclusions. First, data are difficult to collect, and despite efforts to systematize diagnosis, sociocultural differences may complicate the comparability of internationally collected metrics. Second, the lack of standardized data collection instruments, such as a unique patient tracking number, and differing care protocols make it challenging to maintain continuity of care, much less accurate data on trajectory of care or prevalence and incidence.

Health services research aims to be inclusive of all relevant information, both in terms of a grounded appreciation of the positive and negative benefits of a specific therapeutic intervention and a statement of the implications for the service. The need for reliable data on clinical and cost-effectiveness and a range of other contextual information require practitioners and academics to accommodate "research" as part of everyday practice.

In 2009, former President-elect Obama announced that large-scale adoption of health IT was a priority and that all US residents were to have EHR within 5 years. Federal legislation supported the electronic sharing of clinical data among healthcare stakeholders, which includes federal agencies responsible for the collection, analysis, and synthesis of such data. However, a decade after that announcement, the United States has not reached its goal.

There are multiple players, at many levels of government and in the private sector, who collect data and create information designed to answer specific questions or to fulfill reporting requirements. National standards, initiatives, and architecture try to make sense of their concerns and issues, focusing on infrastructure efforts, standards harmonization; certification; nationwide network, privacy, and security issues; and health IT adoption.

However, national data on behavioral health services in the United States remains incomplete at best. Not all behavioral health or behavioral health services data are collected, and in some cases, there are no formal structures or legal requirements in place to capture that data. To effectively handle just the linguistic properties of text, standardized language codes must support document longevity and interoperability of computing and network solutions. The same applies to the creation of network and platform protocols. Standards, whether data, semantic, or syntactic, apply equally to querying, searching, and accessing information from both vendor and the end-user perspectives. However, the issues of sharing information across numerous platforms and the variety of data types have not been made any easier. This is particularly true as we move to an increasingly global reporting on behavioral healthcare, services delivery, and systems design. There is a need to monitor global health regulations, health metrics (by country and perhaps even at a more granular level, such as county or region), disease surveillance systems, architectures, standards, and information systems.

There are numerous issues surrounding just standards development and linguistic congruence for health data. These data have implications on resource allocation, human development, quality of life, regional and economic development, and human security. Add additional issues of disability, functional outcomes, community reintegration, and resiliency. How many ways can these issues be defined and granulized into indicators locally and nationally in the United States, across professional groups, government agencies, consumer and family groups, and advocacy groups? Now consider how we reach consensus on definitions and indicators globally. The possibility of having accurate data, the same comparative indicators, and globally adopted outcomes literally comes back to decades of recommendations leading to the 2030 Sustainable Development Goals and similar national and regional initiatives.

References

Aarons, G. A., Glisson, C., Green, P. D., Hoagwood, K., Kelleher, K. J., Landsverk, J. A., … Schoenwald, S. (2012). The organizational social context of mental health services and clinician attitudes toward evidence-based practice: a United States national study. *Implementation Science, 7*, 56. https://doi.org/10.1186/1748-5908-7-56

Abresch, J., Hanson, A., & Reehling, P. J. (2008). Collection management issues with geospatial information. In J. Abresch, A. Hanson, S. J. Heron, & P. J. Reehling (Eds.), *Integrating geographic information systems into library services: A guide for academic libraries* (pp. 202–238). Hershey, PA: Information Science Publishing.

Allen, J. D., Shelton, R. C., Emmons, K. M., & Linnan, L. A. (2018). Fidelity and its relationship to implementation, effectiveness, adaptation, and dissemination. In R. C. Brownson, G. A. Colditz, & E. K. Proctor (Eds.), *Dissemination and implementation research in health: Translating science to practice* (2nd ed., pp. 267–284). New York, NY: Oxford University Press.

American Psychiatric Association. (1952). Diagnostic and statistical manual: Mental disorders: DSM-I. Washington, DC, US: American Psychiatric Association, Mental Hospital Service.

American Psychiatric Association. (2013). *Diagnostic and statistical manual of mental disorders: DSM-5*. Arlington, VA: Author.

Andrade, L. H., Alonso, J., Mneimneh, Z., Wells, J. E., Al-Hamzawi, A., Borges, G., … Kessler, R. C. (2014). Barriers to mental health treatment: Results from the WHO World Mental Health surveys. *Psychological Medicine, 44*(6), 1303–1317. https://doi.org/10.1017/s0033291713001943

Atkinson, J. A., Page, A., Wells, R., Milat, A., & Wilson, A. (2015). A modelling tool for policy analysis to support the design of efficient and effective policy responses for complex public health problems. *Implementation Science, 10*, 26. https://doi.org/10.1186/s13012-015-0221-5

Bahorik, A. L., Satre, D. D., Kline-Simon, A. H., Weisner, C. M., & Campbell, C. I. (2017). Serious mental illness and medical comorbidities: Findings from an integrated health care system. *Journal of Psychosomatic Research, 100*, 35–45. https://doi.org/10.1016/j.jpsychores.2017.07.004

Berry, N., Lobban, F., Emsley, R., & Bucci, S. (2016). Acceptability of interventions delivered online and through mobile phones for people who experience severe mental health problems: A systematic review. *Journal of Medical Internet Research, 18*(5), e121. https://doi.org/10.2196/jmir.5250

Boerma, T., Eozenou, P., Evans, D., Evans, T., Kieny, M. P., & Wagstaff, A. (2014). Monitoring progress towards universal health coverage at country and global levels. *PLoS Medicine, 11*(9), e1001731. https://doi.org/10.1371/journal.pmed.1001731

Charlson, F. J., Baxter, A. J., Dua, T., Degenhardt, L., Whiteford, H. A., & Vos, T. (2016). Excess mortality from mental, neurological, and substance use disorders in the Global Burden of Disease Study. In V. Patel, D. Chisholm, T. Dua, R. Laxminarayan, & M. E. Medina-Mora (Eds.), *Mental, neurological, and substance use disorders: Disease control priorities* (Vol. 4, 3rd ed., p. 2010). Washington, DC: The International Bank for Reconstruction and Development; The World Bank. https://www.ncbi.nlm.nih.gov/books/NBK361935/

Chaudoir, S. R., Dugan, A. G., & Barr, C. H. (2013). Measuring factors affecting implementation of health innovations: A systematic review of structural, organizational, provider, patient, and innovation level measures. *Implementation Science, 8*, 22. https://doi.org/10.1186/1748-5908-8-22

Clark, L. A., Cuthbert, B., Lewis-Fernandez, R., Narrow, W. E., & Reed, G. M. (2017). Three approaches to understanding and classifying mental disorder: ICD-11, DSM-5, and the National Institute of Mental Health's Research Domain Criteria (RDoC). *Psychological Science in the Public Interest, 18*(2), 72–145. https://doi.org/10.1177/1529100617727266

Escorpizo, R., Kostanjsek, N., Kennedy, C., Nicol, M. M., Stucki, G., & Ustun, T. B. (2013). Harmonizing WHO's International Classification of Diseases (ICD) and International

Classification of Functioning, Disability and Health (ICF): Importance and methods to link disease and functioning. *BMC Public Health, 13*, 742. https://doi.org/10.1186/1471-2458-13-742

Gologorsky, Y., Knightly, J. J., Lu, Y., Chi, J. H., & Groff, M. W. (2014). Improving discharge data fidelity for use in large administrative databases. *Neurosurgical Focus, 36*(6), E2. https://doi.org/10.3171/2014.3.Focus1459

Goodell, S., Druss, B. G., Walker, E. R., & Mat, M. (2011). *Mental disorders and medical comorbidity. The synthesis project.* (Policy Brief No. 21). Princeton, NJ: Robert Wood Johnson Foundation.

Gotham, H. J. (2004). Diffusion of mental health and substance abuse treatments: Development, dissemination, and implementation. *Clinical Psychology: Science and Practice, 11*(2), 160–176. https://doi.org/10.1093/clipsy/bph067

Hanson, A. (2014). Illuminating the invisible voices in mental health policymaking. *Journal of Medicine and the Person, 12*(1), 13–18. https://doi.org/10.1007/s12682-014-0170-9

Hanson, A., & Levin, B. L. (2013). *Mental health informatics.* New York, NY: Oxford University Press.

Health information technology standards, implementation specifications, and certification criteria and certification programs for health information technology, 45 CFR 170 Cong. Rec. (2011).

Hoffman, S. J., Røttingen, J.-A., Bennett, S., Lavis, J. N., Edge, J. S., & Frenk, J. (2012, February 29). *Background paper on conceptual issues related to health systems research to inform a WHO Global Strategy on Health Systems Research: A working paper in progress.* Geneva, CH: World Health Organization. https://www.who.int/alliance-hpsr/alliancehpsr_hsrstrategy_conceptualpaper.pdf

Hosseini Shokouh, S. M., Arab, M., Emamgholipour, S., Rashidian, A., Montazeri, A., & Zaboli, R. (2017). Conceptual models of social determinants of health: A narrative review. *Iranian Journal of Public Health, 46*(4), 435–446.

Hutter, M. F., Rodriguez-Ibeas, R., & Antonanzas, F. (2014). Methodological reviews of economic evaluations in health care: What do they target? *The European Journal of Health Economics, 15*(8), 829–840. https://doi.org/10.1007/s10198-013-0527-7

International Statistical Institute. (1893). *International list of causes of death.* Vienna, Austria: Author.

International Advisory Group for the Revision of ICD-10 Mental and Behavioural Disorders. (2011). A conceptual framework for the revision of the ICD-10 classification of mental and behavioural disorders. *World Psychiatry, 10*(2), 86–92.

Keeley, J. W., Reed, G. M., Roberts, M. C., Evans, S. C., Medina-Mora, M. E., Robles, R., ... Saxena, S. (2016). Developing a science of clinical utility in diagnostic classification systems field study strategies for ICD-11 mental and behavioral disorders. *American Psychologist, 71*(1), 3–16. https://doi.org/10.1037/a0039972

Lutterman, T. C., Phelan, B. E., Berhane, A., Shaw, R., & Rana, V. (2008). *Characteristics of state mental health agency data systems* (DHHS Pub. No.(SMA) 08–4361). Rockville, MD: U.S. Department of Health & Human Services, Center for Mental Health Services. http://purl.fdlp.gov/GPO/gpo60094

Monto, S., Penttila, R., Karri, T., Puolakka, K., Valpas, A., & Talonpoika, A. M. (2016). Improving data collection processes for routine evaluation of treatment cost-effectiveness. *Health Information Management, 45*(1), 45–52. https://doi.org/10.1177/1833358316639451

Murray, C. J. L., Vos, T., Lozano, R., Naghavi, M., Flaxman, A. D., Michaud, C., ... Memish, Z. A. (2012). Disability-adjusted life years (DALYs) for 291 diseases and injuries in 21 regions, 1990-2010: a systematic analysis for the Global Burden of Disease Study 2010. *Lancet, 380*(9859), 2197–2223. https://doi.org/10.1016/s0140-6736(12)61689-4

National Institutes of Health. (2003, February 26). Final NIH statement on sharing research data. *NIH Guide for Grants and Contracts, NOT-OD-03-032*, [HTML]. https://grants.nih.gov/grants/guide/notice-files/NOT-OD-03-032.html

Nesvag, R., Jonsson, E. G., Bakken, I. J., Knudsen, G. P., Bjella, T. D., Reichborn-Kjennerud, T., ... Andreassen, O. A. (2017). The quality of severe mental disorder diagnoses in a national health registry as compared to research diagnoses based on structured interview. *BMC Psychiatry, 17*(1), 93. https://doi.org/10.1186/s12888-017-1256-8

Obama, B. (2009). Memorandum of January 21, 2009: Transparency and open government: Memorandum for the heads of executive departments and agencies. *Federal Register, 74*(15), 4685–4686. https://www.govinfo.gov/content/pkg/FR-2009-01-26/pdf/E9-1777.pdf

President's New Freedom Commission on Mental Health. (2003). *Achieving the promise: Transforming mental health care in America: Final report* (DHHS publication no.). Rockville, MD: U. S. Department of Health and Human Services. http://www.eric.ed.gov/PDFS/ED479836.pdf

Prince, M., Patel, V., Saxena, S., Maj, M., Maselko, J., Phillips, M. R., & Rahman, A. (2007). No health without mental health. *Lancet, 370*(9590), 859–877. https://doi.org/10.1016/s0140-6736(07)61238-0

Rhodes, S. D., Bowie, D. A., & Hergenrather, K. C. (2003). Collecting behavioural data using the world wide web: Considerations for researchers. *Journal of Epidemiology and Community Health, 57*(1), 68–73.

Rosen, L. D., & Weil, M. M. (1997). *The mental health technology bible*. New York, NY: Wiley.

Sujansky, W. V. (1998). The benefits and challenges of an electronic medical record: Much more than a "word-processed" patient chart. *Western Journal of Medicine, 169*(3), 176–183.

Thomsen, S., Ng, N., Biao, X., Bondjers, G., Kusnanto, H., Liem, N. T., … Diwan, V. (2013). Bringing evidence to policy to achieve health-related MDGs for all: Justification and design of the EPI-4 project in China, India, Indonesia, and Vietnam. *Global Health Action, 6*, 19650. https://doi.org/10.3402/gha.v6i0.19650

Vest, J. R., Grannis, S. J., Haut, D. P., Halverson, P. K., & Menachemi, N. (2017). Using structured and unstructured data to identify patients' need for services that address the social determinants of health. *International Journal of Medical Informatics, 107*, 101–106. https://doi.org/10.1016/j.ijmedinf.2017.09.008

Vos, T., Flaxman, A. D., Naghavi, M., Lozano, R., Michaud, C., Ezzati, M., … Memish, Z. A. (2012). Years lived with disability (YLDs) for 1160 sequelae of 289 diseases and injuries 1990-2010: a systematic analysis for the Global Burden of Disease Study 2010. *Lancet, 380*(9859), 2163–2196. https://doi.org/10.1016/s0140-6736(12)61729-2

Whiteford, H., Ferrari, A., & Degenhardt, L. (2016). Global Burden of Disease studies: Implications for mental and substance use disorders. *Health Affairs, 35*(6), 1114–1120. https://doi.org/10.1377/hlthaff.2016.0082

Whiteford, H. A., Degenhardt, L., Rehm, J., Baxter, A. J., Ferrari, A. J., Erskine, H. E., … Vos, T. (2013). Global burden of disease attributable to mental and substance use disorders: Findings from the Global Burden of Disease Study 2010. *Lancet, 382*(9904), 1575–1586. https://doi.org/10.1016/s0140-6736(13)61611-6

Williams, N. J., Ehrhart, M. G., Aarons, G. A., Marcus, S. C., & Beidas, R. S. (2018). Linking molar organizational climate and strategic implementation climate to clinicians' use of evidence-based psychotherapy techniques: Cross-sectional and lagged analyses from a 2-year observational study. *Implementation Science, 13*(1), 85. https://doi.org/10.1186/s13012-018-0781-2

World Health Organization. (2001a). *The world health report 2001: Mental health: New understanding, new hope*. https://www.who.int/whr/2001/en/whr01_en.pdf?ua=1

World Health Organization. (2001b). ICF: *International classification of functioning, disability and health*. Geneva, CH: Author.

World Health Organization. (2010). *Monitoring the building blocks of health systems: A handbook of indicators and their measurement strategies*. Geneva, CH: Author. https://www.who.int/healthinfo/systems/WHO_MBHSS_2010_full_web.pdf

World Health Organization. (2016). *Global monitoring of action on the social determinants of health: A proposed framework and basket of core indicators* [consultation paper]. Geneva, CH: Author. https://www.who.int/social_determinants/consultation-paper-SDH-Action-Monitoring.pdf?ua=1

World Health Organization. (2017). *International classification of functioning, disability and health*. [Interactive Online Web Site]. Geneva, CH: Author. http://apps.who.int/classifications/icfbrowser/Default.aspx

World Health Organization. (2018a). *ICD-11 reference guide*. [Interactive Online Book]. Geneva, CH: Author. https://icd.who.int/browse11/content/refguide.ICD11_en/html/index.html#1.1.0Part1purposeandmultipleusesofICD|part-1-what-is-icd-11|c1

World Health Organization. (2018b). *International classification of diseases and related health problems*. 11th. [Interactive Online Web Site]. Geneva, CH: Author. https://icd.who.int/

Policies and Practices to Support School Mental Health

Katie Eklund, Lauren Meyer, Joni Splett, and Mark Weist

Policies and Practices to Support School Mental Health

Providing mental health services to children and youth in schools has been found to be an effective and innovative approach to reaching at-risk or hard-to-reach youth (Sklarew, Twemlow, & Wilkinson, 2004; Zirkelback & Reese, 2010). A rich history of literature and research supports the use of mental health services in schools. School-based programs that support the mental well-being of children and youth not only promote wellness but have been linked to improved academic achievement and behavioral functioning among school-aged youth (Crespi & Howe, 2002; Owens & Murphy, 2004). The failure of the nation's child mental health system to fully address the mental health needs of children and adolescents has been well documented and highlights the urgency to reconsider current policy and practice (Burns et al., 1995; Kataoka et al., 2003; Simon, Pastor, Reuben, Huang, & Goldstrom, 2015). Furthermore, the need for school mental health services is detailed in special education regulations and national reports indicating that schools should provide services that target the mental health needs of youth (National Academies of Sciences, Engineering, & Medicine, 2018a, 2018b; President's New Freedom Commission on Mental Health, 2003; U.S. Department of Education, 2018).

Research indicates that of the small percentage of children and adolescents who receive mental health services, schools are the most common setting in which children access this care (Carta, Fiandra, Rampazzo, Contu, & Preti, 2015; Demissie,

K. Eklund (✉)
School Psychology Program, University of Arizona, Tucson, AZ, USA
e-mail: keklund@u.arizona.edu

L. Meyer
University of Arizona, Tucson, AZ, USA

J. Splett · M. Weist
University of South Carolina, Columbia, SC, USA

© Springer Nature Switzerland AG 2020
B. L. Levin, A. Hanson (eds.), *Foundations of Behavioral Health*,
https://doi.org/10.1007/978-3-030-18435-3_7

Oarker, & Vernon-Smiley, 2013; Farmer, Burns, Phillips, Angold, & Costello, 2003; Office of the Surgeon General, 2000). Further, data indicate these services are indeed reaching youths, including students from ethnic minority groups and those with less obvious problems, such as depression and anxiety, who are unlikely to access services in specialty mental health settings (Foster & Connor, 2005; Kataoka et al., 2003; Ramos & Alegría, 2014).

School mental health (SMH) services provide youth increased access to services by reducing many of the barriers to seeking traditional services, such as transportation, cost, and stigma (Weist, Lever, Bradshaw, & Sarno Owens, 2013). Providing services within schools can provide a neutral environment whereby youth learn that seeking out help and support is commonplace and exists within a continuum of provided supports (e.g., academic supports, physical health services). Offering a broad range of universal, targeted, and intensive mental health support services to youth in schools has been supported by a public health framework that recognizes the diverse needs of children and families (Kleiver & Cash, 2005; Short, 2003).

Many states have implemented such multitiered systems of support so that children and youth quickly and effectively can access a diverse range of services, requiring individuals other than those solely at the highest level of risk receive attention (Doll & Cummings, 2008). By providing a range of services, schools are able to help address many of the barriers to learning that children and youth may experience at some point throughout their school trajectory.

Evidence indicates that more comprehensive SMH, involving community-based and school staff increasing the intensity and comprehensiveness of services, improves children's outcomes. It increases the likelihood of first appointment after referral (Catron, Harris, & Weiss, 2005), subsequent retention in services (Atkins et al., 2006), and more effective outreach to underserved communities (Anyon, Ong, & Whitaker, 2014; Armbruster & Lichtman, 1999; Atkins et al., 2015), particularly for those children presenting less observable "internalizing" disorders like depression and anxiety (Atkins et al., 2006; Weist, Myers, Hastings, Ghuman, & Han, 1999). There is also an evidence base for research-supported prevention and intervention programs in schools (Durlak, Weissberg, Dymnicki, Taylor, & Schellinger, 2011; Elliott & Mihalic, 2004; Mihalic & Elliott, 2015). However, we must caution there needs to be solid empirical literature showing that mental health services delivered in schools are superior to those delivered in other settings.

Review of the Literature

Children's Mental Health Concerns

Approximately 20% of children experience significant mental, emotional, or behavioral symptoms that would qualify them for a psychiatric diagnosis at both national and global levels (National Research Council & Institute of

Medicine, 2009). Not only does the prevalence of those conditions and indicators increase with age (Perou et al., 2013), behavioral disorders are the leading causes for years lived with a disability for children and adolescents (Baranne & Falissard, 2018; Mokdad et al., 2016).

Furthermore, 9–13% of young people will experience a serious emotional disturbance with substantial functional impairment, while 5–9% will experience a serious emotional disturbance with extreme functional impairment (Friedman, Katz-Leavy, & Sondheimer, 1996). Unfortunately, only 15–30% of the children who demonstrate mental health concerns receive any type of help or support.

In order to address the gap in providing mental health services to children and youth, the President's New Freedom Commission on Mental Health (2003) called for a transformation in the delivery of mental health services in this country. School mental health services were suggested as one strategy in beginning to address many of the unmet mental health needs of children and youth (Atkins, Hoagwood, Kutash, & Seidman, 2010). As children currently receive more services through schools than through any other system, school- and community-employed clinicians are well positioned to provide mental health supports in schools (Larson, Spetz, Brindis, & Chapman, 2017).

History of School Mental Health

The provision of school mental health services originates from four co-occurring initiatives. First was the placement of nurses in schools as a public health approach to detect and treat illness that evolved into the establishment of school-based health centers across the United States. Second was the creation of child guidance clinics that evolved into community mental health centers with the passage of the Community Mental Health Act of 1963 (Public Law 88-164). Third was the passage of Public Law 94-142 in 1975 and its reauthorization as the Individuals with Disabilities Education Act (IDEA) in 1997 that resulted in the hiring of school-employed mental health professionals. The final initiative was the emergence of the expanded school mental health movement which brought community-based mental health professionals into schools to not only consult with teachers but provide direct services to children and families.

School Nursing and School-Based Health Centers

Employing nurses in the school setting largely resulted from the overwhelming number of eastern European immigrants moving to urban areas of the United States in the early part of the twentieth century without access to basic healthcare. In the early years, school nurses were effective at addressing health problems that interfered with student's learning. In fact, rates indicate that the percentage of students who missed school due to illness substantially declined from 10,567 in 1902–1101 in

1903 (Hawkins, Hayes, & Corliss, 1994). However, the school nurses' role was limited to physical health promotion and prevention of illness and injury. At that time, children's emotional well-being in relation to mental disorders was not recognized as affecting student's academic and social functioning.

By the 1960s, school-based health centers (SBHCs) started to emerge from what had previously been termed public health clinics and through the provision of services delivered via school nurses. SBHCs began to flourish in the 1980s, growing from 200 centers in 1990, to 1380 in 2001, and 1909 centers in 45 states by 2010 (U.S. Government Accountability Office, 2010). The SBHCs primarily employed nurse practitioners and/or physician's assistants. With the emerging recognition that many of the visits to the SBHC were related to mental health concerns (Lear, Gleicher, St. Germaine, & Porter, 1991), the SBHCs expanded their role to include mental health counseling provided by a master's level mental health clinician.

Child Guidance Clinics and Community Mental Health Centers

Child guidance clinics began as community-based centers that provided psychological therapeutic and assessment services for children with mental health concerns and their families. Originating in Chicago in 1909, the clinics embraced an interdisciplinary approach to service provision by employing social workers, psychologists, and psychiatrists to best meet the needs of children with mental health concerns (Witmer, 1940). The implementation of the Community Mental Health Centers (sCMHC) Construction Act of 1963 (Pub. Law 88-164) initiated the delivery of mental health consultation and intervention services to children and adolescents via CMHCs. The Walter P. Carter Center in Baltimore, MD, served as a seminal provider of school mental health services by establishing relationships with local schools in the community. The Carter Center provided on-site consultation with educators and discussed children receiving services at the centers' four clinics. These clinics established a foundation for the later development of expanded school mental health (ESMH) programs.

Public Law 94-142 and the Individuals with Disabilities Education Act (IDEA)

Originally passed as Public Law 94-142 in 1975, the IDEA mandates that schools serve all students, including those with learning or emotional disabilities. From its inception, IDEA facilitated the hiring of school mental health professionals, such as psychologists and social workers, to provide mental health supports to students. For example, schools hired school psychologists to conduct IDEA-required student evaluations to determine the degree of disability and necessary educational accommodations (Flaherty & Osher, 2003). The shift of mental health professionals from the community to employment as school staff members included providing services to students with emotional and behavioral challenges (Flaherty & Osher, 2003).

While early provisions of IDEA outlined service provisions to youth who met set criteria, it failed to address an organized and systemic approach to providing school mental health services. For example, students identified as emotionally disturbed (ED) had especially poor outcomes compared to students under other eligibility criteria, which may have been a primary driver in the development and expansion of SMH programming (Osher & Hanley, 1996).

In 1997, IDEA amendments further expanded the educational opportunities and support for students with ED. These revisions provided a broader role for both school- and community-employed practitioners to assist with delivery of services to youth via individualized educational plans. These amendments represent the growing recognition of the need to provide prevention services to intervene when youth display at-risk behaviors rather than postponing intervention until students' symptoms require more intensive placement or supports. IDEA provided a solid foundation for not only expanded service delivery but also expanded school mental health (ESMH) programs.

Expanded School Mental Health Programs

In the 1990s, the concept of "expanded" SMH emerged with early successes defined by the building of the child guidance clinic and CMHC models. This idea involved augmenting pre-existing school-based programs and roles that had been primarily focused on special education and crisis response services, toward a broad-based role of mental health supports (Weist, 1997). CSMH services included individual, family, and group psychotherapy, consultation with teachers and families, as well as mental health promotion and education. Several cities, including Baltimore, Maryland, demonstrated early success related to ESMH and brought about the receipt of significant federal funding in 1995 to establish the Center for School Mental Health (CSMH) at the University of Maryland as a national training and technical assistance center. The CSMH was funded by the Maternal and Child Health Bureau's *Mental Health of School-Age Children and Youth Initiative*, which also provided funding to the University of California at Los Angeles' Center for Mental Health in Schools, as well as five state infrastructure grants to Kentucky, Maine, Minnesota, New Mexico, and South Carolina.

Since 1995, the field of ESMH has grown significantly because of several efforts, including a national conference hosted by the CSMH, collaboration with the IDEA Partnership, and federal investment by the US Department of Education Office of Special Education Programs. These results have created a national Community of Practice on Collaborative School Behavioral Health, as well as 12 practice groups and 17 state groups, and a number of books and journals (Weist et al., 2013).

With this growth, the field came to represent more than just the original conceptualization of community-employed professionals providing mental health services in schools. As the emphases on public health frameworks, prevention science, and interdisciplinary collaboration emerged, the field of ESMH became known simply as school mental health (SMH). The change in acronyms better represented a school- and community-wide approach inclusive of a team of school and community mental health professionals partnering with youth and families to provide a public health continuum of promotion, prevention, early intervention, and treatment services.

Public Health Models that Support a Multitiered Framework

Conversations regarding the provision of school mental health services have been prominent in educational policy dialogues in recent years. Legislative acts continue to address the need for a collaborative focus on mental health in schools, such as the School Safety and Mental Health Services Improvement Act (2018), with an emphasis on preventative measures that deter the seemingly increasing incidence of crisis events in educational settings (Birkland & Lawrence, 2009; Crepeau-Hobson, Sievering, Armstrong, & Stonis, 2012). However, conversations among SMH practitioners examining the importance of an integrated mental health model of service delivery predate contemporary comments by legislators on service implementation methods (Cowen & Lorion, 1976; Windle & Woy, 1983). These early discussions referenced the ineffective nature of traditional reactive methodologies, which are designed to provide services only when concerns arise, echoing a "wait-to-fail" model of service delivery (Albers, Glover, & Kratochwill, 2007). Consequently, students who do not manifest robust externalizing behaviors, for example, may not be identified with missed opportunities for early intervention.

This gap in service has resulted in research to address the short- and long-term deleterious effects (e.g., academic, social, emotional) that may emerge from unmet mental health concerns among children and youth (Perou et al., 2013). The 1999 Surgeon General's Report on Mental Health first highlighted the need for preventative measures to effectively decrease the negative impact mental health concerns may have on youth (Office of the Surgeon General, 1999). Alternative models of service delivery are warranted, including those that reinforce the importance of collaboration between parents, educators, and mental health practitioners in schools and communities (Weist, Lowie, Flaherty, & Pruitt, 2001).

The public health approach incorporates an ecological framework in addressing children's mental health by acknowledging the influence of multiple systems on children's difficulties. This includes integrating systems of care for youth, including but not limited to child welfare, education, health, juvenile justice, mental health, and social services (Blau, Huang, & Mallery, 2010; Stiffman et al., 2010).

Although the public health model is holistic in nature, its goals do not oppose those in public education. The public health model goals are designed to supplement the current educational structure, build a bridge between school- and community-based services, promote partnerships between family systems and the school, and organize formative research that reflects the climate of the school so that the model can be tailored to students' needs (Nastasi, 2004). This approach is strength-based and culturally and environmentally sensitive and prescribes a continuum of mental health services ranging from activities that support and maintain positive mental health to prevention and treatment efforts (Blau et al., 2010; Office of the Surgeon General, 1999). Emerging research highlights a few examples, such as multitiered system of supports, that illustrate the effectiveness of the public health model in children's mental health services (Miles, Espiritu, Horen, Sebian, & Waetzig, 2010).

Similar in design, a multitiered system of support (MTSS) framework aims to provide a continuum of care that combines the efforts of communities, families, and schools. The MTSS framework, however, is defined by the application of high-quality interventions and positive behavioral supports at various levels or "tiers." Extant literature describes response to intervention (RtI) and positive behavioral interventions and supports (PBIS) as MTSS approaches that target specific barriers to learning while amplifying the integration of evidence-based interventions and supports until the obstacles to learning are addressed (Batsche et al., 2005; Sulkowski, Wingfield, Jones, & Alan Coulter, 2011).

These systems underscore the role of prevention and wellness through the activation of multiple tiers (i.e., primary, secondary, tertiary) and progress monitoring. Organizing services in this way allows stakeholders to engage in a systematic data-based decision-making process that promotes the implementation of programming and services that meet the mutable needs of students.

However, despite the multitiered design of PBIS, a common concern in these systems is the insufficient development of Tier 2 and 3 systems and practices, resulting in unaddressed behavioral and emotional needs for students with more complex mental health concerns. In addition, PBIS Tier 1 systems, although showing success in social climate and discipline, do not typically address broader community data and mental health prevention (Barrett et al., 2017). Newer models, whose principles parallel those within the MTSS framework, aim to address these gaps.

The Interconnected Systems Framework (ISF), for example, borrows from the strengths of PBIS, implementation science, and RtI to create a healthy merger with school mental health (Eber, Weist, & Barret, 2014). At its core, ISF capitalizes on the use of (1) effective collaborations between community and mental health providers; (2) data-based decision-making; (3) formal evaluation and implementation of evidence-based practices (EBP); (4) early access via comprehensive screenings; (5) rigorous progress monitoring for both fidelity and effectiveness; and (6) ongoing training and coaching at system and practice levels. The benefits of this model are influential in both economic and social schemes: children and adolescents will gain earlier access to high-quality EBPs; professional roles will be clearly defined, particularly among school- and community-employed mental health staff; and cross-training will endorse common language, communication, and engagement among all parties: students, parents, community members, and school staff.

School Mental Health Services in Multitiered Systems of Support

Within the public health framework of a multitiered system of support, such as the Interconnected Systems Framework, a collaborating team of education and mental health professionals provides a range of services across a continuum of assessment, intervention, and consultation services (Andis et al., 2002). This includes anything from accessing accommodations in the classroom (e.g., extended time, a quiet workspace, break cards) to more targeted and intensive services, such as the provision of individual and small group counseling services.

Universal strategies, often referred to as Tier 1 supports, traditionally provide a platform for promotion and prevention activities. They may also include social-emotional learning programs, welcoming and social support programs for new students and their families, staff development on positive behavior supports, violence prevention, coordination of a universal screening program, efficient referral mechanisms, and/or the development of crisis prevention and response procedures (Elliott & Tolan, 1998).

The second level of support often is referred to as targeted services, or Tier 2 interventions. This may include small group counseling for issues such as social skills, anger control, or depressive symptoms, psychoeducation and consultation with parents and families for issues related to bullying and peer conflicts, and/or daily behavior report cards to teach and reinforce positive replacement behaviors (National Association of School Psychologists, 2015).

The most intensive level of support services are offered at Tier 3 to selected individuals. Services commonly include psychological, psychoeducational, and/or functional behavioral assessments, individual and family counseling, a coordinated system of care, referrals to community service agencies, crisis intervention and response, and/or home-based programs (Andis et al., 2002; Splett, Fowler, Weist, McDaniel, & Dvorsky, 2013).

Across these tiers, SMH services include data-based decision-making, implementation support, and consultation and collaboration. Data-based decision-making includes using data to determine what services are needed and are working for an entire school (Tier 1), small group of students (Tier 2), and individual students (Tier 3). This includes formative and summative evaluation to monitor progress of prevention and intervention activities, as well as evaluate their overall efficacy and implementation fidelity.

Implementing evidence-based programs and practices as intended is an essential, yet often ignored, aspect of delivering an effective continuum of mental health services in schools. Research indicates the need for access to implementation supports such as coaching, training, and technical assistance to promote high-quality implementation of evidence-based programs in "real-world" settings (Fixsen, Naoom, Blase, Friedman, & Wallace, 2005).

Thus, a conduit for providing effective mental health services in schools is certainly access to a strong infrastructure of implementation supports. Similarly, consultation and collaboration with parents, youth, teachers, school administrators, other mental health professionals, and key community stakeholders are critical to effective SMH services (Weist et al., 2005). Consultation and collaboration promote engagement and service quality across the continuum of services.

Critical Issues in School Mental Health

Providing School Mental Health Services

A critical challenge in the field is effectively addressing the question of why mental health services should be provided in schools. Often times, schools may view mental health services as "add-ons" that are not central to the academic mission of schools (School Mental Health Alliance, 2004), and traditional school reform efforts focus on student learning, teaching strategies, and non-cognitive barriers to development (Burke, 2002; Koller & Svoboda, 2002). While educators may be willing to address barriers to student learning, they often do not recognize that social-emotional well-being is essential to academic success (Klem & Connell, 2004). National efforts, such as the No Child Left Behind Act (NCLB, 2001), the President's Commission on Excellence in Special Education (2002), and the Every Student Succeeds Act (ESSA, 2015), place priority on academic goals and may minimize attention to the social-emotional or mental health needs of students. There are provisions in national legislation that focus on health promotion and risk reduction (e.g., safe and drug-free schools in the NCLB Act and reducing risk for serious emotional disturbance in the New Freedom Commission on Mental Health report, 2003). However, policy reform still is needed at the local, state, and federal levels to include a focus on how behavioral and academic outcomes can be highly correlated (Nastasi, 2004).

Providing school mental health services within a public health model differs from traditional service delivery models as the explicit focus is on a community or society as opposed to any one individual. Theoretically, this perspective is well aligned with ecological systems perspectives, as proposed by Bronfenbrenner (1979), in which individuals and systems are mutually influential. Within an ecological framework, each student is at the center of a series of concentric circles, which represent increasingly expanding, mutually influential systems. For lasting impact to occur, change must occur at a broader level than just within an individual.

If the focus of school mental health services is to provide prevention, intervention, and response services to children and youth, the educational context by which services are delivered must also be a core consideration. Namely, teachers spend countless hours with students each day and often become intimately familiar with children's behavior, routines, and abilities. As many disorders often arise for the first time in adolescents or young adults, early recognition and treatment increases the chances of better long-term outcomes. However, identification and help-seeking behaviors can only occur if young people and their support systems (e.g., families, teachers, friends) know about early changes produced by mental disorders and how to access help.

Universal Screening

Universal screening is a proactive approach of using brief and efficient measures to identify students at risk for future difficulties (Eklund & Dowdy, 2014; Jenkins, Hudson, & Johnson, 2007). A primary purpose of universal screening pertains to the identification of individual students who have not responded to universal prevention efforts and are likely in need of targeted or intensive supports (Eklund & Tanner, 2014; Levitt, Saka, Romanelli, & Hoagwood, 2007).

Research suggests schools provide an ideal setting for identifying at-risk students due to the large number of youth in school and the ability to provide follow-up care within schools (Glover & Albers, 2007; Levitt et al., 2007). For example, providing behavioral supports in schools allows for the modification of environmental contingencies toward the disruption of problem behavior development. On the basis of research that shows positive outcomes may be achieved through early identification and intervention, recent educational policy and legislation place an increasing focus on data-based decision-making and universal assessment in schools (IDEA, 2004; (Lane, Robertson Kalberg, Lambert, Crnobori, & Bruhn, 2010; Reschly, 2008). Indeed, children with childhood behavioral difficulties who are identified early and receive intervention are likely to make significant gains in positive emotional and behavioral functioning (Brophy-Herb, Lee, Nievar, & Stollak, 2007; Eklund & Dowdy, 2014).

Despite this research and screening's status as an essential component of MTSS service delivery, many schools have not begun to adopt universal screening (Bruhn, Woods-Groves, & Huddle, 2014; Romer & McIntosh, 2017). Although reasons for such limited implementation of universal screening abound (Chafouleas, Kilgus, & Wallach, 2010), more understanding of how screening is implemented and whether or not they achieve intended outcomes is needed. While initial research demonstrates that screening identifies a group of at-risk students previously unknown to school staff and/or not receiving services (Eklund & Dowdy, 2014), additional research on treatment utility is needed to demonstrate students are receiving improved access to care and ultimately, positive response to early intervention services.

Parent and Community Partnerships

One of the greatest strengths of school mental health models is the emphasis on building an alliance between those who have a shared responsibility for the child, particularly models that invite and encourage parent, school, and community involvement. However, efforts to develop links between stakeholders have illuminated the inadequacy of services and holes in delivery, which subsequently produce a lack of enthusiasm for participation in dialogues on SMH. One qualitative study (Ouellette, Briscoe, & Tyson, 2004) reported that while parents would like to participate in community events and services, the absence of public and private transportation made following through with these commitments difficult. Furthermore, parents reported that too few organizations offer the services they need to build partnerships with the community. The limited availability of after-school programming and tutor services may contribute to this resistance.

Service provider's concerns echoed those of parents, citing the importance of transportation services. An increase in public transportation availability may help address these concerns.

Communication was another noted weakness, as the discourse used by human service workers may fail to convey useful information and strategies for interventions adequately (Ouellette et al., 2004). Faith-based organizations contributed to the conversation as well, expressing concerns for safe home environments and resources for crisis situations (e.g., clothing, employment, food, shelter).

Ecological models designed to facilitate conversation between parents, teachers, and community members are gaining recognition. The Positive Attitudes for Learning in School (PALS) model, for example, encourages clinicians and community members to work collaboratively on school-based teams to address concerns unique to the community, in addition to issues arising in academic achievement, behavior management, and social support for parents, teachers, and children (Frazier, Abdul-Adil, Atkins, Gathright, & Jackson, 2007).

Variations in geographic landscapes may also inform the development of mental health services. The limited availability of services and their proximity to individuals in need, for example, may act as barriers to those in rural communities. Reinforced by restrictions in transportation and the less than desirable fiscal obligations, families residing in these small rural communities may feel less inclined to pursue services, even if needs are demonstrated (Girio-Herrera, Owens, & Langberg, 2013).

Alternatively, researchers examining the bridge between mental health and education in urban communities identified socioeconomic status and disconnects between community resources and school supports as major challenges in the implementation of effective services (Cappella, Jackson, Bilal, Hamre, & Soulé, 2011).

Mobilization of SMH services requires a network of practitioners and researchers who are willing to share jurisdiction over the development, implementation, and evaluation of interventions. Programs like Bridging Education and Mental Health in Urban Schools (BRIDGE) are an example of such a partnership (Cappella, Frazier, Atkins, Schoenwald, & Glisson, 2008). This particular program capitalized on teacher consultation to increase pro-social interactions between students with behavioral difficulties and their classmates. It was designed to connect mental health practitioners with educators so that students receive the most effective form of service delivery possible. Individualized support and teacher observations were at the core of this framework.

School mental health practitioners are in a unique position to connect parents with community services. School psychologists and school counselors, for example, may lead the task of identifying culturally and environmentally sensitive resources that bridge the two contexts for the child (Nastasi, 2004; Nastasi, Varjas, & Moore, 2010). Additionally, SMH providers may find it appropriate to implement training programs for parents, teachers, and community members that prioritize learning goals and address concerns voiced by all parties while empowering each group to contribute to the implementation and monitoring of interventions (Cappella et al., 2008; Nastasi, 2004).

Evidence-Based, Culturally Sensitive Interventions

Building partnerships across settings is critical to balancing evidence-based services with cultural sensitivity. While research has demonstrated positive outcomes when evidence-based interventions are tailored to meet culturally diverse needs (Harachi, Catalano, & Hawkins, 1997; Wang-Schweig, Kviz, Altfeld, Miller, & Miller, 2014), other findings indicate the outcomes can be weakened or reduced when unexpected or ill-advised changes occur (Kumpfer, Alvarado, Tait, & Turner, 2002; Milburn & Lightfoot, 2016).

Evidence-based interventions in SMH that allow for cultural adaptation through partnerships with local communities during the dissemination, planning, and implementation stages have shown positive outcomes and greater buy-in (Ngo et al., 2008). For example, exposure to violence is a significant national concern and particularly prevalent among minority and ethnically diverse youth (Carothers, Arizaga, Carter, Taylor, & Grant, 2016; Weist & Cooley-Quille, 2001). In recognition of this concern, violence prevention and trauma response have been prioritized by national initiatives and federal funding associated with President Obama's Now is the Time Initiative (The White House, 2013, January 16).

One evidence-based intervention focused on treating youth exposed to violence from a culturally sensitive framework is *Cognitive Behavioral Intervention for Trauma in Schools* (CBITS; Jaycox et al., 2007). CBITS prioritizes partnerships with local schools and communities, including stakeholders from parents, clinicians, community organizations, and faith-based groups throughout all stages of the program. It was developed for and with diverse children and families in mind and has shown positive outcomes in randomized control studies and dissemination evaluations with Mexican and Central American youth, urban African American students, Native American children, and children in rural communities (Kataoka et al., 2003).

CBITS includes formal and informal feedback mechanisms, as well as multi-stakeholder planning committees, during local program development and implementation planning to ensure the consultation, outreach, training/supervision, evaluation, and service delivery models meet the cultural context while keeping the core cognitive behavioral therapy components intact (Ngo et al., 2008). Tailoring implementation to be culturally sensitive and respectful of the local community is supported by collaboration with cultural liaisons, who have both knowledge of the cultural context and clinical intervention (Ngo et al., 2008). SMH practitioners implementing CBITS or any other evidence-based practice should (1) develop partnerships across stakeholder groups; (2) familiarize themselves with the local cultural context and any individual issues that may arise; (3) stay vigilant in their attention to the unique needs of their students; and (4) work with others who have cultural knowledge and clinical expertise for collaboration, training, and supervision.

From a research perspective, more efforts are needed to invite open dialogues and use the cultural experiences of youth to inform the development and delivery of culturally sensitive and specific interventions. Dialogue among a wide range of culturally diverse stakeholders in SMH is needed to improve the service delivery, consultation, and evaluation models currently employed in the field. Given issues of disparity and collaboration with parents and families, more dialogues around methods to break through these barriers are needed. Additionally, in developing culturally specific interventions and/or tailoring existing evidence-based interventions to be more culturally sensitive, ethnographic research is needed to better understand the cultural experience of youth (Anyon et al., 2014).

Similar to CBITS, other interventions have been developed because of ethnographic research, which aimed to expand the literature on students' cultural experiences and in what ways these experiences affect behavioral and academic functioning. In one particular study, four culture-specific themes emerged—adult-sanctioned behaviors and practices, adolescents' perspectives about the present, adolescents' aspirations for the future, and societal factors (Varjas, Nastasi, Moore, & Jayasena, 2005). The authors argue these factors should guide the development and implementation of culture-specific interventions and conclude that these factors will intersect in different domains of the ecological framework, including school, family, peer, and community contexts.

Mental Health Literacy

Mental health literacy has been recognized as one strategy in facilitating early intervention for mental health concerns. In this approach, young people and their support systems are taught how to provide appropriate mental health first aid and how to support help-seeking behaviors upon first recognition of a mental health concerns. These interventions can include community campaigns aimed at both youth and adults; school-based interventions that teach help-seeking behavior, mental health literacy, or resilience; and programs training individuals on how to intervene in a mental health encounter or crisis (Kelly, Jorm, & Wright, 2007).

While there is no standardization of mental health education in schools, initial research suggests mental health literacy can be improved with planned interventions. Key components may include campaigns tailored to the specific needs and preferences of the intended community that will appeal to different groups (e.g., youth, teachers, parents); ensuring the availability of trusted and established help-seeking pathways among youth; and providing education and accurate information on what to expect when seeking help and obtaining professional support (Kelly et al., 2007; Rickwood, Deane, Wilson, & Ciarrochi, 2005). Gatekeepers, such as teachers, parents, and other important adults, play an important role in offering help to those who need it most.

Financing for School Mental Health Services

It is estimated that childhood emotional and behavioral disorders cost the public $247 billion annually (National Research Council & Institute of Medicine, 2009). Other estimates suggest that in 2012, $13.9 billion was spent for the treatment of mental disorders in children, which was the highest of any children's healthcare expenditures exceeding asthma, trauma-related disorders, acute bronchitis, and infectious disease (Soni, 2015, April). As an estimated 20% of children have a diagnosable mental, emotional, or behavioral disorder, treatment remains one of the most prevalent and costly of all chronic illness in youth.

Historically, as many as one in seven adolescents have been without health insurance and therefore have been unable to receive third-party reimbursable mental health services in the private sector (Crespi & Howe, 2002). Reports by the US Department of Health and Human Services indicated that a disproportionate number of children with mental health problems in the United States do not receive mental health services due to a lack of insurance (Maternal and Child Health Bureau, 2010, 2018, October). An estimated 2.8 million children are eligible for Medicaid or the Children's Health Insurance Program but are not enrolled currently in either (Kenney, Jennifer, Pan, Lynch, & Buettgens, 2016, May). Sole reliance on providers outside the school environment has placed considerable burden on families without such insurance.

It is projected that implementation of the Patient Protection and Affordable Care Act (PPACA), Public Law 111-148 (June 2010), will have a significant impact on the way that healthcare services are delivered, as many youth who were previously uninsured or underinsured will gain access to services. With the expansion of health insurance coverage, many of the most vulnerable populations, such as young children, youth aging out of foster care, and children living in poverty, will have increased access to preventive services, as well as mental health treatment (English, 2010). In addition, the authorization of funding for home visitation programs to promote improvements in areas such as child development, parenting, and school readiness will provide opportunities for families who are in the greatest need. The provision of the PPACA to authorize funding to establish and expand school-based health centers has the potential to significantly increase and enhance mental health education, prevention, and early intervention efforts within schools.

While school mental health programs have grown over the past two decades, identifying and securing sustainable funding sources continues to be a concern. Recent studies suggest 70% of school districts reported an increase in need for services but saw funding remain stagnant or decreased (Foster & Connor, 2005). As education systems provide limited funding for SMH services, schools traditionally look to grants or other fee for service programs (e.g., Medicaid). However, sole reliance on these mechanisms may not provide sufficient revenue and can be highly bureaucratic and difficult to obtain (Center for Health and Health Care in Schools, 2003; Evans et al., 2013; Freeman, 2011). In addition, fee-for-service approaches have created concerns about overdiagnosis, limited time for prevention activities, and an inability to serve students without Medicaid (Lever, Stephan, Axelrod, & Weist, 2004; Mills et al., 2006). As a result, schools are called upon to explore collaborative and unique funding arrangements to sustain SMH services and programs.

Sustainable funding is needed to support SMH services. Although there are some potential funding sources that are underutilized (e.g., from Early and Periodic Screening, Diagnosis, and Treatment, Safe and Drug-Free Schools, Title I), access to such funds and continued sustainability continue to be a concern for many schools. In order to address these barriers, many programs and services have blended or "braided" funding, by deriving funding from multiple sources, including grants, contracts, and private agencies (Lever et al., 2004). Fee-for-service revenue has served as a primary source of funding for many mental health services provided in schools. Third-party payers (e.g., Medicaid, State Children's Health Insurance Programs, private insurance) provide reimbursement for mental health services provided to children. However, reimbursement is typically limited to those students who have a clinical diagnosis from the *Diagnostic and Statistical Manual of Mental Disorders* (DSM-5; APA, 2013) for traditional mental health services (e.g., individual and group counseling, family counseling) versus broader SMH services (e.g., teacher consultation, parent consultation, prevention services, case management).

Sole or primary reliance on fee-for-service models provides a number of barriers to school districts and agencies, including significant paperwork, administrative duties, and managerial responsibilities. Although larger school districts and agencies may have mechanisms in place to be able to hire and train staff to manage Medicaid billing and services, rural communities and smaller agencies may be at a disadvantage. Many of these same barriers are placed upon clinicians, who face substantial paperwork that can become burdensome when the primary focus should be on providing direct clinical services and preventative care.

Implications for Behavioral Health

The SMH field has grown significantly since its beginning days in child guidance clinics and primary focus on expanded models inclusive only of community providers. The opportunity to provide mental and behavioral health services within the school setting has been an ongoing goal for many mental health professionals (e.g., social workers, psychologists, counselors) who desire to improve access to care by providing evidence-based interventions to a greater number of children and families.

Service delivery models that emphasize teaming and collaboration across school, community, and family stakeholders within the system of a multitiered public health continuum of promotion, prevention, early intervention, and treatment are increasingly showing positive outcomes for children in need. This includes the aforementioned Interconnected Systems Framework that combines implementation science, school-based response to intervention models, and PBIS to streamline services for children, families, and educators. This framework provides concrete examples of interdisciplinary collaboration among school- and community-based mental health providers as being essential to delivering high-quality evidence-based mental and behavioral health services in schools.

Furthermore, schools continue to utilize public health models that emphasize prevention through screening and early intervention practices that can eliminate or reduce the severity of behavioral and emotional symptoms when combined with early intervention. However, more work is needed, and critical issues remain.

The field must continue to emphasize the critical role of mental health in the academic mission of schools and should consider how to intertwine behavioral and academic standards for student success. For example, Illinois Learning Standards now include three social/emotional development standards that students should know and be able to do to varying degrees in grades K-12 (Illinois State Board of Education, 2018). This includes the development of self-awareness and self-management skills, as well as the use of social-awareness and interpersonal skills to establish and maintain positive relationships. These types of educational policies can be instrumental in continuing to advance mental health promotion in the school setting.

References

Albers, C. A., Glover, T. A., & Kratochwill, T. R. (2007). Introduction to the special issue: How can universal screening enhance educational and mental health outcomes? *Journal of School Psychology, 45*(2), 113–116. https://doi.org/10.1016/j.jsp.2006.12.002

American Psychiatric Association. (2013). *Diagnostic and statistical manual of mental disorders: DSM-5*. Arlington, VA: Author.

Andis, P., Cashman, J., Oglesby, D., Praschil, R., Adelman, H., Taylor, L., & Weist, M. (2002). A strategic and shared agenda to advance mental health in schools through family and system partnerships. *International Journal of Mental Health Promotion, 4*(4), 28–35. https://doi.org/1 0.1080/14623730.2002.9721886

Anyon, Y., Ong, S. L., & Whitaker, K. (2014). School-based mental health prevention for Asian American adolescents: Risk behaviors, protective factors, and service use. *Asian American Journal of Psychology, 5*(2), 134–144. https://doi.org/10.1037/a0035300

Armbruster, P., & Lichtman, J. (1999). Are school based mental health services effective? Evidence from 36 inner city schools. *Community Mental Health Journal, 35*(6), 493–504.

Atkins, M. S., Frazier, S. L., Birman, D., Adil, J. A., Jackson, M., Graczyk, P. A., ... McKay, M. M. (2006). School-based mental health services for children living in high poverty urban communities. *Administration and Policy in Mental Health and Mental Health Services Research, 33*(2), 146–159. https://doi.org/10.1007/s10488-006-0031-9

Atkins, M. S., Hoagwood, K. E., Kutash, K., & Seidman, E. (2010). Toward the integration of education and mental health in schools. *Administration and Policy in Mental Health, 37*(1–2), 40–47. https://doi.org/10.1007/s10488-010-0299-7

Atkins, M. S., Shernoff, E. S., Frazier, S. L., Schoenwald, S. K., Cappella, E., Marinez-Lora, A., ... Bhaumik, D. (2015). Redesigning community mental health services for urban children: Supporting schooling to promote mental health. *Journal of Consulting and Clinical Psychology, 83*(5), 839–852. https://doi.org/10.1037/a0039661

Baranne, M. L., & Falissard, B. (2018). Global burden of mental disorders among children aged 5-14 years. *Child and Adolescent Psychiatry and Mental Health, 12*, 19. https://doi.org/10.1186/s13034-018-0225-4

Barrett, S., Eber, L., Weist, M. (2017). *Advancing education effectiveness: interconnecting school mental health and school-wide positive behavior support.* OSEP Technical Assistance Center on Positive Behavioral Interventions and Supports. Retrieved from https://www.pbis.org/school/school-mental-health/interconnectedsystems

Batsche, G., Elliot, J., Graden, J. L., Grimes, J., Kovaleski, J. F., Prasse, D., ... Tilly, W. D., III. (2005). *Response to intervention: Policy considerations and implementation.* Alexandria, VA: National Association of State Directors of Special Education.

Birkland, T. A., & Lawrence, R. G. (2009). Media framing and policy change after Columbine. *American Behavioral Scientist, 52*(10), 1405–1425. https://doi.org/10.1177/0002764209332555

Blau, G. M., Huang, L. N., & Mallery, C. J. (2010). Advancing efforts to improve children's mental health in America: A commentary. *Administration and Policy in Mental Health, 37*(1–2), 140–144. https://doi.org/10.1007/s10488-010-0290-3

Bronfenbrenner, U. (1979). *Ecology of human development: Experiments by nature and design.* Cambridge: Harvard University Press.

Brophy-Herb, H. E., Lee, R. E., Nievar, M. A., & Stollak, G. (2007). Preschoolers' social competence: Relations to family characteristics, teacher behaviors and classroom climate. *Journal of Applied Developmental Psychology, 28*(2), 134–148. https://doi.org/10.1016/j.appdev.2006.12.004

Bruhn, A. L., Woods-Groves, S., & Huddle, S. (2014). A preliminary investigation of emotional and behavioral screening practices in K–12 schools. *Education and Treatment of Children, 37*(4), 611–634. https://doi.org/10.1353/etc.2014.0039

Burke, R. W. (2002). Social and emotional education in the classroom. *Kappa Delta Pi Record, 38*(3), 108–111. https://doi.org/10.1080/00228958.2002.10516354

Burns, B. J., Costello, E. J., Angold, A., Tweed, D., Stangl, D., Farmer, E. M., & Erkanli, A. (1995). Children's mental health service use across service sectors. *Health Affairs, 14*(3), 147–159.

Cappella, E., Frazier, S. L., Atkins, M. S., Schoenwald, S. K., & Glisson, C. (2008). Enhancing schools' capacity to support children in poverty: An ecological model of school-based mental health services. *Administration and Policy in Mental Health and Mental Health Services Research, 35*(5), 395–409. https://doi.org/10.1007/s10488-008-0182-y

Cappella, E., Jackson, D. R., Bilal, C., Hamre, B. K., & Soulé, C. (2011). Bridging mental health and education in urban elementary schools: Participatory research to inform intervention development. *School Psychology Review, 40*(4), 486–508. http://search.ebscohost.com/login.aspx?direct=true&db=psyh&AN=2012-00587-003&site=ehost-liveelise.cappella@nyu.edu

Carothers, K. J., Arizaga, J. A., Carter, J. S., Taylor, J., & Grant, K. E. (2016). The costs and benefits of active coping for adolescents residing in urban poverty. *Journal of Youth and Adolescence, 45*(7), 1323–1337. https://doi.org/10.1007/s10964-016-0487-1

Carta, M. G., Fiandra, T. D., Rampazzo, L., Contu, P., & Preti, A. (2015). An overview of international literature on school interventions to promote mental health and well-being in children and adolescents. *Clinical Practice and Epidemiology in Mental Health, 11*(Suppl 1 M1), 16–20. https://doi.org/10.2174/1745017901511010016

Catron, T., Harris, V. S., & Weiss, B. (2005). Post-treatment results after 2 years of services in the Vanderbilt School-Based Counseling Project. In M. H. Epstein, K. Kutash, & A. J. Duchnowski (Eds.), *Outcomes for children and youth with emotional and behavioral disorders and their families: Programs and evaluations, best practices* (pp. 633–656). Austin, TX: PRO-ED.

Center for Health and Health Care in Schools. (2003). *School-based health centers: Surviving a difficult economy.* Washington, DC: George Washington University.

Chafouleas, S. M., Kilgus, S. P., & Wallach, N. (2010). Ethical dilemmas in school-based behavioral screening. *Assessment for Effective Intervention, 35*(4), 245–252. https://doi.org/10.1177/1534508410379002

Community Mental Health Centers Construction Act, Pub. L. No. 88-164 (1963). https://www.gpo.gov/fdsys/pkg/STATUTE-77/pdf/STATUTE-77-Pg282.pdf

Cowen, E. L., & Lorion, R. P. (1976). Changing roles for the school mental health professional. *Journal of School Psychology, 14*(2), 131–138. https://doi.org/10.1016/0022-4405(76)90048-0

Crepeau-Hobson, F., Sievering, K. S., Armstrong, C., & Stonis, J. (2012). A coordinated mental health crisis response: Lessons learned from three Colorado school shootings. *Journal of School Violence, 11*(3), 207–225. https://doi.org/10.1080/15388220.2012.682002

Crespi, T. D., & Howe, E. A. (2002). Families in Crisis: Considerations for special service providers in the schools. *Special Services in the Schools, 18*(1–2), 43–54. https://doi.org/10.1300/J008v18n01_03

Demissie, Z., Oarker, t., & Vernon-Smiley, M. (2013). Mental health and social services. In Centers for Disease Control and Prevention (Ed.), *Results from the school health policies and practices study* (Vol. 2012, pp. 65–70). Atlanta, GA: U.S. Department of Health and Human Services, Centers for Disease Control and Prevention.

Doll, B., & Cummings, J. A. (2008). Why population-based services are essential for school mental health, and how to make them happen in your school. In B. Doll & J. A. Cummings (Eds.), *Transforming school mental health services: Population-based approaches to promoting the competency and wellness of children*. Thousand Oaks, CA: Corwin Press.

Durlak, J. A., Weissberg, R. P., Dymnicki, A. B., Taylor, R. D., & Schellinger, K. B. (2011). The impact of enhancing students' social and emotional learning: A meta-analysis of school-based universal interventions. *Child Development, 82*(1), 405–432. https://doi.org/10.1111/j.1467-8624.2010.01564.x

Eber, L., Weist, M. D., & Barret, S. (2014). *An introduction to the interconnected systems framework*. s.l.: OSEP Technical Assistance Center on Positive Behavioral Interventions and Supports. https://www.pbis.org/school/school-mental-health/interconnected-systems

Eklund, K., & Dowdy, E. (2014). Screening for behavioral and emotional risk versus traditional school identification methods. *School Mental Health, 6*(1), 40–49. https://doi.org/10.1007/s12310-013-9109-1

Eklund, K., & Tanner, N. (2014). Providing multi-tiered systems of support for behavior: Conducting behavior screening at school. *Principal Leadership, 10*, 50–52.

Elliott, D. S., & Mihalic, S. (2004). Issues in disseminating and replicating effective prevention programs. *Prevention Science, 5*(1), 47–53.

Elliott, D. S., & Tolan, P. H. (1998). Youth violence, prevention, intervention, and social policy. In D. J. Flannery & C. R. Huff (Eds.), *Youth violence: Prevention, intervention, and social policy* (pp. 3–46). Washington, DC: American Psychiatric Press.

English, A. (2010). *The Patient Protection and Affordable Care Act of 2010: How does it help adolescents and young adults*. Chapel Hill, NC: NAHIC. http://nahic.ucsf.edu/downloads/HCR_Issue_Brief_Aug2010_Final_Aug31.pdf

Evans, A., Glass-Siegel, M., Frank, A., Van truren, R., Lever, N. A., & Weist, M. D. (2013). Overcoming the challenges of funding school mental health programs. In M. D. Weist, N. A. Lever, C. P. Bradshaw, & J. Sarno Owens (Eds.), *Handbook of school mental health: Research, training, practice, and policy* (pp. 73–86). New York, NY: Springer.

Every Student Succeeds Act [ESSA], Pub. L. No. 114–95 (2015). https://www.gpo.gov/fdsys/pkg/PLAW-114publ95/pdf/PLAW-114publ95.pdf

Farmer, E. M. Z., Burns, B. J., Phillips, S. D., Angold, A., & Costello, E. J. (2003). Pathways into and through mental health services for children and adolescents. *Psychiatric Services, 54*(1), 60–66. https://doi.org/10.1176/appi.ps.54.1.60

Fixsen, D. L., Naoom, S. F., Blase, K. A., Friedman, R. M., & Wallace, F. (2005). *Implementation research: A synthesis of the literature*. Tampa, FL: University of South Florida, Louis de la Parte Florida Mental Health Institute, National Implementation Research Network.

Flaherty, L. T., & Osher, D. (2003). History of school-based mental health services. In M. D. Weist, S. W. Evans, & N. A. Lever (Eds.), *Handbook of school mental health research, training, practice, and policy* (pp. 11–22). New York, NY: Kluwer Academic.

Foster, E. M., & Connor, T. (2005). Public costs of better mental health services for children and adolescents. *Psychiatric Services, 56*(1), 50–55. https://doi.org/10.1176/appi.ps.56.1.50

Frazier, S. L., Abdul-Adil, J., Atkins, M. S., Gathright, T., & Jackson, M. (2007). Can't have one without the other: Mental health providers and community parents reducing barriers to services for families in urban poverty. *Journal of Community Psychology, 35*(4), 435–446. https://doi.org/10.1002/jcop.20157

Freeman, E. V. (2011). *What are some strategies to sustain school mental health programs?* (School mental health sustainability: Funding strategies to build sustainable school mental health programs, 4). Washington, DC. https://www.air.org/sites/default/files/downloads/report/Sustaining%20School%20Mental%20Health%20Programs_4.pdf

Friedman, R. M., Katz-Leavy, J. W., & Sondheimer, D. L. (1996). Prevalence of serious emotional disturbance in children and adolescents. In R. W. Manderscheid & M. A. Sonnenschein (Eds.), *Mental health, United States, 1996* (pp. 71–89). Rockville, MD: U.S. Department of Health and Human Services, Public Health Services, Substance Abuse and Mental Health Services Administration, Center for Mental Health Services.

Girio-Herrera, E., Owens, J. S., & Langberg, J. M. (2013). Perceived barriers to help-seeking among parents of at-risk kindergarteners in rural communities. *Journal of Clinical Child and Adolescent Psychology, 42*(1), 68–77. https://doi.org/10.1080/15374416.2012.715365

Glover, T. A., & Albers, C. A. (2007). Considerations for evaluating universal screening assessments. *Journal of School Psychology, 45*(2), 117–135. https://doi.org/10.1016/j.jsp.2006.05.005

Harachi, T. W., Catalano, R. F., & Hawkins, J. D. (1997). Effective recruitment for parenting programs within ethnic minority communities. *Child & Adolescent Social Work Journal, 14*(1), 23–39. https://doi.org/10.1023/A:1024540829739

Hawkins, J. W., Hayes, E. R., & Corliss, C. P. (1994). School nursing in America–1902-1994: A return to public health nursing. *Public Health Nursing, 11*(6), 416–425.

Illinois State Board of Education. (2018). *Social/emotional learning standards.* [Web page]. Springfield, IL: Author. https://www.isbe.net/pages/social-emotional-learning-standards.aspx

Individuals with Disabilities Education, Pub. L. No. 94–142 (2004). https://www.govinfo.gov/content/pkg/STATUTE-89/pdf/STATUTE-89-Pg773.pdf

Jaycox, L. H., Tanielian, T. L., Sharma, P., Morse, L., Clum, G., & Stein, B. D. (2007). Schools' mental health responses after Hurricanes Katrina and Rita. *Psychiatric Services, 58*(10), 1339–1343. https://doi.org/10.1176/appi.ps.58.10.1339

Jenkins, J. R., Hudson, R. F., & Johnson, E. S. (2007). Screening for at-risk readers in a response to intervention framework. *School Psychology Review, 36*(4), 582–600. http://search.ebscohost.com/login.aspx?direct=true&db=psyh&AN=2008-00698-005&site=ehost-live

Kataoka, S. H., Stein, B. D., Jaycox, L. H., Wong, M., Escudero, P., Tu, W., ... Fink, A. (2003). A school-based mental health program for traumatized Latino immigrant children. *Journal of the American Academy of Child and Adolescent Psychiatry, 42*(3), 311–318. https://doi.org/10.1097/00004583-200303000-00011

Kelly, C. M., Jorm, A. F., & Wright, A. (2007). Improving mental health literacy as a strategy to facilitate early intervention for mental disorders. *Medical Journal of Australia, 187*(7 Suppl), S26–S30.

Kenney, G. M., Haley Jennifer, Pan, C., Lynch, V., & Buettgens, M. (2016, May). *Children's coverage climb continues: Uninsurance and Medicaid/CHIP eligibility and participation under the ACA.* Washington, DC: Urban Institute. http://www.urban.org/sites/default/files/publication/80536/2000787-Childrens-Coverage-Climb-Continues-Uninsurance-and-Medicaid-CHIP-Eligibility-and-Participation-Under-the-ACA.pdf

Kleiver, A., & Cash, R. E. (2005). Characteristics of a public health model of a mental health service delivery. *Communiqué, 34*(3), 19.

Klem, A. M., & Connell, J. P. (2004). Relationships matter: Linking teacher support to student engagement and achievement. *Journal of School Health, 74*(7), 262–273.

Koller, J. R., & Svoboda, S. K. (2002). The application of a strengths-based mental health approach in schools. *Childhood Education, 78*(5), 291–294. https://doi.org/10.1080/00094056.2002.10 522744

Kumpfer, K. L., Alvarado, R., Tait, C., & Turner, C. (2002). Effectiveness of school-based family and children's skills training for substance abuse prevention among 6-8-year-old rural children. *Psychology of Addictive Behaviors, 16*(4, Suppl), S65–S71. https://doi.org/10.1037/0893-164X. 16.4S.S65

Lane, K. L., Robertson Kalberg, J., Lambert, E. W., Crnobori, M., & Bruhn, A. L. (2010). A comparison of systematic screening tools for emotional and behavioral disorders: A replication. *Journal of Emotional and Behavioral Disorders, 18*(2), 100–112. https://doi.org/10. 1177/1063426609341069

Larson, S., Spetz, J., Brindis, C. D., & Chapman, S. (2017). Characteristic differences between school-based health centers with and without mental health providers: A review of national trends. *Journal of Pediatric Health Care, 31*(4), 484–492. https://doi.org/10.1016/j.pedhc. 2016.12.007

Lear, J. G., Gleicher, H. B., St. Germaine, A., & Porter, P. J. (1991). Reorganizing health care for adolescents: The experience of the school-based adolescent health care program. *Journal of Adolescent Health, 12*(6), 450–458. https://doi.org/10.1016/1054-139X(91)90022-P

Lever, N. A., Stephan, S. H., Axelrod, J., & Weist, M. D. (2004). Fee-for-service revenue for school mental health through a partnership with an outpatient mental health center. *Journal of School Health, 74*(3), 91–94.

Levitt, J. M., Saka, N., Romanelli, L. H., & Hoagwood, K. (2007). Early identification of mental health problems in schools: The status of instrumentation. *Journal of School Psychology, 45*(2), 163–191. https://doi.org/10.1016/j.jsp.2006.11.005

Maternal and Child Health Bureau. (2010). *The mental and emotional well-being of children: A portrait of States and the nation 2007.* Rockville, MD: U.S. Dept. of Health and Human Services, Health Resources and Services Administration, Maternal and Child Health Bureau.

Maternal and Child Health Bureau. (2018, October). *National Survey of Children's Health NSCH fact sheet.* Washington, DC: Data Resource Center for Child and Adolescent Health. https:// mchb.hrsa.gov/sites/default/files/mchb/Data/NSCH/NSCH-factsheet-2017-release.pdf

Mihalic, S. F., & Elliott, D. S. (2015). Evidence-based programs registry: Blueprints for healthy youth development. *Evaluation and Program Planning, 48*, 124–131. https://doi.org/10.1016/j. evalprogplan.2014.08.004

Milburn, N. G., & Lightfoot, M. (2016). Improving the participation of families of color in evidence-based interventions: Challenges and lessons learned. In N. Zane, G. Bernal, & F. T. L. Leong (Eds.), *Evidence-based psychological practice with ethnic minorities: Culturally informed research and clinical strategies* (pp. 273–287). Washington, DC: American Psychological Association.

Miles, J., Espiritu, R. C., Horen, N., Sebian, J., & Waetzig, E. (2010). *A public health approach to children's mental health: A conceptual framework.* Washington, DC. https://gucchdtacenter. georgetown.edu/publications/PublicHealthApproach.pdf

Mills, C., Stephan, S. H., Moore, E., Weist, M. D., Daly, B. P., & Edwards, M. (2006). The President's New Freedom Commission: capitalizing on opportunities to advance school-based mental health services. *Clinical Child and Family Psychology Review, 9*(3–4), 149–161. https:// doi.org/10.1007/s10567-006-0003-3

Mokdad, A. H., Forouzanfar, M. H., Daoud, F., Mokdad, A. A., El Bcheraoui, C., Moradi-Lakeh, M., ... Murray, C. J. (2016). Global burden of diseases, injuries, and risk factors for young people's health during 1990-2013: A systematic analysis for the Global Burden of Disease Study 2013. *Lancet, 387*(10036), 2383–2401. https://doi.org/10.1016/s0140-6736(16)00648-6

Nastasi, B. K. (2004). Meeting the challenges of the future: Integrating public health and public education for mental health promotion. *Journal of Educational and Psychological Consultation, 15*(3–4), 295–312. https://doi.org/10.1080/10474412.2004.9669519

Nastasi, B. K., Varjas, K. M., & Moore, R. B. (2010). *School-based mental health services: Creating comprehensive and culturally specific programs*. Washington, DC: American Psychological Association.

National Academies of Sciences, Engineering, & Medicine. (2018a). *Exploring early childhood care and education levers to improve population health: Proceedings of a workshop*. Washington, DC: The National Academies Press.

National Academies of Sciences, Engineering, & Medicine. (2018b). *Opportunities for improving programs and services for children with disabilities*. Washington, DC: The National Academies Press.

National Association of School Psychologists. (2015). *NASP position statement: Early childhood services*. Bethesda, MD: Author. https://www.nasponline.org/x32403.xml

National Research Council, & Institute of Medicine. (2009). *Preventing mental, emotional, and behavioral disorders among young people: Progress and possibilities*. Washington, DC: The National Academies Press. https://www.nap.edu/catalog/12480/preventing-mental-emotional-and-behavioral-disorders-among-young-people-progress

Ngo, V., Langley, A., Kataoka, S. H., Nadeem, E., Escudero, P., & Stein, B. D. (2008). Providing evidence-based practice to ethnically diverse youths: Examples from the Cognitive Behavioral Intervention for Trauma in Schools (CBITS) program. *Journal of the American Academy of Child and Adolescent Psychiatry, 47*(8), 858–862. https://doi.org/10.1097/CHI.0b013e3181799f19

No Child Left Behind Act [NCLB], Pub. L. No. 107-110. (2001). https://www.gpo.gov/fdsys/pkg/PLAW-107publ110/html/PLAW-107publ110.htm

Office of the Surgeon General. (1999). *Mental health: A report of the Surgeon General*. Rockville, MD: Department of Health and Human Services, U.S. Public Health Service.

Office of the Surgeon General. (2000). *Report of the Surgeon General's Conference on Children's Mental Health: A national action agenda*. Washington, DC: US Department of Health and Human Services. http://www.ncbi.nlm.nih.gov/bookshelf/br.fcgi?book=mhch

Osher, D., & Hanley, T. V. (1996). Implications of the national agenda to improve results for children and youth with or at risk of serious emotional disturbance. *Special Services in the Schools, 10*(2), 7–36. https://doi.org/10.1300/J008v10n02_02

Ouellette, P. M., Briscoe, R., & Tyson, C. (2004). Parent-school and community partnerships in children's mental health: Networking challenges, dilemmas, and solutions. *Journal of Child and Family Studies, 13*(3), 295–308. https://doi.org/10.1023/B:JCFS.0000022036.44808.ad

Owens, J. S., & Murphy, C. E. (2004). Effectiveness research in the context of school-based mental health. *Clinical Child and Family Psychology Review, 7*(4), 195–209. https://doi.org/10.1007/s10567-004-6085-x

Perou, R., Bitsko, R. H., Blumberg, S. J., Pastor, P., Ghandour, R. M., Gfroerer, J. C., … Huang, L. N. (2013). Mental health surveillance among children: United States, 2005-2011. *Morbidity and Mortality Weekly Report. Surveillance Summaries, 62*(Suppl 2), 1–35.

President's Commission on Excellence in Special Education. (2002). *A new era: Revitalizing special education for children and their families*. Washington, DC: U.S. Department of Education.

President's New Freedom Commission on Mental Health. (2003). *Achieving the promise: transforming mental health care in America: Final report* (DHHS publication no.). Rockville, MD: U. S. Department of Health and Human Services. http://www.eric.ed.gov/PDFS/ED479836.pdf

Ramos, Z., & Alegría, M. (2014). Cultural adaptation and health literacy refinement of a brief depression intervention for Latinos in a low-resource setting. *Cultural Diversity and Ethnic Minority Psychology, 20*(2), 293–301. https://doi.org/10.1037/a0035021

Reschly, D. J. (2008). School psychology paradigm shift and beyond. In A. Thomas & J. Grimes (Eds.), *Best practices in school psychology* (5th ed.). Washington, DC: National Association of School Psychologists.

Rickwood, D., Deane, F. P., Wilson, C. J., & Ciarrochi, J. (2005). Young people's help-seeking for mental health problems. *AeJAMH (Australian e-Journal for the Advancement of Mental Health), 4*(3). https://doi.org/10.5172/jamh.4.3.218

Romer, D., & McIntosh, M. (2017). The roles and perspectives of school mental health professionals in promoting adolescent mental health. In D. L. Evans, E. B. Foa, R. E. Gur, H. Hendin, C. P. O'Brien, M. E. P. Seligman, & B. T. Walsh (Eds.), *Treating and preventing adolescent mental health disorders: What we know and what we don't know: A research agenda for improving the mental health of our youth* (pp. 597–616). New York, NY: Oxford University Press.

School Mental Health Alliance. (2004). *Working together to promote learning, social-emotional competence and mental health for all children.* New York, NY, US: Columbia University.

School Safety and Mental Health Services Improvement Act [S.2513], (2018).

Short, R. J. (2003). Commentary: School psychology, context, and population-based practice. *School Psychology Review, 32*(2), 181–184.

Simon, A. E., Pastor, P. N., Reuben, C. A., Huang, L. N., & Goldstrom, I. D. (2015). Use of mental health services by children ages six to 11 with emotional or behavioral difficulties. *Psychiatric Services, 66*(9), 930–937. https://doi.org/10.1176/appi.ps.201400342

Sklarew, B., Twemlow, S. W., & Wilkinson, S. M. (2004). The school-based mourning project: A preventive intervention in the cycle of inner-city violence. In B. Sklarew, S. W. Twemlow, & S. M. Wilkinson (Eds.), *Analysts in the trenches: Streets, schools, war zones* (1st ed., pp. 195–210). Hillsdale, NJ: Analytic Press.

Soni, A. (2015, April). *Top five most costly conditions among children, ages 0–17, 2012: Estimates for the U.S. Civilian noninstitutionalized population* (Statistical brief #472). Rockville, MD. https://meps.ahrq.gov/data_files/publications/st472/stat472.shtml

Splett, J. W., Fowler, J., Weist, M. D., McDaniel, H., & Dvorsky, M. (2013). The critical role of school psychology in the school mental health movement. *Psychology in the Schools, 50*(3), 245–258. https://doi.org/10.1002/pits.21677

Stiffman, A. R., Stelk, W., Horwitz, S. M., Evans, M. E., Outlaw, F. H., & Atkins, M. (2010). A public health approach to children's mental health services: Possible solutions to current service inadequacies. *Administration and Policy in Mental Health, 37*(1–2), 120–124. https://doi.org/10.1007/s10488-009-0259-2

Sulkowski, M. L., Wingfield, R. J., Jones, D., & Alan Coulter, W. (2011). Response to intervention and interdisciplinary collaboration: Joining hands to support children's healthy development. *Journal of Applied School Psychology, 27*(2), 118–133. https://doi.org/10.1080/15377903.2011.565264

The White House. (2013, January 16). *Now is the time: The president's plan to protect our children and our communities by reducing gun violence.* Washington, D.C.: The White House. http://purl.fdlp.gov/GPO/gpo33229

U.S. Department of Education. (2018, January). *39th annual report to Congress on the Individuals with Disabilities Education Act, 2017.* Washington, DC, U.S. Department of Education. https://www2.ed.gov/about/reports/annual/osep/2017/parts-b-c/39th-arc-for-idea.pdf

U.S. Government Accountability Office. (2010, October 8). *School-based health centers: Available information on federal funding* (GAO-11-18R). Washington, DC. http://purl.fdlp.gov/GPO/gpo8486

Varjas, K., Nastasi, B. K., Moore, R. B., & Jayasena, A. (2005). Using ethnographic methods for development of culture-specific interventions. *Journal of School Psychology, 43*(3), 241–258. https://doi.org/10.1016/j.jsp.2005.04.006

Wang-Schweig, M., Kviz, F. J., Altfeld, S. J., Miller, A. M., & Miller, B. A. (2014). Building a conceptual framework to culturally adapt health promotion and prevention programs at the deep structural level. *Health Promotion Practice, 15*(4), 575–584. https://doi.org/10.1177/1524839913518176

Weist, M. D. (1997). Expanded school mental health services: A national movement in progress. In T. H. Ollendick & R. J. Prinz (Eds.), *Advances in clinical child psychology.* New York, NY: Plenum.

Weist, M. D., & Cooley-Quille, M. (2001). Advancing efforts to address youth violence involvement. *Journal of Clinical Child Psychology, 30*(2), 147–151. https://doi.org/10.1207/S15374424JCCP3002_2

Weist, M. D., Lever, N. A., Bradshaw, C. P., & Sarno Owens, J. (2013). *Handbook of school mental health: Research, training, practice, and policy.* http://proxy.library.carleton.ca/login? url=http://books.scholarsportal.info/viewdoc.html?id=/ebooks/ebooks3/springer/2014-02-13/1/9781461476245

Weist, M. D., Lowie, J. A., Flaherty, L. T., & Pruitt, D. (2001). Collaboration among the education, mental health, and public health systems to promote youth mental health. *Psychiatric Services, 52*(10), 1348–1351. https://doi.org/10.1176/appi.ps.52.10.1348

Weist, M. D., Myers, C. P., Hastings, E., Ghuman, H., & Han, Y. L. (1999). Psychosocial functioning of youth receiving mental health services in the schools versus community mental health centers. *Community Mental Health Journal, 35*(1), 69–81. https://doi.org/10.1023/A:10 18700126364

Weist, M. D., Sander, M. A., Walrath, C., Link, B., Nabors, L., Adelsheim, S., … Carrillo, K. (2005). Developing principles for best practice in expanded school mental health. *Journal of Youth and Adolescence, 34*(1), 7–13. https://doi.org/10.1007/s10964-005-1331-1

Windle, C., & Woy, J. R. (1983). From programs to systems: Implications for program evaluation illustrated by the community mental health centers program experience. *Evaluation and Program Planning, 6*(1), 53–68. https://doi.org/10.1016/0149-7189(83)90045-9

Witmer, H. L. (1940). *Psychiatric clinics for children.* New York, NY: Commonwealth Fund.

Zirkelback, E. A., & Reese, R. J. (2010). A review of psychotherapy outcome research: Considerations for school-based mental health providers. *Psychology in the Schools, 47*(10), 1084–1100. https://doi.org/10.1002/pits.20526

Behavioral Health and the Juvenile Justice System

Richard Dembo, Jessica Faber, Jennifer Cristiano, Ralph J. DiClemente, and Asha Terminello

Introduction

Adolescents' involvement in the juvenile justice system represents a significant public health problem. Annually, over a one million youth under the age of 18 are arrested in the United States (Office of Juvenile Justice and Delinquency Prevention, 2014), with most cases disposed in juvenile courts annually (Furdella & Puzzanchera, 2015). Of those cases, more than a quarter involve females. In 2013, juveniles younger than age 16 at the time of referral to court accounted for 53% of all delinquency cases handled.

Approximately 83% of all delinquency cases referred to juvenile court are made by law enforcement (Sickmund & Puzzanchera, 2015). In most states, the juvenile court has jurisdiction over all youth younger than age 18 who were charged with a violation of the law at the time of the offense, arrest, or referral to court. Once a juvenile is adjudicated delinquent in juvenile court, the probation staff develop a disposition plan which takes into account available support systems and programs, as well as existing assessments conducted on the youth, and may include additional

The original version of this chapter was revised. The correction to this chapter is available at https://doi.org/10.1007/978-3-030-18435-3_18

R. Dembo (✉)
Criminology Department, University of South Florida, Tampa, FL, USA
e-mail: dembo@usf.edu

J. Faber · J. Cristiano · A. Terminello
Agency for Community Treatment Services, Inc., Tampa, FL, USA

R. J. DiClemente
Emory University, Atlanta, GA, USA

New York University, New York, NY, USA

© Springer Nature Switzerland AG 2020
B. L. Levin, A. Hanson (eds.), *Foundations of Behavioral Health*,
https://doi.org/10.1007/978-3-030-18435-3_8

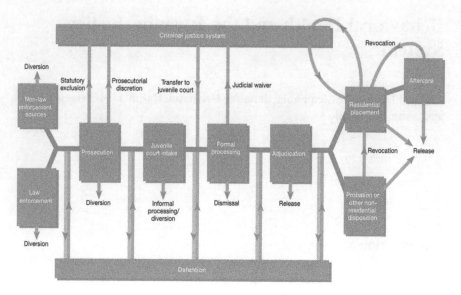

Fig. 1 Stages of delinquency case processing in the juvenile justice system (Sickmund & Puzzanchera, 2015)

psychological evaluations or diagnostic tests (Fig. 1 shows the stages of delinquency case processing in the juvenile justice system).

Youth involved in the juvenile justice system experiences a disproportionate prevalence of serious mental health issues, including substance use and depression. Youths with substance use disorders are more likely to continue to offend and are less likely to spend time in employment or attending school (Sickmund & Puzzanchera, 2015). For example, Teplin et al. observed that among juvenile justice-involved youth, two-thirds of males and almost three-quarters of females met diagnostic criteria for one or more psychiatric disorders. Further, half of the males and nearly half of the females had a substance use disorder. Affective disorders were also prevalent, especially among females, 20% of whom met diagnostic criteria for a major depressive episode (Teplin, Abram, McClelland, Dulcan, & Mericle, 2002).

Youths involved with the juvenile justice system also have a high prevalence of sexually transmitted diseases (e.g., CDC, 2010; Freudenberg, 2009; Hendershot, Magnan, & Bryan, 2010; Schmiege, Levin, Broaddus, & Bryan, 2009; Teplin, Mericle, McClelland, & Abram, 2003). Involvement in sexual risk behaviors and STD acquisition are also associated with depressive symptoms among youth in the general population (e.g., Hallfors et al., 2004; Shrier, Harris, Sternberg, & Beardslee, 2001). Similar data for juvenile justice-involved youth is equivocal. Some research has observed relationships between depression and involvement in sexual risk behavior (e.g., Teplin et al., 2005); other studies have identified null findings (e.g., Chen, Stiffman, Cheng, & Dore, 1997).

Hence, the direction of association between sexual risk behaviors and depressive symptoms remains unclear. For instance, analyses of National Longitudinal Study of Adolescent Health data by Hallfors, Waller, Bauer, Ford, and Halpern (2005) indicated engaging in sexual risk behavior and drug use increased the likelihood of future depression among adolescents, especially girls, but depression itself did not predict risky sexual and drug behaviors. In an earlier study using the same data source, however, Shrier et al. (2001) reported depressive symptoms predicted sexual risk behaviors (lack of condom use) and STD infection among boys, but not among girls (see also, Lehrer, Shrier, Gortmaker, & Buka, 2006; Shrier, Harris, & Beardslee, 2002). More research is needed to clarify the association between sexual risk behavior and depression.

Research has also linked marijuana and other drug use with mental health problems among adolescents (e.g., Bovasso, 2001; Chen, Wagner, & Anthony, 2002; McGee, Williams, Poulton, & Moffitt, 2000), including depression (Rao, 2006) and other mental disorders (Brook, Zhang, Rubenstone, Primack, & Brook, 2016). For example, in a longitudinal study of adolescents, Horwood et al. (2012) found increased frequency of marijuana use was related to more symptoms of anxiety and depression, with the association declining in adulthood. Patton et al. (2002) also examined longitudinal data on marijuana use and mental health problems from adolescence into adulthood. Their results indicated the prevalence of depression and anxiety increased with increased use of marijuana, with the effects being most prominent for females; females using cannabis daily had a fivefold greater increase in the odds of experiencing anxiety and depression. Studies of justice-involved youth have also identified comorbidity in marijuana use and depression (e.g., Abram, Teplin, McClelland, & Dulcan, 2003; Stein et al., 2011).

Informed by the above reported research, providing sexual disease and related health screening with indicated service follow-up to youth entering the juvenile justice system is urgently needed for several reasons. First, sexually transmitted diseases, such as chlamydia and gonorrhea, are asymptomatic and, if left untreated, can have profound adverse medical consequences. Second, most youths following arrest are released back to the community, not placed in secure detention. Statistics indicate approximately 80% of arrested youths are not detained (Snyder & Sickmund, 2006). Arrested youths whose sexual disease infections are not identified and treated are at risk of becoming "core transmitters" of STDs upon their return to the community (Office of National Drug Control Policy, 2016). Further, urban factors, such as income inequalities, education, and per capita income, also may affect core transmitters adversely since these factors are well-known barriers to treatment and service utilization (Patterson-Lomba, Goldstein, Gómez-Liévano, Castillo-Chavez, & Towers, 2015). Third, it is cost-effective to provide medical treatment to infected youth at the early stages of disease rather than after the diseases have developed into more serious medical conditions.

The purpose of this chapter is to describe a case study conducted within an innovative juvenile assessment facility that examined the relationships among depression, age, race/ethnicity, age at first arrest, drug involvement, and sexual behaviors among youth in the criminal justice system. After a thorough discussion of the results, we consider larger service and practice implications.

Serving Youth Within the Juvenile Justice System: The Juvenile Assessment Center (JAC)

Brief History of JACs

Following a 15-month development period involving extensive discussions and collaboration with various community stakeholders, the first JAC was established in Hillsborough County (Tampa), Florida, in 1993 (Dembo & Brown, 1994). Funds for the JAC were obtained via competition from the Drug Abuse Act of 1998 (Byrne Grant) Funds. The Tampa JAC opened its doors to truant youth in January 1993; in May 1993, the JAC began accepting youth arrested on felony, and weapons misdemeanor, charges. In July 1994, the JAC opened its doors to all arrested youth.

In June 1993, a special session of the Florida Legislature was held to address the issue of prison overcrowding. Prior to this special session, the head of the Florida House of Representatives, Appropriations Committee, visited the Tampa JAC with his wife. Impressed with the center, he was instrumental in including $1.2 million in the special appropriations budget, resulting from this special session, to establish three additional JACs. In 1994, the Florida Legislature established the Florida Department of Juvenile Justice and added an additional $two million to the budget to set up eight more JACs in the state.

In the mid to late 1990s, word about the Tampa and other Florida JACs (e.g., Orlando, Tallahassee) spread, and several other states expressed an interest in opening similar facilities in their jurisdictions (e.g., Colorado and Kansas). In contrast to Colorado, where JACs were established in a number of different counties, the Kansas Legislature included these programs as part of the Kansas Youth Authority that was established in 1997. Following this early period, JACs spread throughout the United States. In 2003, there were approximately 60 operating JACs in the United States, the last date for which we have these data. Currently, there are 18 operating JACs in Florida.

In 1995, the Office of Juvenile Justice and Delinquency Prevention (OJJDP) became interested in the concept and held a focus group meeting to review the potential of JACs to serve at-risk youth around the United States. The Florida experience was an important component of this discussion. Although positive about the JAC concept, the group expressed concern over their "net widening" potential, overrepresentation of minorities, and the limited knowledge about the level and type of community support needed for JACs to succeed (OJJDP, 1995; Oldenettel & Wordes, 2000). In response to these issues, OJJDP sponsored a fact-finding study conducted by Roberta Cronin. Ms. Cronin's effort involved visiting a number of JACs as well as a mail survey of juvenile justice and youth service personnel nationally and extensive telephone networking (Cronin, 1996).

Based on the results of Cronin's inquiry (1996), OJJDP established a Community Assessment Center (CAC) initiative in 1996 to explore the usefulness of the concept. The CAC demonstration effort involved funding several communities. Denver, Colorado, and Lee County, Florida, were designated "planning sites" and received funds to develop new CACs. Jefferson County, Colorado, and Orlando, Florida, were designated "enhancement sites," in which funds were to be used to improve their current assessment centers.

In the mid-1990s, the Center for Substance Abuse Treatment (CSAT) also became interested in JACs as an effective approach to intervene with juvenile offenders with drug abuse problems. CSAT commissioned James Rivers to complete a report on JACs. Rivers (1997) visited five JACs: (1) Orlando, Florida; (2) Tallahassee, Florida; (3) Tampa, Florida; (4) Golden, Colorado; and (5) Olathe, Kansas (serving Orlando, Leon, Hillsborough, Jefferson, and Johnson Counties, respectively). He also reviewed available reports and statistics. In his report, Rivers concluded that funding JACs could make a contribution to the mission of CSAT, particularly in the area of knowledge development.

Key Elements of JACs

Although JACs may differ in a number of ways (e.g., organizational structures, staffing patterns, operating schedules), they generally share a number of common elements (also see Oldenettel & Wordes, 2000):

1. *Single point of entry:* There is a 24-h centralized point of intake and screening for juveniles who have come or are likely to come into contact with the juvenile justice system.
2. *Immediate and comprehensive screening:* Service providers associated with the JAC make an initial broad-based screening, followed, if necessary, by a later, in-depth assessment of youths' circumstances and treatment needs.
3. *Management information systems:* Needed to manage and monitor youth, they help to ensure the provision of appropriate treatment services and to avoid the duplication of services.
4. *Integrated case management services:* JAC staff use information obtained from the screening process, and the management information systems, to develop recommendations to improve access to services, to complete follow-ups of referred youth, and to periodically reassess youth placed in various services.

Health Coach Services

The Health Coach service is housed at a JAC located in a southeastern US city, where all arrested youth are brought for justice system processing, psychosocial screening, and determination of release status (e.g., secure detention, home arrest, recommended for placement in a diversion program) (Dembo, DiClemente, & Brown, 2015). The JAC meets statutory requirements, as well as identifies and responds to the results of psychosocial screening indicating a need for follow-up evaluation and services (Dembo & Brown, 1994; Dembo & Walters, 2012).

Health Coaches are Department of Health (DOH)-trained, undergraduate degree holders working under the direction of a project manager. Health Coaches are selected based on their ability to interact with youth and to nonjudgmentally discuss sexual behavior issues. They are on duty 11 a.m. to midnight, Monday to Friday, during which period most youths enter the JAC and are on call on weekends to serve JAC-processed youth.

County Sheriff Office detention deputies operate the secure wing at the JAC. In addition to providing for facility security, deputies complete a booking process for each youth that occurs immediately after youth enter the JAC secure wing, which includes the collection of basic demographic and contact information (e.g., address), electronic fingerprints, and a photograph. After this required process, each youth is approached by a Health Coach and invited to participate in the new service.

Each youth is informed the Health Coach service will involve the following information gathering and service activities: (1) sociodemographic (e.g., age, living arrangement); (2) alcohol and other substance use (Texas Christian University Drug Screen V (Institute of Behavioral Research, 2014)) as well as collecting a urine specimen for substance use analysis; (3) split testing of the urine specimen for STD testing (i.e., chlamydia and gonorrhea) with free confidential follow-up treatment by the DOH if indicated; (4) screening for HIV, with follow-up, DOH confirmatory testing and treatment; (5) completion of a screen to identify a need for hepatitis C testing and treatment of all positive youth is available; (6) sexual behavior; (7) depression (Melchior, Huba, Brown, & Reback, 1993); (8) linking youth with a primary healthcare physician, if they do not have one, at a local family healthcare center; (9) completion of an online sexually transmitted disease risk-reduction intervention; (10) follow-up phone calls by Health Coaches to monitor their health behavior and need for additional services; and (11) randomly selected youth will receive a 6-month follow-up assessment. Youths testing positive for any drug or with an elevated depression score (7+) are promptly referred to an on-site therapist for follow-up care. Each participating youth is informed he/she will be eligible for one of five $100 gift cards to be determined before Christmas each year.

Male and female youths interested in receiving Health Coach services complete a consent form and receive Health Coach pre-counseling. The DOH has trained the Health Coaches to administer health department standard pre- and post-counseling to youth, as well as follow other department protocols, such as post-JAC contact procedures.

STD Risk-Reduction Interventions

Gender-specific interventions are planned for use among youth receiving Health Coach services. Intervention videos are in multimedia, digital format. The female video, Horizons, based on social cognitive theory and the theory of gender and power, is a CDC evidence-based intervention designed to reduce sexually transmitted diseases (STDs), increase condom use, increase communication with male partners about safer sex and STDs, and increase male partners accessing STD services (DiClemente et al., 2009). Initially developed for use among heterosexually active African American adolescent girls, it has been adapted for use among diverse cultural groups of girls. The male STD risk-reduction intervention video, designed for use among diverse cultural groups, is currently in development. It is based on information collected in focus group discussions with behavioral health agency clients in treatment. A shortened version of each intervention video is planned for viewing on laptops while the youth is at the JAC, with a full-length version of the video being accessible via the Internet following release.

Community Collaborating Agencies

Collaborating community-based family health centers are key partners in this new service system. The Tampa Family Health Centers receive referrals from the DOH and JAC-based Health Coaches. Health Coach referrals are made to a designated family health center staff member, who contacts the youth and assigns her/him to a health center near their home. (The Tampa Family Health Centers are federally recognized and funded to provide services to low-income families.)

Health Coach Service MIS

Referral, treatment engagement), retention, and service outcome (e.g., treatment received) information are shared with the Health Coaches for inclusion in a comprehensive medical information system (MIS established for this new service, which includes the information described earlier. With the routine collection of individual data (e.g., drug use, STD and HIV status) and community-level data (e.g., increases in medical services delivered to youth in family health centers located in zip codes where JAC-processed Health Coach youths are heavily concentrated), the MIS will permit the study of multilevel outcomes).

Case Study

This case study involving arrested youth entering JAC Health Coach services explored the relationship between depression and age, race/ethnicity, age at first arrest, reported past year drug involvement, reported number of sexual partners, and biological data on the youth's marijuana use and sexually transmitted diseases (chlamydia and gonorrhea). Based on previous research (Dembo, Belenko, Childs, & Wareham, 2009), it was expected that (1) female youth level of depression would be higher, than that of males; (2) female rates of sexually transmitted diseases would be greater than that of male youth; and (3) male and female youth would experience multiple, overlapping behavioral health issues, with females being more affected by these issues than males. Following a psychometric assessment of the depression measure across the male and female youth groups, a cross gender, multigroup regression analysis was performed to examine these empirical expectations.

Project Setting: JAC Health Coach Service

The Health Coach data used in this study were collected in the innovative, comprehensive health service for youth entering the JAC, described earlier. Given the disproportionate risk of STD and HIV among girls (CDC, 2013, 2015; Dembo et al., 2009), Health Coach services initially focused on this gender group. However, on February 4, 2016, the service was expanded to include boys. Participation in the service is voluntary. The data were routinely collected by Health Coaches from the youth clients they served. The Health Coaches were trained to follow a data collection and service delivery protocol, and their data entry was monitored for integrity and quality by the program manager (a co-author of this paper).

Following informed consent, 241 females and 102 males received Health Coach services from October 19, 2015 (project implementation date), through March 21, 2016 (Florida Public Health law does not require youth 12 years and over to obtain parental consent for STD or HIV testing or treatment). Among male and female youth approached to participate in this voluntary service, 57% of males and 75% of females agreed. Sociodemographic information (age, race/ethnicity), and data on age at first arrest, and post-JAC placement (secure detention, home detention, outright release) were available for all youth declining Health Coach services. Comparison of youth participating or declining to participate in Health Coach services identified only one significant difference between them: participating youth were slightly older than nonparticipating youth (15.5 vs 15.8, respectively, $p < 0.05$). (Due to space concerns, detailed results are not presented. A copy of the results can be obtained from the senior author upon request.)

Measures

The data the authors collected came from a number of sources and were important in understanding empirical and correlational relationships among the youth being served in the JAC and the factors (e.g., sociodemographic, drug use, at-risk sexual behaviors, and depression) that may contribute to their current involvement with the juvenile justice system. As shown in the literature, low rates of engagement in mental health services are found for juveniles subsequent to their first contact with juvenile justice (Burke, Mulvey, & Schubert, 2015).

SocioDemographic Characteristics

Several demographic characteristics on the youth were used in this study: (1) age (in number of years), (2) gender (0 = male; 1 = female), and (3) information on the youths' race/ethnicity (described in more detail in the results section) which was coded as race (1 = African American; 0 = other race) and ethnicity (1 = Hispanic; 0 = non-Hispanic).

Age at First Arrest

Drawing on the literature indicating early contact with law enforcement resulting in arrest is associated with long-term problem behavior outcomes (Farrington & Hawkins, 1991; Farrington, Ttofi, & Coid, 2009; Moffitt, 1993), we included a measure of age of first arrest for the youths in this case study. These data were obtained from official records.

Drug Use

Measuring drug use using self-report and drug screen measures allows us to appropriately estimate the amount of use by the youth electing to participate in the Health Coach program. Geared to DSM-V criteria, the *TCUDS V (TCU Drug Screen V)* (TCU Institute of Behavioral Research, 2014) is a detailed, self-report instrument probing use of various drugs and consequences of use during the 12 months prior to JAC entry. Responses to this instrument are scored to produce a single total score ranging from 0 to 11, which is, then, converted to three severity categories corresponding to DSM-5 criteria: 1 = mild disorder, score of 2–3 points (presence of 2–3 symptoms); 2 = moderate disorder, score of 4–5 points (presence of 4–5 symptoms); and 3 = severe disorder, score of 6 or more points (presence of 6 or more symptoms). In addition, we added another "severity" category, corresponding to the presence of fewer than 2 points: 0 = no disorder.

Youth also agreed to drug screens. At the DOH testing lab, the urine specimens were split with half the specimen being tested for the following seven drugs using the EMIT procedure: (1) methamphetamines, (2) cocaine, (3) opiates, (4) marijuana, (5) spice (UR144 metabolite), (6) alcohol (4 days use), and (7) benzodiazepines. Few youths were found to be drug positive for any drug other than marijuana (range 0% to 3%); hence, these drugs were excluded from further analysis. The cutoff level for a positive for marijuana is 50 ng/ml of urine. The UA results for marijuana were dichotomized (0 = negative, 1 = positive) for analysis.

STD Status

A noninvasive, FDA-approved, urine-based nucleic acid test, Gen-Probe APTIMA Combo 2 Assay, was used to test for chlamydia and gonorrhea in the second half of the split urine specimen. The sensitivity of Gen-Probe's test has been shown to be superior to culture and direct specimen tests. For chlamydia, the sensitivity and specificity of the Gen-Probe urine-based test are 95.9% and 98.2%, respectively, and for gonorrhea, they are 97.8% and 98.9%, respectively (Chacko, Barnes, Wiemann, & DiClemente, 2004). For analysis purposes, each youth's STD results were recoded into a dichotomous variable representing positive (coded as 1) for any STD (i.e., chlamydia, gonorrhea, or both) or negative (coded as 0) for both STDs. While a more detailed breakdown of the youth's specific STDs is given in the results section, it is important to note that Florida STD rates are quite high among male and female youth. Florida DOH data indicate males aged 10–19 accounted for 17% of all male recorded STDs and females aged 10–19 accounted for 33% of all female STDs, in 2012 (the latest year for which these data are available; www.floridahealth. gov accessed April 14, 2016).

Lifetime Number of Sexual Partners

Number of sexual partners is widely used as a sexual risk behavior measure (e.g., Komro, Tobler, Maldonado-Molina, & Perry, 2010). We selected a question from the high school version of the Centers for Disease Control and Prevention, Youth Risk Behavior Survey (2015), to measure the youths' number of sexual partners. The question asked of each youth was: During your life, with how many people have you had sexual intercourse? Response choices were the following: A. I have never had sexual intercourse; B. 1 person; C. 2 people; D. 3 people; E. 4 people; F. 5 people; or G. 6 or more people.

Depression

We used the 8-item, shortened version of the widely used 20-item Center for Epidemiological Studies Depression Scale (CES-D) (Radloff, 1977). The 8-item measure resulted from the psychometric work of Melchior et al. (1993), in which they found the 8-item CES-D correlated 0.93 with the full 20-item CES-D. The following items were used: '(1) I felt I could not shake off the blues even with the help from my family and friends; (2) I felt sad; (3) I felt depressed; (4) I thought my life had been a failure; (5) I felt fearful; (6) My sleep was restless; (7) I felt lonely; and (8) I had crying spells (time frames, the past week). Each item was scored as follows: 0 = less than 1 day, 1 = 1–2 days, 2 = 3–4 days, and 3 = 5–7 days. Although the 8-item measure was originally developed among a community sample of women, we wished to assess its usefulness among female and male youth receiving Health Coach services.

Data Analysis

The analyses proceeded in several stages. First, descriptive comparisons were made between male and female youth on the variables analyzed in this study. Second, a confirmatory factor analysis (CFA) was performed in the depression items to determine if their psychometric properties were the same for both gender groups. Third, a regression analysis was completed to determine the significant predictors of the male and female youths' depression involving the above discussed variables. Steps 2 and 3 involved multigroup analysis.

Since we have complete data in the depression measure for the youths, missing data on the predictor variables can be considered as missing at random (Enders, 2010). The depression CFA and regression analyses were performed using Mplus Version 7.4 (Muthèn & Muthèn, 1998–2012).

Results

Descriptive Statistics and Variable Comparisons Across Gender Groups

Most of the youths were female (70%). Female youth averaged 15.2 (SD = 1.46), and the males averaged 16.1 (SD = 0.85) years in age. This difference was, in part, a consequence of the decision to provide Health Coach services to older adolescent males, aged 15–17, who are at greater risk of contracting sexually transmitted diseases (CDC, 2012, 2014a, 2014b, 2014c), than younger males. The youth were racially and ethnically diverse. A majority of male (69.9%) and female (52.3%) youth were African American, but sizable percentages of Hispanic and Anglo youth are represented in the study, as Table 1 shows.

Age at first arrest was similar for the male and female youth. The average age was 14 years for each gender group.

The TCU drug screen results indicated most males (87%) and females (78%) were in the no drug use group. However, more females than males were in the mild and moderate severity groups. Similar percentages of both gender groups were in the severe drug use category.

As noted earlier, few youths were UA positive for methamphetamines, cocaine, opiates, spice (UR144 metabolite), alcohol, or benzodiazepines. However, among tested male and female youth, 74% of the males and 36% of the females were drug positive for marijuana.

Table 1 Male and female comparison covariates

	Male (n = 90–102)	Female (n = 192–241)	Significance
Sociodemographic:			
Age	16.1 (SD = 0.845)	15.2 (SD = 1.464)	N.S.
Ethnicity/race			
African American	69.9%	52.3%	
Hispanic	10.8%	16.2%	p < 0.05
Anglo	19.6%	30.7%	
Others	–	0.8%	
	100.0%	100.0%	
Risk/problem factors:			
Age at first arrest	14.02 (SD = 2.243)	14.35 (SD = 1.773)	
Depression (mean)	2.81 (SD = 5.308)	5.20 (SD = 6.350)	p < 0.001
Depression of 7 or more	14.7%	30.7%	p < 0.001
UA marijuana positive	74.4%	35.7%	p < 0.001
TCU drug severity category			
None	87.3%	77.6%	
Mild	5.9%	10.8%	N.S.
Moderate	1.0%	6.6%	
Severe	4.9%	5.0%	
	100.0%	100.0%	
Number of sexual partners (lifetime) mean	3.99 (SD = 2.150)	1.77 (SD = 1.913)	p < 0.001
STD positive	8.4%	14.6%	N.S

In regard to STD status, 15% of females and 8% of males were positive for chlamydia or gonorrhea or both STDs. The prevalence of chlamydia among females (11.8%) was nearly double that for males (6.2%). The observed STD prevalence is markedly higher than found among youth aged 10–19 in the general Hillsborough County population. In 2014, for example, 1.8% of females, compared to 0.4% of males, were diagnosed with chlamydia; and 0.2% of females, versus 0.1% of males, were diagnosed with gonorrhea (Florida Department of Health in Hillsborough County, private communication on 4/11/2016).

Number of sexual partners also differed between the two gender groups. Females reported 1.77 lifetime partners compared to 3.99 partners for males, with 43% of the males, compared to 8% of the females, reporting 6+ lifetime sexual partners. Thirty-five percent of the females, versus 7% of the males, reported no sexual partners. Comparison of these results with findings reported in the Centers for Disease Control and Prevention's 2013 Youth Risk Behavior Surveillance System ([YRBSS] CDC, 2014a, 2014b, 2014c) indicates a much higher rate of ever having had sexual intercourse among youths in the present study (73%), than that reported by youths in the YRBSS nationally (47%) or in Florida (overall, 44%).

Many youth reported depressive symptomatology. Overall, females had a CES-D summary score of 5.20, compared to 2.81 for the males (F = 11.14, df = 1341, $p < 0.001$). Importantly, 31% of females, versus 15% of males, had a depression score of seven or higher (the designated threshold score), a level indicative of potentially needing clinical intervention (Brown et al., 2014; Santor & Coyne, 1997).

Confirmatory Factor Analysis (CFA) of the Depression Items

A multigroup, male-female, one-factor CFA involving Mplus version 7.4 (Muthèn & Muthèn, 1998–2012) was conducted on the eight depression items, using WLSMV estimation. Specification involved equal factor loadings and thresholds. Results indicated a less than acceptable fit of the model to the data (chi-square = 86.695, df = 62, $p = 0.029$, RMSEA = 0.048, CFI = 0.997, TLI = 0.997). A modification index review indicated model fit could be improved by freeing the thresholds for the item "I felt lonely." When this adjustment was made, a good, partial invariant model fit was obtained (chi-square = 74.346, df = 59, $p = 0.086$, RMSEA = 0.038, CFI = 0.998, TLI = 0.998) across the two gender groups. (Due to space concerns, detailed results are not presented. A copy of the results can be obtained from the senior author upon request.)

Predictors of Depression Among Female and Male Youth

Among males, sparse numbers of cases in some predictor variable cells (e.g., 7 with STD-positive results), as well as missing data on predictor variables, precluded meaningful multigroup regression model analysis using Bayesian or WLSMV estimation. Instead, we decided to use an overall measure of depression, involving the sum of responses across the eight items. The scores ranged from 0 to 24. The overall, summed measure had acceptable skewness (1.32) and kurtosis values (0.619) (Fabrigar, Wegener, MacCallum, & Strahan, 1999). Further, the summed depression measure was highly correlated with the depression latent variable resulting from the CFA of the eight items ($r = 0.905$).

The results of the multigroup (gender) regression analysis are presented in Table 2. For males a significant positive relationship was observed between age and depression, and a significant negative relationship was found between number of sexual partners and depression. Among females, significant positive relationships were found between TCU level of drug use severity, and number of reported sexual partners, and depression.

Table 2 Maximum likelihood regression (MLR) of depression score on covariate predictors among male ($n = 83$) and female ($n = 187$) youth (unstandardized estimates)

	Males			Females		
	Estimate	S.E.	Critical ratio	Estimate	S.E.	Critical ratio
Depression on						
Age	1.548	0.596	2.597**	0.375	0.365	1.029
African American (=1)	−0.030	1.373	−0.022	−2.093	1.049	−1.995*
Hispanic (=1)	1.141	2.278	0.501	−0.273	1.436	−0.190
Age at first arrest	−0.019	0.289	−0.065	−0.026	0.255	−0.105
TCU drug involvement level	1.354	1.301	1.041	1.154	0.551	2.094*
# of sexual partners (lifetime)	−0.620	0.284	−2.181*	0.830	0.302	2.747**
STD status (positive =1)	0.713	1.742	0.409	−1.680	1.276	−1.317
UA marijuana result (positive =1)	−1.776	1.351	−1.314	−1.050	0.985	−1.066
Intercept for depression	−18.783	9.812	−1.914	−0.093	4.969	−0.019
Residual variance for depression	23.107	5.566	4.152***	35.176	3.975	8.850***
***R^2	0.161	0.076	2.119*	0.137	0.046	2.949**

Two-tailed p-values: *$p > 0.05$; **$p < 0.01$; ***$p < 0.001$

Discussion

This case study examined the relationship between depression and age, race/ethnicity, age at first arrest, severity of reported past year drug involvement, reported number of sexual partners, and biological data on the youth's marijuana use and sexually transmitted diseases (chlamydia and gonorrhea). The case study and data analyses were informed by several research questions. Question 1, female youth level of depression would be higher than that of males. Prior to answering this question, the authors conduced CFA analyses to assess if the depression measures were invariant across the male and female youth. The authors found the eight-item depression measure was partially invariant across the gender groups. Based on these results, the authors compared the mean depression scores across the gender groups and found, consistent with previous studies on depression among youth, that females had significantly higher depression scores than the males (e.g., Lehrer et al., 2006; Shrier et al., 2001, 2002). In addition, a significantly larger percent of females, than males, had an CES-D summary score above the threshold of seven.

Question 2, informing this case study related to our expectation, based on the research reported earlier, that the prevalence of sexually transmitted diseases would be higher among females than males. This was the case, with the prevalence of STD among females (15%) being almost twice that observed among males (8%).

Our third expectation, reflected in research question 3, was that male and female youth would experience multiple, overlapping behavioral health issues, with females being more impacted by these issues. To address this question, we conducted a cross gender, multigroup maximum likelihood regression analysis. The results of the regression analysis highlighted, among male youth, a significant positive relationship between age and depression and a significant negative relationship between reported number of sexual partners and depression.

In contrast, among females (1) a significant negative relationship was found between depression and being African American, and (2) significant positive relationships were found between reported number of sexual partners and depression and between TCU drug involvement level and depression, with females having more serious levels of drug involvement reporting a higher level of depression. These results provide evidence of behavioral health differences between the two gender groups and highlight that females are more adversely impacted. In particular, a larger number of sexual partners among males seem to enhance their sense of well-being, while the opposite is the case among females.

Another interesting finding in our analysis is that females who are non-African American (mainly Anglo) have higher depression scores, than African American girls. This finding can, perhaps, be explained by the concept of relative deviance (Dembo & Shern, 1982). According to this view, youths who are "deviant" from the norms of their social and cultural setting are more likely to be involved in problem behavior than youths who follow these norms. Since Anglo youth are less likely to enter the juvenile justice system, those that do are more likely to be experiencing emotional/psychological issues. Future research should explore this relationship, particularly among other at-risk racial/ethnic populations.

Our results highlight that screening for depression at intake into the juvenile justice system is important, especially among females. Youth with elevated depression should be linked promptly with additional evaluative and clinical services. This is an ongoing component of the Health Coach service, with all youth having depression scores of seven or higher being referred to an on-site therapist for further evaluation. Relatedly, intervention programs should be aware of possible differential gender group effects of drug use and having multiple sexual partners on youth depression.

A particular strength of the Health Coach project is its use of biological markers to assess STDs and drug use. Studies on the topic of this chapter among justice-involved youth often rely on self-report data, which often reflect social desirability biases yielding systematic underreporting (Dembo et al., 1999).

There are several limitations to our research. First, it is important to note that the regression analysis was conducted on cross-sectional data. Hence, no causal interpretations of our findings are possible. Second, the results of the study may not generalize to male and female youth arrested in other jurisdictions, reflecting different sociodemographic circumstances. Third, the data on number of sexual partners and depression, although reflecting relationships that are consistent with other studies noted earlier, were based on self-reports.

The results of this case study indicate there is a crucial need to provide quality behavioral health and public health screening assessment of youth entering the justice system, with special attention to females who bear a greater burden of these problems. Implementing interventions targeting substance use, depression, and sexual risk behavior is needed to help these youths, who often lack access to quality health services, engage in healthier behavior and avoid adverse outcomes such as HIV/AIDS.

Implications for Behavioral Health

This case study results document the serious need for front-end, juvenile justice intake facilities to provide behavioral and public health screening and treatment follow-up on newly arrested youth. These youths represent the high-risk end of the community, and most arrested youths are soon returned to the community (in our case study, 70% were placed on nonsecure home detention or released outright). This service need is reflected, for example, in the high urine tested prevalence rate for marijuana, the high STD prevalence rates, and the high level of depression among these youths.

The authors found gender differences in behavioral health and public health needs among the youth. Female youth had a higher prevalence rates for STDs, than males. A higher percentage of males tested positive for recent marijuana use than females. Further, higher percentage of females scored 7+ on our evidence-based depression measure, than the males. And, as discussed earlier, multigroup regression analysis highlighted male and female youth experience multiple, overlapping behavioral health issues, with females being more impacted by these issues.

JACs, or similar centralized intake facilities, are ideal places to conduct these screening and service linkage activities. They can serve as a critical community resource to identify and respond to the service needs of arrested youth, whose families often lack the resources to access these services on their own.

Vision for the Future

The authors plan to continue current efforts to serve as a public health monitoring station. Our efforts include (1) collaboration with the University of Maryland's Community Drug Early Warning System project to identify new drugs of abuse and include testing for new metabolites in our UA testing protocol, as the authors have done for the synthetic spice metabolite UR-144 (Wish, Billing, & Artigiani, 2015) and (2) collaboration with other scientists to identify, test, and evaluate the efficacy and feasibility of collecting microbiological markers to assess depression.

The authors are currently working with other jurisdictions in Florida to expand the Health Coach service model the authors have implemented; hopefully, out-of-state jurisdictions will be interested in adopting this service as well. The authors plan to provide training and implementation support to requesting jurisdictions, so they can better identify and address the behavioral and public health needs of justice-involved youth.

Acknowledgments The authors are grateful for the support of the Florida Department of Children and Families and the Central Florida Behavioral Care Network and thank Ms. Julie Krupa for helping in preparing the tables for this manuscript and editing the references.

References

Abram, K. M., Teplin, L. A., McClelland, G. M., & Dulcan, M. K. (2003). Comorbid psychiatric disorders in youth in juvenile detention. *Archives of General Psychiatry, 60*(11), 1097–1108. https://doi.org/10.1001/archpsyc.60.11.1097

Bovasso, G. (2001). Cannabis abuse as a risk factor for depressive symptoms. *American Journal of Psychiatry, 158*(12), 2033–2037. https://doi.org/10.1176/appi.ajp.158.12.2033

Brook, J. S., Zhang, C., Rubenstone, E., Primack, B. A., & Brook, D. W. (2016). Comorbid trajectories of substance use as predictors of antisocial personality disorder, major depressive episode, and generalized anxiety disorder. *Addictive Behaviors, 62*, 114–121. https://doi.org/10.1016/j.addbeh.2016.06.003

Brown, J. L., Sales, J. M., Swartzendruber, A. L., Eriksen, M. D., DiClemente, R. J., & Rose, E. S. (2014). Added benefits: Reduced depressive symptom levels among African-American female adolescents participating in an HIV prevention intervention. *Journal of Behavioral Medicine, 37*(5), 912–920. https://doi.org/10.1007/s10865-013-9551-4

Burke, J. D., Mulvey, E. P., & Schubert, C. A. (2015). Prevalence of mental health problems and service use among first-time juvenile offenders. *Journal of Child and Family Studies, 24*(12), 3774–3781. https://doi.org/10.1007/s10826-015-0185-8

Centers for Disease Control and Prevention (CDC). (2010). *STDs in persons entering corrections facilities*. Retrieved from http://www.cdc.gov/std/stats10/corrections.htm. Accessed 7/24/2015.

Centers for Disease Control and Prevention (CDC). (2012). Estimated HIV incidence in the United States, 2007–2010. *HIV Surveillance Supplemental Report, 17*(4), 1–26. Retrieved from http://www.cdc.gov/hiv/pdf/statistics_hssr_vol_17_no_4.pdf

Centers for Disease Control and Prevention (CDC). (2013). *STDs in Adolescents and Young Adults*. Retrieved from http://www.cdc.gov/std/stats13/adol.htm. Accessed 6-4-2015.

Centers for Disease Control and Prevention (CDC). (2014a). *STDs in adolescents and young adults*. Retrieved from http://www.cdc.gov/std/stats13/adol.htm

Centers for Disease Control and Prevention (CDC). (2014b). *Sexually transmitted disease surveillance 2013*. Atlanta, GA: U.S. Department of Health and Human Services, Centers for Disease Control and Prevention.

Centers for Disease Control and Prevention (CDC). (2014c). *Youth online-high school youth risk behavior survey*. Retrieved from www.cdc.gov/yrbs

Centers for Disease Control and Prevention (CDC). (2015). *2015 State and local youth risk behavior survey*. Retrieved from ftp://ftp.cdc.gov/pub/data/yrbs/2015/2015_hs_questionnaire.pdf

Chacko, M., Barnes, C., Wiemann, C., & DiClemente, R. (2004). Implementation of urine testing for chlamydia (CT) and gonorrhea (NGC) in a community clinic. *Journal of Adolescent Health, 34*, 146–153. https://doi.org/10.1016/j.jadohealth.2003.11.041

Chen, C., Wagner, F., & Anthony, J. (2002). Marijuana use and the risk of major depressive episode: Epidemiological evidence from the United States National Comorbidity Survey. *Social Psychiatry and Psychiatric Epidemiology, 37*(5), 199–203. https://doi.org/10.1007/s00127-002-0541-z

Chen, Y.-W., Stiffman, A. R., Cheng, L.-C., & Dore, P. (1997). Mental health, social environment and sexual risk behaviors of adolescent service users: A gender comparison. *Journal of Child and Family Studies, 6*(1), 9–25. https://doi.org/10.1023/A:1025064522258

Cronin, R. (1996). *Fact-finding report on Community Assessment Centers (CACs): Final report.* Washington, DC: U. S. Department of Justice, Office of Justice Programs, Office of Juvenile Justice and Delinquency Prevention.

Dembo, R., Belenko, S., Childs, K., & Wareham, J. (2009). Drug use and sexually transmitted diseases among female and male arrested youths. *Journal of Behavioral Medicine, 32*(2), 129–141. https://doi.org/10.1007/s10865-008-9183-2

Dembo, R., & Brown, R. (1994). The Hillsborough County juvenile assessment center. *Journal of Child and Adolescent Substance Abuse, 3*(2), 25–43. https://doi.org/10.1300/J029v03n02_03

Dembo, R., Di Clemente, R. J., & Brown, R. (2015). *Health coaches: An innovative and effective approach for identifying and addressing health needs of justice involved youth.* Tampa, FL: University of South Florida, Department of Criminology.

Dembo, R., Shemwell, M., Guida, J., Schmeidler, J., Baumgartner, W., Ramirez-Garnica, G., & Seeberger, W. (1999). A comparison of self-report, urine sample, and hair sample testing for drug use: A longitudinal study. In T. Mieczkowski (Ed.), *Drug testing methods: Assessment and evaluation* (pp. 91–108). New York, NY: CRC Press.

Dembo, R., & Shern, D. (1982). Relative deviance and the process(es) of drug involvement among inner-city youths. *International Journal of the Addictions, 17*(8), 1373–1399. https://doi.org/10.3109/10826088209064069

Dembo, R., & Walters, W. (2012). Juvenile assessment centers: Early intervention with youth involved in drug use. In N. Jainchill (Ed.), *Understanding and treating adolescent substance use disorders* (pp. 15-2–15-8). Kingston, NJ: Civic Research Institute.

DiClemente, R. J., Wingood, G. M., Rose, E. S., Sales, J. M., Lang, D. L., … Crosby, R. A. (2009). Efficacy of STD/HIV sexual risk-reduction intervention for African American adolescent females seeking sexual health services: A randomized controlled trial. *Archives of Pediatrics & Adolescent Medicine, 163*(12), 1112–1121. https://doi.org/10.1001/archpediatrics.2009.205

Enders, C. K. (2010). *Applied missing data analysis.* New York, NY: Guilford Press.

Fabrigar, L. R., Wegener, D. T., MacCallum, R. C., & Strahan, E. J. (1999). Evaluating the use of exploratory factor analysis in psychological research. *Psychological Methods, 4*(3), 272–299. https://doi.org/10.1037/1082-989X.4.3.272

Farrington, D. P., & Hawkins, J. D. (1991). Predicting participation, early onset and later persistence in officially recorded offending. *Criminal Behavior and Mental Health, 1*(1), 1–33.

Farrington, D. P., Ttofi, M. M., & Coid, J. W. (2009). Development of adolescence-limited, late-onset, and persistent offenders from age 8 to age 48. *Aggressive Behavior, 35*(2), 150–163. https://doi.org/10.1002/ab.20296

Florida Department of Health in Hillsborough County. (2016). Personal communication 04/11/2016

Freudenberg, N. (2009). Incarcerated and delinquent youth. In R. J. DiClemente, J. S. Santelli, & R. A. Crosby (Eds.), *Adolescent health: Understanding and preventing risk behaviors* (pp. 339–358). San Francisco, CA: Jossey-Bass.

Furdella, J., & Puzzanchera, C. (2015). *Delinquency cases in juvenile court* (Juvenile Offenders and Victims National Report Series Fact Sheet, October). Washington, DC: OJJDP. Retrieved from http://www.ojjdp.gov/pubs/248899.pdf

Hallfors, D. D., Waller, M. W., Bauer, D., Ford, C. A., & Halpern, C. T. (2005). Which comes first in adolescence – Sex and drugs or depression? *American Journal of Preventive Medicine, 29*(3), 163–170. https://doi.org/10.1016/j.amepre.2005.06.002

Hallfors, D. D., Waller, M. W., Ford, C. A., Halpern, C. T., Brodish, P. H., & Iritani, B. (2004). Adolescent depression and suicide risk: Association with sex and drug behavior. *American Journal of Preventive Medicine, 27*(3), 224–230. https://doi.org/10.1016/j.amepre.2004.06.001

Hendershot, C. S., Magnan, R. E., & Bryan, A. D. (2010). Associations of marijuana use and sex-related marijuana expectancies with HIV/STD risk behavior in high-risk adolescents. *Psychology of Addictive Behaviors, 24*(3), 404–414. https://doi.org/10.1037/a0019844

Horwood, L. J., Fergusson, D. M., Coffey, C., Patton, G. C., Tait, R., Smart, D., … Hutchinson, D. M. (2012). Cannabis and depression: An integrative data analysis of four Australasian cohorts. *Drug and Alcohol Dependence, 126*(3), 369–378. https://doi.org/10.1016/j.drugalcdep.2012.06.002

Institute of Behavioral Research. (2014). *TCU drug screen V (TCUDS V)*. Ft. Worth, TX: Texas Christian University, Institute of Behavioral Research.

Komro, K. A., Tobler, A. L., Maldonado-Molina, M. M., & Perry, C. L. (2010). Effects of alcohol use initiation patterns on high-risk behaviors among urban, low-income, young adolescents. *Prevention Science, 11*(1), 14–23. https://doi.org/10.1007/s11121-009-0144-y

Lehrer, J. A., Shrier, L. A., Gortmaker, S., & Buka, S. (2006). Depressive symptoms as a longitudinal predictor of sexual risk behaviors among US middle and high school students. *Pediatrics, 118*(1), 189–200.

McGee, R., Williams, S., Poulton, R., & Moffitt, T. E. (2000). A longitudinal study of cannabis use and mental health from adolescence to early adulthood. *Addiction, 95*(4), 491–503. https://doi.org/10.1046/j.1360-0443.2000.9544912.x

Melchior, L. A., Huba, G. J., Brown, V. B., & Reback, C. J. (1993). A short depression index for women. *Educational and Psychological Measurement, 53*(4), 1117–1125. https://doi.org/10.1177/0013164493053004024

Moffitt, T. E. (1993). Adolescence-limited and life–course–persistent antisocial behavior: A developmental taxonomy. *Psychological Review, 100*(4), 674–701. https://doi.org/10.1037/0033-295X.100.4.674

Muthèn, L. K., & Muthèn, B. O. (1998–2012). *Mplus user's guide, 7th version*. Los Angeles, CA: Muthèn & Muthèn.

Office of Juvenile Justice and Delinquency Prevention. (1995). *Community assessment centers: A discussion of the concept's efficacy* (Issue Overview).Washington, DC: Author.

Office of Juvenile Justice and Delinquency Prevention. (2014). Law enforcement and juvenile crime. In *OJJDP statistical briefing book*. Washington, DC: OJJDP. [Web page]. Retrieved from http://www.ojjdp.gov/ojstatbb/crime/qa05101.asp?qaDate=2014

Office of National Drug Control Policy. (2016). *2016 National Drug Control Strategy*. [Web page]. Retrieved from https://obamawhitehouse.archives.gov/sites/default/files/ondcp/policy-and-research/2016_ndcs_final_report.pdf

Oldenettel, D., & Wordes, M. (2000, March). *The community assessment center concept. OJJDP Juvenile Justice Bulletin* (NCJ 178942). Washington, DC: U.S. Department of Justice, Office of Justice Programs, Office of Juvenile Justice and Delinquency Prevention.

Patterson-Lomba, O., Goldstein, E., Gómez-Liévano, A., Castillo-Chavez, C., & Towers, S. (2015). Per capita incidence of sexually transmitted infections increases systematically with urban population size: A cross-sectional study. *Sexually Transmitted Infections, 91*(8), 610–614. https://doi.org/10.1136/sextrans-2014-051932

Patton, G. C., Coffey, C., Carlin, J. B., Degenhardt, L., Lynskey, M., & Hall, W. (2002). Cannabis use and mental health in youth people: Cohort study. *The BMJ, 325*(7374), 1195–1198. https://doi.org/10.1136/bmj.325.7374.1195

Radloff, L. S. (1977). The CES-D scale: A self-report depression scale for research in the general population. *Applied Psychological Measurement, 1*(3), 385–401. https://doi.org/10.1177/014662167700100306

Rao, U. (2006). Links between depression and substance abuse in adolescents. *American Journal of Preventive Medicine, 31*(6, Suppl 1), S161–S174. https://doi.org/10.1016/j.amepre.2006.07.002

Rivers, J. (1997). *Juvenile assessment centers site visits: Executive summary and final report* (prepared for the Center for Substance Abuse Treatment). Miami, FL: University of Miami School of Medicine, Comprehensive Drug Research Center.

Santor, D. A., & Coyne, J. C. (1997). Shortening the CES-D to improve its ability to detect cases of depression. *Psychological Assessment, 9*(3), 223–243. https://doi.org/10.1037/1040-3590.9.3.233

Schmiege, S., Levin, M., Broaddus, M., & Bryan, A. (2009). Randomized trial of group interventions to reduce HIV/STD risk and change theoretical mediators among detained adolescents. *Journal of Consulting and Clinical Psychology, 77*(1), 38–50. https://doi.org/10.1037/a0014513

Shrier, L. A., Harris, S. K., & Beardslee, W. R. (2002). Temporal associations between depressive symptoms and self-reported sexually transmitted disease among adolescents. *Archives of Pediatrics & Adolescent Medicine, 156*(6), 599–606. https://doi.org/10.1001/archpedi.156.6.599

Shrier, L. A., Harris, S. K., Sternberg, M., & Beardslee, W. R. (2001). Associations of depression, self-esteem, and substance use with sexual risk among adolescents. *Preventive Medicine, 33*(3), 179–189. https://doi.org/10.1006/pmed.2001.0869

Sickmund, M., & Puzzanchera, C. (2015). *Juvenile offenders and victims: 2014 national report*. Pittsburgh, PA: National Center for Juvenile Justice. Retrieved from http://www.ojjdp.gov/ojstatbb/nr2014/downloads/NR2014.pdf

Snyder, H. N., & Sickmund, M. (2006). *Juvenile offenders and victims: 2006 national report*. Washington, DC: US Dept. of Justice, Office of Juvenile Justice and Delinquency Prevention.

Stein, L. A. R., Lebeau, R., Colby, S. M., Barnett, N. P., Golembeske, C., & Monti, P. M. (2011). Motivational interviewing for incarcerated adolescents: Effects of depressive symptoms on reducing alcohol and marijuana use after release. *Journal of Studies on Alcohol and Drugs, 72*(3), 497–506. https://doi.org/10.15288/jsad.2011.72.497

Teplin, L. A., Abram, K. M., McClelland, G. M., Dulcan, M. K., & Mericle, A. A. (2002). Psychiatric disorders in youth in detention. *Archives of General Psychiatry, 59*(12), 1133–1143. https://doi.org/10.1001/archpsyc.59.12.1133

Teplin, L. A., Elkington, K. S., McClelland, G. M., Abram, K. M., Mericle, A. A., & Washburn, J. J. (2005). Major mental disorders, substance use disorders, comorbidity, and HIV-AIDS risk behaviors in juvenile detainees. *Psychiatric Services, 56*(7), 823–828. https://doi.org/10.1176/appi.ps.56.7.823

Teplin, L. A., Mericle, A. A., McClelland, G. M., & Abram, K. M. (2003). HIV and AIDS risk behaviors in juvenile detainees: Implications for public health policy. *American Journal of Public Health, 93*, 906–912.

Wish, E. D., Billing, A. S., & Artigiani, E. E. (2015). *Community drug early warning system: The CDEWS-2 replication study. Office of National Drug Control Policy*. Washington, DC: Executive Office of the President.

Women's Behavioral Health Needs

Marion Ann Becker and Vickie Ann Lynn

Introduction

Historically, teaching and research are structured around specific disciplines, each with its own nomenclature, conceptual approaches, literature base, target audiences, and application strategies. However, thus far, outside the field of public health, minimal efforts have been devoted to an interdisciplinary approach to solving health-care problems. One of the core concepts underlining a public health approach or perspective is a focus on the health of an entire population. Accordingly, a public health approach involves an emphasis on health promotion and disease prevention throughout the lifespan. It takes into consideration an interdisciplinary framework for examining both physical and behavioral health problems. The World Health Organization suggests a public health approach should include the following four steps:

1. "*Surveillance*: To define the problem through the systematic collection of information about the magnitude, scope, characteristics and consequences of the problem.
2. *Identify risk and protective factors*: To establish what the problem is and why it occurs using research to determine the causes and correlates, the factors that increase or decrease the risk of, and the factors that could be modified through interventions.
3. *Develop and evaluate interventions*: To find out what works to prevent the health issue by designing, implementing and evaluating interventions.

The original version of this chapter was revised. The correction to this chapter is available at https://doi.org/10.1007/978-3-030-18435-3_18

M. A. Becker (✉)
School of Social Work and Louis de la Parte Florida Mental Health Institute, University of South Florida, Tampa, FL, USA
e-mail: mbecker2@usf.edu

V. A. Lynn
Department of Community and Family Health, College of Public Health, University of South Florida, Tampa, FL, USA

4. *Implementation*: To implement effective and promising interventions in a wide range of settings. The effects of these interventions on risk factors and the target outcome should be monitored, and their impact and cost-effectiveness should be evaluated." (Violence Prevention Alliance, 2018, p. 11).

Hence, we suggest that a public health framework that encompasses an interdisciplinary approach to behavioral disorders and emphasizes opportunities for prevention, early detection, and intervention will be more likely to reduce the burden of both physical and behavioral health illnesses (Becker, Levin, & Hanson, 2010). Since a public health approach is population-based, it encompasses important social, cultural, economic, and environmental factors that affect women's health.

This chapter examines critical issues in women's behavioral health from an interdisciplinary public health perspective. The content focuses on the essential elements of a public health perspective and discusses some of the major concerns in improving women's health outcomes. This chapter has two objectives: (1) to discuss behavioral health (alcohol, drug abuse, and mental) problems of concern to women and (2) to review services delivery and services research issues related to women's behavioral health. We also include a discussion of current challenges in prevention and treatment for three selected areas: (1) HIV; (2) postpartum depression; and (3) trauma-informed care, which are significant public health concerns. The chapter concludes with an *Implications for Behavioral Health* section, discussing the relevance of each issue to the overall field of women's behavioral health and health-care policy.

The material in this chapter is particularly timely in that it provides new information from current research findings and discusses important reimbursement policy and service delivery challenges that must be addressed if women's health-care outcomes are to be improved. The chapter is also very comprehensive. Among other things, in addition to the major topics mentioned above, it includes a discussion of the global burden of disease, health disparities, comorbidity, trauma-informed services, and health literacy. In addition to examination of the relevant issues in women's mental health, this chapter emphasizes the importance of maintaining a public health perspective and using an interdisciplinary approach for the study of women's behavioral health. An interdisciplinary public health approach is preferred because it will encourage individuals from diverse disciplines to work together in future research to improve health-care outcomes for women.

Epidemiology

Behavioral health problems, which include mental health and substance use disorders, are major contributors to the global burden of disease. Worldwide, approximately 450 million people live with a behavioral disorder (GBD 2016 DALYs and HALE Collaborators, 2017). In developing countries, behavioral disorders are second only to cardiovascular diseases in contributing to lost years of life (World Health Organization, 2017). Although behavioral disorders have a serious impact upon all individuals, it is important to recognize gender differences in the rates, experience, and course of these disorders. For example, women are twice as likely as men to suffer from major depression and rates of anxiety disorders, including post-traumatic stress disorder (PTSD), which are two to three times higher in women compared to men (Kessler, Berglund, et al., 2005; Office on Women's Health, 2009). Women also are at greater risk of poor self-care and poor adherence to treat (Rapaport, Clary, Fayyad, & Endicott, 2005).

To explore gender differences in health, researchers (Pratt & Brody, 2014) analyzed data from the National Health and Nutrition Examination Survey (NHANES), which is a continuous cross-sectional survey of the civilian, non-institutionalized US population, designed to assess the health and nutrition of Americans. Not only did females have higher rates of depression than males in every age group; the rate of depression increased by age, from 5.7% among girls aged 12–17 to 9.8% among women aged 40–59. Women aged 40–59 also had the highest rate of depression (12.3%) among all age groups and gender. The lowest rates of depression were for males aged 12–17 (4.0%) and for males 60 and over (3.4%). Nearly 90% of persons with depressive symptoms reported difficulty with work, home, or social activities. Just one-third of persons with severe depressive symptoms sought care from a behavioral health professional (Pratt & Brody, 2014).

Women with behavioral disorders not only have higher morbidity and mortality rates but are also at higher risk for underdiagnosis of major physical disorders (Becker et al., 2010; McCabe & Leas, 2008), while women who have depressive symptoms or anxiety are at higher risk for cardiovascular disease, which is the leading cause of death in women in developed countries (O'Neil et al., 2016).

The Global Burden of Disease Study (Whiteford et al., 2013) found behavioral disorders are one of the leading causes of disease burden. They are responsible for 7.4% of global disability-adjusted life years (DALYs) and 22.9% of global years lived with a disability (YLDs). Depression is the most predominant mental health problem followed by anxiety, schizophrenia, and bipolar disorder. Despite increased attention and promising advances in the science and practice of women's behavioral health, disparities based upon gender, race, ethnicity, age, and socioeconomic status persist, and women continue to have a higher risk than men for most behavioral disorders (Warner & Brown, 2011).

While there is now a greater recognition of the important role of behavioral health in the overall well-being of individuals and considerable progress in our understanding and treatment of behavioral disorders, there is an increased prevalence of behavioral disorders reported by women in the United States. Data show that almost one-half (48.5%) of American women report a lifetime experience of a mental disorder, and about a third (30.9%) report a disorder in the prior year (Kessler, Berglund, et al., 2005; Kessler, Chiu, Demler, Merikangas, & Walters, 2005).

Although the presence of multiple chronic conditions increases with age for both genders, women have a higher prevalence of multiple chronic conditions than men (Buttoroff, Ruder, & Bauman, 2017). In the most recent National Comorbidity Replication study, the individual profile for persons with any mental or substance use disorder in the prior year was being female, Hispanic, or African American; with less than a college education and low income; not currently cohabitating; and living in a rural area (Kessler, Berglund, et al., 2005). Behavioral disorders are among the leading causes of mortality and morbidity for women and men. Furthermore, the negative impact of mental disorders on overall health and life is reported to be similar worldwide (Beaglehole, Irwin, & Prentice, 2004; Murray & Lopez, 1996).

According to the Substance Abuse and Mental Health Services Administration (SAMHSA, 2014a, 2014b), about 44.7 million adults and 13.7 million children had diagnosable behavioral disorders in 2016 (Ahrnsbrak, Bose, Hedden, Lipari, & Park-Lee, 2017). Most individuals with behavioral health needs do not receive treatment, even though 80–90% of these disorders are treatable using medication and other evidence-based therapies (Kessler, Chiu, et al., 2005). Access and utilization barriers include lack of perceived need, lack of health insurance coverage, financial barriers, lack of transportation (Andrade et al., 2014), stigma (Brohan, Slade, Clement, & Thornicroft, 2010; Kakuma et al., 2011), lack of provider reimbursement, and other structural barriers (e.g., system fragmentation) (Corrigan, Druss, & Perlick, 2014). Since untreated behavioral health conditions are a serious public health concern, efforts are needed to reduce individual, community, and system level barriers to treatment.

Although prevalence rates for behavioral disorders vary depending upon the study, the age of the population, presence of co-occurring diagnosis such as HIV, and research methods used across the life span, researchers consistently report higher rates of behavioral disorders for females compared with males (Centers for Disease Control and Prevention (CDC), 2017). Researchers also note that starting in early adolescence, rates of these disorders increase for both genders, but the rates for adolescent females double and continue throughout women's lives (Kessler, Berglund, et al., 2005). Although gender differences might be attributed to women being more willing than men to report symptoms of depression and be more willing than men to seek treatment when they do have symptoms, studies have shown this is not the case and that gender differences do exist (Girgus & Yang, 2015). Depression in women is correlated with genes, hormonal changes, stress, and other factors and is pronounced during puberty, pregnancy, and perimenopause (Albert, 2015).

Substance Abuse

In recent years, there has been growing attention to the importance of gender in the treatment of substance use disorders in women. While past medical research mainly focused on men, there is now growing recognition that biologic and psychosocial differences between men and women influence the prevalence, presentation, comorbidity, and treatment of substance use disorders (Greenfield et al., 2007).

In the recent past, alcohol and substance dependence and abuse have predominately been seen as a male problem, as the research shows higher prevalence rates of drug and alcohol use disorders among men. The National Institute on Alcohol Abuse and Alcoholism's National Epidemiologic Survey on Alcohol and Related Conditions (NESARC) found that men are twice as likely as women to meet lifetime DSM-V criteria for any drug use disorder (12.3% of men vs. 7.7% of women)

(Grant et al., 2016). Twelve-month prevalence rates of alcohol abuse are almost twice as high among men as they are among women (17.6% of men vs 10.4% of women) (Grant et al., 2015). On the other hand, research also shows the prevalence rates of prescription drug abuse in women closely approach that of men. The Office of the Surgeon (2016) reported 12.5 million Americans reported misusing prescription pain relievers in the past year. Twelve-month prevalence rates of abuse or dependence for non-medical use of pain relievers were 20.5% for men and 15.3% for women (Office of the Surgeon General, 2016).

Women and men differ in substance abuse etiology, disease progression, and adherence to treatment. Alcohol is the most common substance abused by both men and women. Although men have higher rates of use, women have more severe health consequences and are more likely to overdose due to continued use and higher rates of illicit drugs (Fernandez-Montalvo, Lopez-Goni, Azanza, Arteaga, & Cacho, 2017; Greenfield, Back, Lawson, & Brady, 2010; Greenfield et al., 2007; Picci et al., 2012; Substance Abuse and Mental Health Services Administration, 2014a).

Given the aging of the "baby boomer" generation who uses alcohol and other drugs at a higher rate than past generations, and longer lifespans overall, it is anticipated that society will need additional specialized screenings, interventions, and treatments for addiction. This is noteworthy and concerning; women have greater medical vulnerability and social consequences associated as their behavioral disorders continue across age groups. Women carry additional risks during pregnancy because of the effects medication, alcohol, and illicit drugs have on the developing fetus (Erol & Karpyak, 2015). Since explanations for gender, racial, and age differences in behavioral disorders are evolving, continued research is required.

Comorbidity

Co-occurring physical disorders may lead to an increased risk of mental disorders, and mental disorders may increase a person's risk for a medical disorder, yet many comorbidities often go undetected (Goodell, Druss, Walker, & Mat, 2011). Comorbidity, having more than one chronic health condition at a time, is a growing public health concern, with one in four adults in the United States having two or more chronic health conditions and disorders and complex comorbidities.

The NCS-R reported approximately 74% of adults having one or more disorders in the previous 12 months (Druss et al., 2009). Despite the prevalence and clinical importance of comorbid disorders, relatively little is known about the etiology of these disorders, and most of the epidemiological research on comorbidity is relatively recent. Additional research is clearly needed as comorbidity is increasingly associated with worse health outcomes, more complex clinical management, and increased health-care costs. Understanding the nature of comorbidity through research has great potential value, as it could help identify the targets for prevention and treatment interventions. If comorbidity arises because different mental and physical disorders share the same risk factors, then interventions addressing these risk factors should help to reduce the prevalence and disability from frequently occurring comorbidities.

Mental and Substance Abuse Disorders

There are several gender differences in the relationship between mental and substance use disorders. Epidemiologic studies of treatment-seeking women indicate that gender differences in the patterns of comorbid mental disorders in substance users follow the same patterns experienced by women in the general population. Women with comorbid mental disorders are more likely to meet criteria for anxiety, depression, eating disorders, and borderline personality disorder and men more likely to meet criteria for antisocial personality disorder (Anker & Carroll, 2010; Grant et al., 2015; Grant et al., 2016; Greenfield et al., 2010; Lieber, 2000). A number of studies also indicate that for women, the onset of the mental disorder is more likely to antedate the onset of their substance use disorder (Back, Contini, & Brady, 2007; Greenfield et al., 2007; Mann et al., 2005).

Co-occurring Physical Illnesses

The typical woman with a behavioral disorder often has a co-occurring physical health condition (Becker & Gatz, 2005; Larson et al., 2005). Since co-occurring physical health disorders are more common in women than men, successful treatment requires an interdisciplinary approach to health care as well as health-care providers who are competent in recognizing, referring, and treating common co-occurring physical and behavioral disorders. Untreated or undertreated physical and behavioral health conditions can result in premature death, functional limitations, increased service utilization, and lowered quality of life for women with dual and triple diagnoses. The literature shows that women with behavioral disorders are at higher risk for both acute and chronic physical disorders (De Hert et al., 2011).

Despite the high prevalence and negative impact of co-occurring physical and behavioral disorders, many primary care providers fail to detect these conditions, and some believe that women with behavioral disorders will not make good use of health-care services. This is unfortunate because women have a higher risk for a number of physical health conditions including cardiovascular disease and cancer. Thus, primary care clinicians should carefully screen for physical health conditions among women with a behavioral disorder. As a result of higher rates of serious physical illness and underdiagnoses of physical health conditions, women with behavioral disorders have higher rates of premature death (Olfson, Gerhard, Huang, Crystal, & Stroup, 2015).

Research shows that for up to half of all primary care patients, there are no physical explanations for their symptoms (Edwards, Stern, Clarke, Ivbijaro, & Kasney,

2010; Institute of Medicine, 2006; Lipsitt, Joseph, Meyer, & Notman, 2015). Data from the Medical Outcomes Study suggest that primary care clinicians fail to recognize 50% of patients with depression (Katon, 2003), a failing that continues today (Knickman et al., 2016). In addition, gynecologic care, pregnancy, family planning, and contraception are issues that deserve special attention in women with behavioral disorders. Treatment of behavioral disorders during pregnancy requires careful thought, as there is scant data on the use of psychotropic medication in this population (Byatt et al., 2018). Decisions about medication during pregnancy are complicated further due to the small number of adequate studies and relative absence of randomized control trials.

In response to current epidemiologic data, the principle that "there is no health without mental health" is gaining ground. Efforts to transform America's public behavioral health delivery systems to systems that are more person-centered, recovery-focused, evidenced-based, and quality-driven are intensifying. Due, in part, to the Surgeon General's reports on mental health and addiction (Office of the Surgeon General, 1999, 2016), the efforts of the World Health Organization (GBD 2016 DALYs and HALE Collaborators, 2016), and the President's New Freedom Commission on Mental Health (2003), a broader framework for health has been advocated which emphasizes the idea that disease extends beyond its clinical dimensions. This broader framework makes it essential that public health practitioners, policy makers, consumers, and advocates understand the extent and distribution of behavioral disorders and disability, so they can develop policies and practices that reduce health disparities and contribute to people's daily activities and participation in society (President's New Freedom Commission on Mental Health, 2003).

Health Disparities

Despite current efforts to close the gap between socioeconomic status between majority and minority populations, health disparities continue to exist (Peck & Denney, 2012; Primm et al., 2010). Health disparities occur across intersecting identities; include race/ethnicity, age, gender, socioeconomic status, disability status, sexual identify, and sexual orientation; and refer to differences between groups in health insurance coverage, access to and use of care, and quality of care (Chen, Vargas-Bustamante, Mortensen, & Ortega, 2016). *Healthy People 2020* defines a health disparity as:

> A particular type of health difference that is closely linked with social, economic, and/or environmental disadvantage. Health disparities adversely affect groups of people who have systematically experienced greater obstacles to health based on their racial or ethnic group; religion; socioeconomic status; gender; age; mental health; cognitive, sensory, or physical disability; sexual orientation or gender identity; geographic location; or other characteristics historically linked to discrimination or exclusion. (The Secretary's Advisory Committee on National Health Promotion and Disease Prevention Objectives for 2020, 2008, October 28, p. 4646)

Data show that women from different ethnic and cultural groups, as well as other minority populations, such as LGBTQ (lesbian, gay, bisexual, transgender, queer/questioning), have multiple intersecting identities increasing health disparities and negative health outcomes (Adepoju, Preston, & Gonzales, 2015; National Academies of Sciences, Engineering, & Medicine, 2017). For example, over the past few decades, the gap in life expectancy between men and women is narrowing and is due, in part, to an increase in mortality for women (Arias, 2016; Chetty et al., 2016).

The challenges faced by women from minority and other underserved groups are well documented and include lower socioeconomic status, poorer health conditions, lower use of services, higher rates of premature death, disease, and disability status (Jang, Chiriboga, & Becker, 2010). The complex relationships among biological, physical, and social environmental factors influence access to care and affect population and individual health outcomes (Institute of Medicine, 2010). These challenges and the devalued status of minority and underserved women have important implications for behavioral health services provided to minority populations.

Women from an underserved population may present with somatic complaints or other symptoms not traditionally associated with a behavioral health diagnosis (Kohrt et al., 2014). In addition, women from an underserved population may be less trusting, less adherent, and more skeptical. Further, chronic physical illnesses may result in depression and or anxiety, and patients from minority populations may respond differently to medications. Since each patient's culture and ethnic background must be addressed when they present for behavioral health services, clinicians should always ask about cultural issues and determine if they are of concern in the treatment of their client (Kohrt et al., 2014). Good communication, clarity, and collaboration are key to successful patient-provider relationships and positive behavioral health treatment outcomes across diverse groups (Kohrt et al., 2014).

Location also is an important consideration, as there are significant differences in access to care for women who live in rural and urban areas, as the majority of behavioral health providers work in high population metropolitan areas (Ellis, Konrad, Thomas, & Morrissey, 2009). Women living in rural areas are more likely to be poor, lack health insurance, and often travel longer distances to access medical, dental, and behavioral health specialty services (Buzza et al., 2011). Rural women are also more likely than urban women to experience stressors related to behavioral health, yet they are less likely to receive behavioral health services (Weaver & Himle, 2017).

Barriers to behavioral health care are a major concern. An estimated 40% of women in rural areas seek mental health treatment in a primary care setting rather than a behavioral health-care setting, yet stigma is a significant barrier when living in small communities (Smalley et al., 2010). Rural populations have higher rates of behavioral and somatic health conditions (i.e., substance abuse, smoking, and obesity) compared to urban populations. Further, up to 40% of rural women have comorbid substance use and mental disorders and higher rates of suicide (Smalley et al., 2010). While there have been some policy changes to improve health services delivery, outcomes have not been sufficient in meeting the health needs of this population. Additional policies need to be developed to address the needs of underserved populations (Smalley et al., 2010).

Selected Issues in Women's Behavioral Health

Understanding, preventing, and managing women's health involve understanding their unique health needs in relation to specific physical and behavioral health conditions. The next section discusses issues related to women diagnosed with human immunodeficiency virus (HIV), postpartum depression (PPD), and women who have experienced trauma. These three conditions have a major impact on women's behavioral health, and they are a particular problem for women living in poverty. Despite their prevalence and association with poorer health-care outcomes, they are an under-researched population and require more attention and additional research.

Women and HIV

The burden of behavioral health conditions among women living with human immunodeficiency virus (WLHIV) is a significant public health concern. Innovative methods of detecting and treating the complex physical and behavioral health conditions of WLHIV are needed to improve health outcomes and women's quality of life. Over the past 35 years, public health has made tremendous accomplishments in the prevention and treatment of HIV and acquired immunodeficiency syndrome (AIDS). In the early days of the epidemic, HIV was seen as a death sentence. Today, HIV is considered a chronic health condition that can be controlled with medications (Brooks et al., 2017; Cohen et al., 2016; Rodger et al., 2016).

Although HIV in women is life changing and significantly increases morbidity and mortality (Quinlivan et al., 2015), access to highly active antiretroviral therapy (HAART) for the treatment of HIV increases life expectancy, improves quality of life, and has the potential to reduce transmission of HIV (Rodger et al., 2016). However, women are less likely to use or have access to HAART, and WLHIV often face an array of co-occurring physical and mental health conditions as well as socioeconomic hardships that impede their ability to maintain access to care and treatment (Beer, Mattson, Bradley, & Skarbinski, 2016).

Globally, women account for more than 50% of the 36.7 million persons living with HIV (PLHIV), with approximately 380,000 new HIV infections occurring among girls and women aged 15–24 each year (UNAIDS, 2017). In the United States, women represent approximately 25% of the 1.2 million PLHIV, and women of color are disproportionately affected by HIV (CDC, 2017). Even though women of color account for less than 30% of the US population, they represent nearly 80% of all WLHIV (CDC, 2015). Not only are they less likely to engage in care; women of color are at a higher risk for morbidity and mortality compared with men and white women (Quinlivan et al., 2015).

Although many WLHIV are living longer healthier lives, an HIV diagnosis impacts physical, psychological, and social well-being, and WLHIV experience an increased prevalence of behavioral health conditions when compared to men (Orza et al., 2015) and the general population (Chapin-Bardales, Rosenberg, & Sullivan, 2017). WLHIV have high levels of emotional distress and report more psychological and psychosocial problems including fear, loss, grief, hopelessness, guilt, low self-esteem, anxiety, depression, denial, and anger (Fabianova, 2011). In addition, WLHIV are affected by high rates of sexual and physical trauma in childhood and as adults. A recent meta-analysis reports the estimated rate of recent post-traumatic stress disorder (PTSD) in WLHIV is 30.0%, over five times the national rate for women. In addition, intimate partner violence (IPV) among WLHIV was estimated at 55%, twice the national rate (Machtinger, Wilson, Haberer, & Weiss, 2012).

A large-scale study conducted in the southeastern United States found as high as 60% of PLHIV report symptoms of mental illness, 32% report substance use problems, and 23% are triply diagnosed with HIV, substance abuse, and a mental health problem, with women reporting a higher number of mental illness symptoms (Whetten et al., 2005). Clinical management of HIV for these triple diagnoses requires integrated treatment services that address both mitigation of substance use and psychiatric and medical symptoms and other health behaviors (Durvasula & Miller, 2014).

Health-care systems around the world are now making an effort to integrate behavioral health services with primary health care. Integration can increase access to mental health and substance abuse services and improve adherence to lifesaving HIV treatment. There is a need to educate both primary care and HIV specialists about the importance of routine screening of WLHIV for depression, anxiety, substance use, and other mental health conditions.

Postpartum Depression

Postpartum depression (PPD) is a serious mental health condition and a major concern for women. About half of postpartum women experience the "baby blues," whereas about 10%–15% of new mothers experience PPD (Yim, Tanner Stapleton, Guardino, Hahn-Holbrook, & Dunkel Schetter, 2015). PPD, also called postnatal or perinatal depression, is a type of mood disorder associated with childbirth. The postpartum period begins immediately following childbirth and continues for 6 weeks. The exact cause of PPD is unclear; however, it is believed to be a combination of physical and emotional factors that may include hormonal changes in addition to sleep deprivation and other stressors associated with a new infant in the family (Jevitt, Groer, Crist, Gonzalez, & Wagner, 2012). Risk factors include prior episodes of PPD, bipolar disorder, a family or personal history of depression, psychological stress, complications of childbirth, lack of social support, history of violence, or a drug use disorder (Dennis & Vigod, 2013).

Symptoms of PPD can include extreme sadness, low energy, anxiety, crying episodes, irritability, and changes in sleeping or eating patterns. PPD can affect the health of the mother as well as the health and development of her child(ren). Maternal bonding with her new infant may be impaired, leading to attachment and developmental delays for the child (Howard et al., 2014). Onset is typically between 1 week and 3 months following childbirth and affects up to 15% of women around childbirth and, in some women, leads to postpartum psychosis (Pearlstein, Howard, Salisbury, & Zlotnick, 2009; Spinelli, 2004).

Postpartum psychosis is a more severe form of postpartum mood disorder that occurs in about 1–2 women per 1000 following childbirth. Postpartum psychosis is one of the leading causes of the murder of children less than 1 year of age. In the United States, this occurs in about 8 per 100,000 births (Spinelli, 2004).

Review of antidepressant medication use during pregnancy suggests these medications increase perinatal disorders, including congenital malformations and neurologic injury (Yaeger, Smith, & Altshuler, 2006), and women often stop their use during pregnancy (Petersen, Gilbert, Evans, Man, & Nazareth, 2011). Research on PPD also suggests that serotonin reuptake inhibitors (SSRIs) can increase the risk of congenital heart defects (Chambers, Moses-Kolko, & Wisner, 2007). There are fewer studies on postpartum psychosis, so clinicians know less about the health outcomes of antipsychotic medication use during pregnancy among women with PPD. Both pharmacological and non-pharmacological treatment options (e.g., interpersonal therapy and cognitive behavioral therapy) are important because, without treatment, PPD can last for months or years. In addition to its effects on the mother's health, PPD can interfere with the mother's ability to nurture and connect with her baby, which may cause the baby to have problems with sleeping, eating, and behavior as he or she grows.

Trauma-Informed Services

Trauma, stigma, and discrimination are also factors that influence health-care outcomes for women. There is ample evidence regarding the high prevalence of trauma, violence, and abuse against women, which increases the prevalence of behavioral disorders and the need for trauma-informed services. Trauma-informed care (TIC) is an intervention and approach to services that focuses on how trauma may affect a women's life and her response to behavioral health services from prevention through treatment. Trauma refers to extreme stress that overwhelms a person's ability to cope. Clinicians meet with various clients in a wide range of settings, and while each client has different needs and goals and requires different care approaches, the common thread is awareness of the need for trauma-informed care (Muskett, 2014).

According to SAMHSA (2014a, 2014b), trauma-informed services are based on an understanding of the vulnerabilities or triggers of trauma survivors that traditional service delivery approaches may exacerbate. Thus, trauma-informed services are designed to be very supportive and avoid any potential re-traumatization of the client. Trauma-informed care can also be viewed as an overarching philosophy and approach, or a set of universal precautions, designed to be both preventive and rehabilitative in nature, in which the relationship among environment, triggers, and perceived dangers are noted and addressed.

Trauma-informed care is based on the understanding that many clients have suffered traumatic experiences, and the provider is responsible for being sensitive to this fact, regardless of whether a person is being treated specifically for the trauma (Huckshorn & LeBel, 2013). Therefore, all clinicians should approach their clients as if they have a trauma history, regardless of the services for which the clients are being seen.

Women of special concern who require trauma-informed services include the growing population of incarcerated women, female veterans, and active female military personnel who are often exposed to trauma, violence, and abuse (Friedman, Collier, & Hall, 2016; Lehavot, O'Hara, Washington, Yano, & Simpson, 2015; Mustillo et al., 2015). Unfortunately, these women frequently have limited access to behavioral health services and often suffer from post-traumatic stress disorder (PTSD). For example, it has been reported that as many as 30 percent of women were raped during their military services; this compounds the heavy burden already experienced by female veterans and their families (Zinzow, Grubaugh, Monnier, Suffoletta-Maierle, & Frueh, 2007). Thus, there is a critical need for new initiatives to address both the short- and long-term effects of trauma, violence, and abuse experienced by female veterans and women suffering from interpersonal violence.

Services Delivery

Community behavioral health-care programs face many challenges and incur skyrocketing costs. Persons with behavioral health problems often do not receive the behavioral health-care services they need and those with serious chronic disorders die, on average, 25 years earlier than persons without behavioral health problems (Olfson et al., 2015). The seminal US President's New Freedom Commission on Mental Health (2003) identified fragmentation of health delivery systems as one of the three major obstacles impeding the treatment of behavioral disorders in the United States. The observed system fragmentation that characterizes the American health-care systems has direct implications for access to services and the utilization of effective health care for both primary and behavioral health-care consumers.

Successful models of behavioral health care most often use a "strengths-based" model or approach to service delivery that promotes the well-being of both clients and society (Tse et al., 2016). In a strength-based approach, the professional tells the client to think about problems, responses, or situations they solved in the past. This reflective approach promotes the well-being of the client because it helps the client realize their strength(s) and the possibilities they have to deal with their problems.

The strength-based approach helps the client identify successful solutions to cope with their behavioral health problems and assists communities and individuals to solve their behavioral health service delivery challenges.

Integrated health care is another model or approach to services delivery promoted to improve health-care outcomes and reduce costs. Integrated care is the systematic coordination of physical and behavioral health care. Since physical and behavioral health problems often occur simultaneously, integrating services to treat both will yield the best results and be the most acceptable and effective approach for those being served (Kuramoto, 2014). In addition to service system fragmentation, health literacy affects health outcomes for women and is an issue of increasing concern, as clients are expected to take more responsibility for their own treatment outcomes.

Health Literacy

Title V of the Patient Protection and Affordable Care Act of 2010 is "the degree to which an individual has the capacity to obtain, communicate, process, and understand health information and services in order to make appropriate health decisions" (§5002(b)(21), p. 473). Low health literacy is associated with poorer health outcomes and poorer use of health-care services which is why health literacy and health literacy skills are important and should be developed (Berkman, Sheridan, Donahue, Halpern, & Crotty, 2011). Health literacy skills are used by people to realize their potential in health situations. Anyone who needs health information and services needs health literacy skills to obtain needed behavioral health information and services. Therefore, health literacy is vital to improving behavioral health outcomes for women.

In general, health literacy in America is quite low; approximately 80 million adults have low basic health literacy (Berkman et al., 2011). Basic health literacy allows women to understand information (e.g., diagnostic, treatment, medication, and lifestyle change) provided by a health and behavioral health-care professional (e.g., physician, social worker, nurse practitioner, pharmacist, and rehabilitation specialist). An expanded model of health literacy includes the ability of consumers to generate questions about their health, understand the health information provided, and be able to engage effectively with treatment protocols and procedures. As treatment becomes more complex with the adoption of evidence-based practices, such as new psychopharmacological agents, health literacy will become even more important in the treatment of both physical and behavioral disorders.

Making information useful to particular clients begins with identifying the intended users of the health information and services. Clinicians should evaluate users' understanding before, during, and after providing health information and services. They should also be sure the materials and messages reflect the age, social and cultural diversity, language, and literacy skills of the intended users. Other components to consider are patients' economic contexts, access to services, and life experiences.

Beyond demographics, culture, and language, clinicians must consider the communication capacities of the intended users. Approximately one in six Americans has a communication disorder (Black, Vahratian, & Hoffman, 2015). These individuals require communication strategies tailored to their specific needs. Hence, clinicians should determine what information patients need to know and how they will be used. Clinicians can then pretest the information, receive feedback, and refine the information so that it is useful for the client. Plain language helps patients understand the information communicated to them and how they should proceed or continue with an effective treatment plan.

Implications for Behavioral Health

In the United States, attention to improving women's behavioral health outcomes is recent. Collaborative efforts by federal agencies to effect positive changes and promote progress to improve the overall health of the nation's women and girls were detailed first in *Action Steps for Improving Women's Mental Health* (Office on Women's Health, 2009). This comprehensive groundbreaking report, issued by the National Mental Health Information Center, foreshadow international action plans suggested by the World Health Organization (World Health Organization, 2015, 2017). Among other things, the action steps encouraged nations to "Promote a recovery-oriented, strengths-based approach to treatment for women…" and "Build resilience and protective factors to promote the mental health of girls and women and aid recovery" (Office on Women's Health, 2009, p. iiiiii). These action steps support the goals of the World Health Organization (World Health Organization, 2015, p. 1111) to (1) "provide comprehensive, integrated and responsive mental health and social care services in community-based settings" and (2) "implement strategies for promotion and prevention in mental health." Both of these documents are a response to research that documented low rates of health-care services available to women with behavioral disorders and evidence that medical care for women needed to be improved.

To improve health-care outcomes for women with behavioral health needs, health-care policies and delivery systems around the world need to integrate behavioral and physical health services. Integrated care would not only increase access to behavioral and physical health-care services but could also improve adherence to lifesaving physical and behavioral health treatment.

Despite the increase in life expectancy and development of new medications for more effective treatment of behavioral disorders, women continue to face increased vulnerability and gender-based risks for major depression, PTSD, anxiety, and eating disorders. In addition, women with behavioral disorders face significant social stigma and discrimination.

Overcoming the stigma and discrimination associated with behavioral disorders must become a national priority. Research suggests that women may neglect care for their mental disorder because of stigma and discrimination associated with these disorders (Corrigan et al., 2014). In an effort to avoid being shamed, or because of self-doubt brought on by shaming, women with a mental or substance use disorder may try to hide their disorder from family or avoid disclosing their symptoms to their doctor. The signs of alcohol and other drug abuse, anorexia, bulimia, anxiety, and depression often are concealed until a life-threatening incident occurs. Therefore, delaying behavioral health care can have serious negative conse-quences. Designing health-care systems to integrate behavioral health into physical or primary health care could reduce stigma and free women with behavioral disor-ders from any shame or discrimination from their conditions that they or their fam-ily may have experienced. Integrated health care can break through the barrier of stigma and help clients know that help is available without criticism or blame. Although much outreach needs to be done to overcome mental health stigma, the growing adoption of integrated care is making real gains in reducing stigma in the communities we serve.

Lastly, to improve both access and quality of health-care services, a radical trans-formation of health-care systems will be needed to eliminate disparities in health-care outcomes that currently exist in both behavioral and physical health-care services. To provide essential behavioral health education and disease prevention, an integrated information technology and communications infrastructure is critical. An effective communication infrastructure, at a minimum, would include the inte-gration of medical records, the use of interdisciplinary teams, and use of surveil-lance systems for tracking health-care progress and treatment outcomes.

Since behavioral disorders begin in childhood and adolescence, successful behavioral health policy and efforts in prevention and early intervention should be targeted toward this critical period. Currently, there is also a growing need for the provision of behavioral health policies and services for women who are incarcerated in jails and prisons as well as the increasing number of women in the military. These at-risk populations create an increased demand for communities, states, and federal health-care systems to provide greater access to effective and affordable behavioral health-care services for women.

As acknowledged by the multiple World Health Organization reports cited in this chapter and discussed in *Action Steps for Improving Women's Mental Health* (2009), there is an opportunity and an urgent need to improve access, utilization, and quality of behavioral health services for women in the United States and worldwide. However, given global budgets for health care and the dramatic reductions in state and federal (financial) support for health, education, and social services in the United States, it remains to be seen if the opportunity will be realized. Nevertheless, the recommendations of the *President's New Freedom Commission* (2003), the *Action Steps for Improving Women's Mental Health* (2009), and the recent National Academies workshop on *Women's Mental Health Across the Life Course Through a Sex-Gender Lens* (National Academies of Sciences, Engineering, & Medicine, 2018) provide a blueprint for progress in improving women's behavioral and physi-cal health that could be realized with adequate leadership and financial support.

In support of integrated care, there is a need for reimbursement policies that provide for care management services which are needed by women with complex co-occurring disorders. Finally, providing quality health care for women with complex health-care needs requires additional training, collaboration between specialists, and the provision of case management services, which will increase the costs of care and require additional reimbursement policy to pay for these services.

References

Adepoju, O. E., Preston, M. A., & Gonzales, G. (2015). Health care disparities in the post-affordable care act era. *American Journal of Public Health, 105*(Suppl 5), S665–S667. https://doi.org/10.2105/ajph.2015.302611

Ahrnsbrak, R., Bose, J., Hedden, S. L., Lipari, R. N., & Park-Lee, E. (2017). *Key substance use and mental health indicators in the United States: Results from the 2016 National Survey on Drug Use and Health* (DHHS Publication No. SMA 17–5044, NSDUH Series). Rockville, MD: Center for Behavioral Health Statistics and Quality, Substance Abuse and Mental Health Services Administration. https://www.samhsa.gov/data/sites/default/files/NSDUH-FFR1-2016/NSDUH-FFR1-2016.pdf

Albert, P. R. (2015). Why is depression more prevalent in women? *Journal of Psychiatry and Neuroscience, 40*(4), 219–221.

Andrade, L. H., Alonso, J., Mneimneh, Z., Wells, J. E., Al-Hamzawi, A., Borges, G., … Kessler, R. C. (2014). Barriers to mental health treatment: Results from the WHO World Mental Health surveys. *Psychological Medicine, 44*(6), 1303–1317. https://doi.org/10.1017/s0033291713001943

Anker, J. J., & Carroll, M. E. (2010). Females are more vulnerable to drug abuse than males: Evidence from preclinical studies and the role of ovarian hormones. In *Biological basis of sex differences in psychopharmacology* (pp. 73–96). Berlin: Springer.

Arias, E. (2016). *Changes in life expectancy by race and Hispanic origin in the United States, 2013–2014*. Atlanta, GA: US Department of Health and Human Services, Centers for Disease Control and Prevention, National Center for Health Statistics.

Back, S. E., Contini, R., & Brady, K. T. (2007). Substance abuse in women: Does gender matter? *Women, 24*(1), 1–2. http://www.psychiatrictimes.com/substance-use-disorder/substance-abuse-women-does-gender-matter

Beaglehole, R., Irwin, A., & Prentice, T. (2004). Annex table 3: Burden of disease in DALYs by cause, sex, and mortality stratum in WHO regions, estimates for 2002. In R. Beaglehole, A. Irwin, & T. Prentice (Eds.), *The world health report 2004: Changing history* (p. 126). Bellegarde-sur-Valserine: SADAG Imprimerie. Retrieved from http://www.who.int/whr/2004/en/

Becker, M. A., & Gatz, M. (2005). Introduction to the impact of co-occurring disorders and violence on women: Findings from the SAMHSA women, co-occurring disorders and violence study. *Journal of Behavioral Health Services and Research, 32*(2), 111–112.

Becker, M. A., Levin, B. L., & Hanson, A. (2010). Public health and women's mental health. In B. L. Levin & M. A. Becker (Eds.), *A public health perspective of women's mental health*. New York, NY: Springer.

Beer, L., Mattson, C. L., Bradley, H., & Skarbinski, J. (2016). Understanding cross-sectional racial, ethnic, and gender disparities in antiretroviral use and viral suppression among HIV patients in the United States. *Medicine, 95*(13), e3171. https://doi.org/10.1097/md.0000000000003171

Berkman, N. D., Sheridan, S. L., Donahue, K. E., Halpern, D. J., & Crotty, K. (2011). Low health literacy and health outcomes: An updated systematic review. *Annals of Internal Medicine, 155*(2), 97–107. https://doi.org/10.7326/0003-4819-155-2-201107190-00005

Black, L. I., Vahratian, A., & Hoffman, H. J. (2015). Communication disorders and use of intervention services among children aged 3–17 years: United States, 2012. *NCHS Data Brief*(205), 1–8.

Brohan, E., Slade, M., Clement, S., & Thornicroft, G. (2010). Experiences of mental illness stigma, prejudice and discrimination: A review of measures. *BMC Health Services Research, 10*, 80. https://doi.org/10.1186/1472-6963-10-80

Brooks, J. T., Kawwass, J. F., Smith, D. K., Kissin, D. M., Lampe, M., Haddad, L. B., … Jamieson, D. J. (2017). Effects of antiretroviral therapy to prevent HIV transmission to women in couples attempting conception when the man has HIV infection - United States, 2017. *MMWR Morbidity and Mortality Weekly Report, 66*(32), 859–860. https://doi.org/10.15585/mmwr.mm 6632e1

Buttoroff, C., Ruder, T., & Bauman, M. (2017). *Multiple chronic conditions in the United States* (TL-221-PFCD). Santa Monica, CA: RAND Health. https://www.rand.org/content/dam/rand/pubs/tools/TL200/TL221/RAND_TL221.pdf

Buzza, C., Ono, S. S., Turvey, C., Wittrock, S., Noble, M., Reddy, G., … Reisinger, H. S. (2011). Distance is relative: Unpacking a principal barrier in rural healthcare. *Journal of General Internal Medicine, 26*(Suppl 2), 648–654. https://doi.org/10.1007/s11606-011-1762-1

Byatt, N., Cox, L., Moore Simas, T. A., Kini, N., Biebel, K., Sankaran, P., … Weinreb, L. (2018). How obstetric settings can help address gaps in psychiatric care for pregnant and postpartum women with bipolar disorder. *Archives of Women's Mental Health, 21*(5), 543–551. https://doi.org/10.1007/s00737-018-0825-2

Centers for Disease Control and Prevention. (2015). *HIV infection, risk, prevention, and testing behaviors among heterosexuals at increased risk of HIV infection—National HIV Behavioral Surveillance, 20 U.S. Cities, 2013* (HIV Surveillance Special Report 13). Atlanta, GA: Author. https://www.cdc.gov/hiv/pdf/library/reports/surveillance/cdc-hiv-HSSR_NHBS_HET_2013.pdf

Centers for Disease Control and Prevention. (2017). *Diagnoses of HIV infection in the United States and dependent areas, 2016* (HIV Surveillance Report). Atlanta, GA: Author. https://www.cdc.gov/hiv/pdf/library/reports/surveillance/cdc-hiv-surveillance-report-2016-vol-28.pdf

Chambers, C., Moses-Kolko, E., & Wisner, K. L. (2007). Antidepressant use in pregnancy: New concerns, old dilemmas. *Expert Review of Neurotherapeutics, 7*(7), 761–764. https://doi.org/10.1586/14737175.7.7.761

Chapin-Bardales, J., Rosenberg, E. S., & Sullivan, P. S. (2017). Trends in racial/ethnic disparities of new AIDS diagnoses in the United States, 1984-2013. *Annals of Epidemiology, 27*(5), 329–334.e322. https://doi.org/10.1016/j.annepidem.2017.04.002

Chen, J., Vargas-Bustamante, A., Mortensen, K., & Ortega, A. N. (2016). Racial and ethnic disparities in health care access and utilization under the affordable care act. *Medical Care, 54*(2), 140–146. https://doi.org/10.1097/mlr.0000000000000467

Chetty, R., Stepner, M., Abraham, S., Lin, S., Scuderi, B., Turner, N., … Cutler, D. (2016). The association between income and life expectancy in the United States, 2001-2014. *JAMA, 315*(16), 1750–1766. https://doi.org/10.1001/jama.2016.4226

Cohen, M. S., Chen, Y. Q., McCauley, M., Gamble, T., Hosseinipour, M. C., Kumarasamy, N., … Fleming, T. R. (2016). Antiretroviral therapy for the prevention of HIV-1 transmission. *New England Journal of Medicine, 375*(9), 830–839. https://doi.org/10.1056/NEJMoa1600693

Corrigan, P. W., Druss, B. G., & Perlick, D. A. (2014). The impact of mental illness stigma on seeking and participating in mental health care. *Psychological Science in the Public Interest, 15*(2), 37–70. https://doi.org/10.1177/1529100614531398

De Hert, M., Cohen, D., Bobes, J., Cetkovich-Bakmas, M., Leucht, S., Ndetei, D. M., … Correll, C. U. (2011). Physical illness in patients with severe mental disorders. II. Barriers to care, monitoring and treatment guidelines, plus recommendations at the system and individual level. *World Psychiatry, 10*(2), 138–151. https://doi.org/10.1002/j.2051-5545.2011.tb00036.x

Dennis, C. L., & Vigod, S. (2013). The relationship between postpartum depression, domestic violence, childhood violence, and substance use: Epidemiologic study of a large community sample. *Violence Against Women, 19*(4), 503–517. https://doi.org/10.1177/1077801213487057

Druss, B. G., Hwang, I., Petukhova, M., Sampson, N. A., Wang, P. S., & Kessler, R. C. (2009). Impairment in role functioning in mental and chronic medical disorders in the United States: Results from the National Comorbidity Survey Replication. *Molecular Psychiatry, 14*(7), 728–737. https://doi.org/10.1038/mp.2008.13

Durvasula, R., & Miller, T. R. (2014). Substance abuse treatment in persons with HIV/AIDS: Challenges in managing triple diagnosis. *Behavioral Medicine, 40*(2), 43–52. https://doi.org/10.1080/08964289.2013.866540

Edwards, T. M., Stern, A., Clarke, D. D., Ivbijaro, G., & Kasney, L. M. (2010). The treatment of patients with medically unexplained symptoms in primary care: A review of the literature. *Mental Health in Family Medicine, 7*(4), 209–221. https://www.ncbi.nlm.nih.gov/pmc/articles/PMC3083260/pdf/MHFM-07-209.pdf

Ellis, A. R., Konrad, T. R., Thomas, K. C., & Morrissey, J. P. (2009). County-level estimates of mental health professional supply in the United States. *Psychiatric Services, 60*(10), 1315–1322. https://doi.org/10.1176/ps.2009.60.10.1315

Erol, A., & Karpyak, V. M. (2015). Sex and gender-related differences in alcohol use and its consequences: Contemporary knowledge and future research considerations. *Drug and Alcohol Dependence, 156*, 1–13. https://doi.org/10.1016/j.drugalcdep.2015.08.023

Fabianova, L. (2011). Psychosocial aspects of people living with HIV/AIDS. In G. Letamo (Ed.), *Social and psychological aspects of HIV/AIDS and their ramifications* (pp. 175–204). London: InTechOpen Limited. https://doi.org/10.5772/1145

Fernandez-Montalvo, J., Lopez-Goni, J. J., Azanza, P., Arteaga, A., & Cacho, R. (2017). Gender differences in treatment progress of drug-addicted patients. *Women & Health, 57*(3), 358–376. https://doi.org/10.1080/03630242.2016.1160967

Friedman, S. H., Collier, S., & Hall, R. C. W. (2016). PTSD behind bars: Incarcerated women and PTSD. In C. R. Martin, V. R. Preedy, & V. B. Patel (Eds.), *Comprehensive guide to posttraumatic stress disorders* (pp. 1497–1512). Cham: Springer International Publishing.

GBD 2016 DALYs and HALE Collaborators. (2016). Global, regional, and national disability-adjusted life-years (DALYs) for 315 diseases and injuries and healthy life expectancy (HALE), 1990-2015: A systematic analysis for the Global Burden of Disease Study 2015. *Lancet, 388*(10053), 1603–1658. https://doi.org/10.1016/s0140-6736(16)31460-x

GBD 2016 DALYs and HALE Collaborators. (2017). Global, regional, and national disability-adjusted life-years (DALYs) for 333 diseases and injuries and healthy life expectancy (HALE) for 195 countries and territories, 1990-2016: A systematic analysis for the Global Burden of Disease Study 2016. *Lancet, 390*(10100), 1260–1344. https://doi.org/10.1016/s0140-6736(17)32130-x

Girgus, J. S., & Yang, K. (2015). Gender and depression. *Current Opinion in Psychology, 4*(August), 53–60. https://doi.org/10.1016/j.copsyc.2015.01.019

Goodell, S., Druss, B. G., Walker, E. R., & Mat, M. (2011). *Mental disorders and medical comorbidity*. The Synthesis Project (Policy Brief No. 21). Princeton, NJ: Robert Wood Johnson Foundation.

Grant, B. F., Goldstein, R. B., Saha, T. D., Chou, S. P., Jung, J., Zhang, H., … Hasin, D. S. (2015). Epidemiology of DSM-5 alcohol use disorder: Results from the National Epidemiologic Survey on Alcohol and Related Conditions III. *JAMA Psychiatry, 72*(8), 757–766. https://doi.org/10.1001/jamapsychiatry.2015.0584

Grant, B. F., Saha, T. D., Ruan, W. J., Goldstein, R. B., Chou, S. P., Jung, J., … Hasin, D. S. (2016). Epidemiology of DSM-5 drug use disorder: Results from the National Epidemiologic Survey on Alcohol and Related Conditions-III. *JAMA Psychiatry, 73*(1), 39–47. https://doi.org/10.1001/jamapsychiatry.2015.2132

Greenfield, S. F., Back, S. E., Lawson, K., & Brady, K. T. (2010). Substance abuse in women. *Psychiatric Clinics of North America, 33*(2), 339–355. https://doi.org/10.1016/j.psc.2010.01.004

Greenfield, S. F., Brooks, A. J., Gordon, S. M., Green, C. A., Kropp, F., McHugh, R. K., … Miele, G. M. (2007). Substance abuse treatment entry, retention, and outcome in women: A review of the literature. *Drug and Alcohol Dependence, 86*(1), 1–21. https://doi.org/10.1016/j.drugalcdep.2006.05.012

Howard, L. M., Molyneaux, E., Dennis, C. L., Rochat, T., Stein, A., & Milgrom, J. (2014). Non-psychotic mental disorders in the perinatal period. *Lancet, 384*(9956), 1775–1788. https://doi.org/10.1016/s0140-6736(14)61276-9

Huckshorn, K., & LeBel, J. L. (2013). Trauma-informed care. In K. Yeager, D. Cutler, D. Svendsen, & G. M. Sills (Eds.), *Modern community mental health work: An interdisciplinary approach* (pp. 62–83). New York, NY: Oxford University Press.

Institute of Medicine. (2006). *Improving the quality of health care for mental and substance-use conditions*. Washington, DC: The National Academic Press.

Institute of Medicine. (2010). *Women's health research: Progress, pitfalls, and promise*. Washington, DC: The National Academies Press.

Jang, Y., Chiriboga, D. A., & Becker, M. A. (2010). Racial and ethnic disparities. In M. A. Becker & B. L. Levin (Eds.), *A public health perspective of women's mental health* (pp. 347–357). New York, NY: Springer.

Jevitt, C. M., Groer, M. W., Crist, N. F., Gonzalez, L., & Wagner, V. D. (2012). Postpartum stressors: A content analysis. *Issues in Mental Health Nursing, 33*(5), 309–318. https://doi.org/10.3109/01612840.2011.653658

Kakuma, R., Minas, H., van Ginneken, N., Dal Poz, M. R., Desiraju, K., Morris, J. E., … Scheffler, R. M. (2011). Human resources for mental health care: Current situation and strategies for action. *Lancet, 378*(9803), 1654–1663. https://doi.org/10.1016/s0140-6736(11)61093-3

Katon, W. J. (2003). Clinical and health services relationships between major depression, depressive symptoms, and general medical illness. *Biological Psychiatry, 54*(3), 216–226. https://doi.org/10.1016/S0006-3223(03)00273-7

Kessler, R. C., Berglund, P., Demler, O., Jin, R., Merikangas, K. R., & Walters, E. E. (2005). Lifetime prevalence and age-of-onset distributions of DSM-IV disorders in the National Comorbidity Survey Replication. *Archives of General Psychiatry, 62*(6), 593–602. https://doi.org/10.1001/archpsyc.62.6.593

Kessler, R. C., Chiu, W. T., Demler, O., Merikangas, K. R., & Walters, E. E. (2005). Prevalence, severity, and comorbidity of 12-month DSM-IV disorders in the National Comorbidity Survey Replication. *Archives of General Psychiatry, 62*(6), 617–627. https://doi.org/10.1001/archpsyc.62.6.617

Knickman, J., Rama Krishnan, K. R., Pincus, H. A., Blanco, C., Blazer, D. G., Coye, M. J., … Vitiello, B. (2016, September 19). *Improving access to effective care for people who have mental health and substance use disorders: Discussion paper. A vital direction for health and health care series*. Washington, DC: National Academies Press. https://nam.edu/wp-content/uploads/2016/09/Improving-Access-to-Effective-Care-for-People-Who-Have-Mental-Health-and-Sustance-Use-Disorders.pdf

Kohrt, B. A., Rasmussen, A., Kaiser, B. N., Haroz, E. E., Maharjan, S. M., Mutamba, B. B., … Hinton, D. E. (2014). Cultural concepts of distress and psychiatric disorders: Literature review and research recommendations for global mental health epidemiology. *International Journal of Epidemiology, 43*(2), 365–406. https://doi.org/10.1093/ije/dyt227

Kuramoto, F. (2014). The affordable care act and integrated care. *Journal of Social Work in Disability & Rehabilitation, 13*(1–2), 44–86. https://doi.org/10.1080/1536710x.2013.870515

Larson, M. J., Miller, L., Becker, M. A., Richardson, E., Kammerer, N., Thom, J., … Savage, A. (2005). Physical health burdens of women with trauma histories and co-occurring substance abuse and mental disorders. *Journal of Behavioral Health Services and Research, 32*(2), 128–140. https://doi.org/10.1097/00075484-200504000-00003

Lehavot, K., O'Hara, R., Washington, D. L., Yano, E. M., & Simpson, T. L. (2015). Posttraumatic stress disorder symptom severity and socioeconomic factors associated with veterans health administration use among women veterans. *Women's Health Issues, 25*(5), 535–541. https:// doi.org/10.1016/j.whi.2015.05.003

Lieber, C. S. (2000). Ethnic and gender differences in ethanol metabolism. *Alcoholism: Clinical and Experimental Research, 24*(4), 417–418.

Lipsitt, D. R., Joseph, R., Meyer, D., & Notman, M. T. (2015). Medically unexplained symptoms: Barriers to effective treatment when nothing is the matter. *Harvard Review of Psychiatry, 23*(6), 438–448. https://doi.org/10.1097/hrp.0000000000000055

Machtinger, E. L., Wilson, T. C., Haberer, J. E., & Weiss, D. S. (2012). Psychological trauma and PTSD in HIV-positive women: A meta-analysis. *AIDS and Behavior, 16*(8), 2091–2100. https://doi.org/10.1007/s10461-011-0127-4

Mann, K., Ackermann, K., Croissant, B., Mundle, G., Nakovics, H., & Diehl, A. (2005). Neuroimaging of gender differences in alcohol dependence: Are women more vulnerable? *Alcoholism: Clinical and Experimental Research, 29*(5), 896–901.

McCabe, M. P., & Leas, L. (2008). A qualitative study of primary health care access, barriers and satisfaction among people with mental illness. *Psychology, Health & Medicine, 13*(3), 303–312. https://doi.org/10.1080/13548500701473952

Murray, C. J. L., & Lopez, A. D. (1996). *The global burden of disease: A comprehensive assessment of mortality and disability from diseases, injuries, and risk factors in 1990 and projected to 2020.* Cambridge, MA: Harvard School of Public Health on behalf of the World Health Organization and the World Bank.

Muskett, C. (2014). Trauma-informed care in inpatient mental health settings: A review of the literature. *International Journal of Mental Health Nursing, 23*(1), 51–59. https://doi.org/10.1111/inm.12012

Mustillo, S. A., Kysar-Moon, A., Douglas, S. R., Hargraves, R., Wadsworth, S. M., Fraine, M., & Frazer, N. L. (2015). Overview of depression, post-traumatic stress disorder, and alcohol misuse among active duty service members returning from Iraq and Afghanistan, self-report and diagnosis. *Military Medicine, 180*(4), 419–427. https://doi.org/10.7205/milmed-d-14-00335

National Academies of Sciences, Engineering, & Medicine. (2017). *Communities in action: Pathways to health equity.* Washington, DC: The National Academies Press.

National Academies of Sciences, Engineering, & Medicine. (2018). *Women's mental health across the life course through a sex-gender lens: Proceedings of a workshop–in brief.* Washington, DC: The National Academies Press.

O'Neil, A., Fisher, A. J., Kibbey, K. J., Jacka, F. N., Kotowicz, M. A., Williams, L. J., ... Pasco, J. A. (2016). Depression is a risk factor for incident coronary heart disease in women: An 18-year longitudinal study. *Journal of Affective Disorders, 196*, 117–124. https://doi.org/10.1016/j.jad.2016.02.029

Office of the Surgeon General. (1999). *Mental health: A report of the Surgeon General.* Rockville, MD: Department of Health and Human Services, U.S. Public Health Service.

Office of the Surgeon General. (2016). *Facing addiction in America: The Surgeon General's report on alcohol, drugs, and health* (Reports of the Surgeon General). Washington, DC: US Department of Health and Human Services. https://addiction.surgeongeneral.gov/surgeon-generals-report.pdf

Office on Women's Health. (2009). *Action steps for improving women's mental health.* Rockville, MD: Office on Women's Health, Substance Abuse and Mental Health Services Administration. https://store.samhsa.gov/shin/content/OWH09-PROFESSIONAL/OWH09-PROFESSIONAL.pdf

Olfson, M., Gerhard, T., Huang, C., Crystal, S., & Stroup, T. S. (2015). Premature mortality among adults with schizophrenia in the United States. *JAMA Psychiatry, 72*(12), 1172–1181. https:// doi.org/10.1001/jamapsychiatry.2015.1737

Orza, L., Bewley, S., Logie, C. H., Crone, E. T., Moroz, S., Strachan, S., ... Welbourn, A. (2015). How does living with HIV impact on women's mental health? Voices from a global survey.

Journal of the International AIDS Society, 18(Suppl 5), 20289. https://doi.org/10.7448/ias.18.6.20289

Patient Protection and Affordable Care Act, U.S.C. 42 §18001, Pub. L. No. 111–148. (2010). https://www.congress.gov/111/plaws/publ148/PLAW-111publ148.pdf

Pearlstein, T., Howard, M., Salisbury, A., & Zlotnick, C. (2009). Postpartum depression. *American Journal of Obstetrics and Gynecology, 200*(4), 357–364. https://doi.org/10.1016/j.ajog.2008.11.033

Peck, B. M., & Denney, M. (2012). Disparities in the conduct of the medical encounter: The effects of physician and patient race and gender. *SAGE Open, 2*(3), 1–14. https://doi.org/10.1177/2158244012459193

Petersen, I., Gilbert, R. E., Evans, S. J., Man, S. L., & Nazareth, I. (2011). Pregnancy as a major determinant for discontinuation of antidepressants: An analysis of data from The Health Improvement Network. *Journal of Clinical Psychiatry, 72*(7), 979–985. https://doi.org/10.4088/JCP.10m06090blu

Picci, R. L., Vigna-Taglianti, F., Oliva, F., Mathis, F., Salmaso, S., Ostacoli, L., … Furlan, P. M. (2012). Personality disorders among patients accessing alcohol detoxification treatment: Prevalence and gender differences. *Comprehensive Psychiatry, 53*(4), 355–363. https://doi.org/10.1016/j.comppsych.2011.05.011

Pratt, L. A., & Brody, D. J. (2014). Depression in the U.S. household population, 2009-2012. *NCHS Data Brief*(172), 1–8. https://www.cdc.gov/nchs/data/databriefs/db172.pdf

President's New Freedom Commission on Mental Health. (2003). *Achieving the promise: transforming mental health care in America: Final report* (DHHS publication no.). Rockville, MD: U. S. Department of Health and Human Services. http://www.eric.ed.gov/PDFS/ED479836.pdf

Primm, A. B., Vasquez, M. J., Mays, R. A., Sammons-Posey, D., McKnight-Eily, L. R., Presley-Cantrell, L. R., … Perry, G. S. (2010). The role of public health in addressing racial and ethnic disparities in mental health and mental illness. *Preventing Chronic Disease, 7*(1), A20.

Quinlivan, E. B., Fletcher, J., Eastwood, E. A., Blank, A. E., Verdecias, N., & Roytburd, K. (2015). Health status of HIV-infected women entering care: Baseline medical findings from the women of color initiative. *AIDS Patient Care and STDs, 29*(Suppl 1), S11–S19. https://doi.org/10.1089/apc.2014.0277

Rapaport, M. H., Clary, C., Fayyad, R., & Endicott, J. (2005). Quality-of-life impairment in depressive and anxiety disorders. *American Journal of Psychiatry, 162*(6), 1171–1178. https://doi.org/10.1176/appi.ajp.162.6.1171

Rodger, A. J., Cambiano, V., Bruun, T., Vernazza, P., Collins, S., van Lunzen, J., … Lundgren, J. (2016). Sexual activity without condoms and risk of HIV transmission in serodifferent couples when the HIV-positive partner is using suppressive antiretroviral therapy. *JAMA, 316*(2), 171–181. https://doi.org/10.1001/jama.2016.5148

Smalley, K. B., Yancey, C. T., Warren, J. C., Naufel, K., Ryan, R., & Pugh, J. L. (2010). Rural mental health and psychological treatment: A review for practitioners. *Journal of Clinical Psychology, 66*(5), 479–489. https://doi.org/10.1002/jclp.20688

Spinelli, M. G. (2004). Maternal infanticide associated with mental illness: Prevention and the promise of saved lives. *American Journal of Psychiatry, 161*(9), 1548–1557. https://doi.org/10.1176/appi.ajp.161.9.1548

Substance Abuse and Mental Health Services Administration. (2014a). *Results from the 2013 National Survey on Drug Use and Health: Summary of national findings* (NSDUH Series H-48; DHHS Publication no.). Rockville, MD: Author. https://www.samhsa.gov/data/sites/default/files/NSDUHresultsPDFWHTML2013/Web/NSDUHresults2013.pdf

Substance Abuse and Mental Health Services Administration. (2014b). *Trauma-informed care in behavioral health services. A treatment improvement protocol.* Rockville, MD: Author. https://store.samhsa.gov/shin/content//SMA14-4816/SMA14-4816.pdf

The Secretary's Advisory Committee on National Health Promotion and Disease Prevention Objectives for 2020. (2008, October 28). Section IV. Advisory Committee findings and recommendations. In The Secretary's Advisory Committee (Ed.), *Phase I report: Recommendations for the framework and format of healthy people 2020* (pp. 19–36). Washington, DC: U. S. Department of Health and Human Services. Retrieved from https://www.healthypeople.gov/sites/default/files/PhaseI_0.pdf

Tse, S., Tsoi, E. W., Hamilton, B., O'Hagan, M., Shepherd, G., Slade, M., ... Petrakis, M. (2016). Uses of strength-based interventions for people with serious mental illness: A critical review. *International Journal of Social Psychiatry, 62*(3), 281–291. https://doi.org/10.1177/0020764015623970

UNAIDS. (2017). *When women lead, change happens: Women advancing the end of AIDS.* Geneva: Author.

Violence Prevention Alliance. (2018). *The public health approach.* [Web page]. Geneva: World Health Organization. http://www.who.int/violenceprevention/approach/public_health/en/

Warner, D. F., & Brown, T. H. (2011). Understanding how race/ethnicity and gender define age-trajectories of disability: An intersectionality approach. *Social Science and Medicine, 72*(8), 1236–1248. https://doi.org/10.1016/j.socscimed.2011.02.034

Weaver, A., & Himle, J. A. (2017). Cognitive–behavioral therapy for depression and anxiety disorders in rural settings: A review of the literature. *Journal of Rural Mental Health, 41*(3), 189–221. https://doi.org/10.1037/rmh0000075

Whetten, K., Reif, S. S., Napravnik, S., Swartz, M. S., Thielman, N. M., Eron, J. J., Jr., ... Soto, T. (2005). Substance abuse and symptoms of mental illness among HIV-positive persons in the southeast. *Southern Medical Journal, 98*(1), 9–14. https://doi.org/10.1097/01.Smj.0000149371.37294.66

Whiteford, H. A., Degenhardt, L., Rehm, J., Baxter, A. J., Ferrari, A. J., Erskine, H. E., ... Vos, T. (2013). Global burden of disease attributable to mental and substance use disorders: Findings from the Global Burden of Disease Study 2010. *Lancet, 382*(9904), 1575–1586. https://doi.org/10.1016/s0140-6736(13)61611-6

World Health Organization. (2015). *Mental health atlas 2014.* Geneva: Author. http://apps.who.int/iris/bitstream/10665/178879/1/9789241565011_eng.pdf?ua=1&ua=1

World Health Organization. (2017). *World health statistics 2017: Monitoring health for the SDGs.* Geneva: Author. http://apps.who.int/iris/bitstream/10665/255336/1/9789241565486-eng.pdf?ua=1

Yaeger, D., Smith, H. G., & Altshuler, L. L. (2006). Atypical antipsychotics in the treatment of schizophrenia during pregnancy and the postpartum. *American Journal of Psychiatry, 163*(12), 2064–2070. https://doi.org/10.1176/ajp.2006.163.12.2064

Yim, I. S., Tanner Stapleton, L. R., Guardino, C. M., Hahn-Holbrook, J., & Dunkel Schetter, C. (2015). Biological and psychosocial predictors of postpartum depression: Systematic review and call for integration. *Annual Review of Clinical Psychology, 11*, 99–137. https://doi.org/10.1146/annurev-clinpsy-101414-020426

Zinzow, H. M., Grubaugh, A. L., Monnier, J., Suffoletta-Maierle, S., & Frueh, B. C. (2007). Trauma among female veterans: A critical review. *Trauma, Violence & Abuse, 8*(4), 384–400. https://doi.org/10.1177/1524838007307295

The Behavioral Health of American Indian/Alaska Native Populations: Risk and Resiliency

Julie A. Baldwin, Emery R. Eaves, Betty G. Brown, Kristan Elwell, and Heather J. Williamson

Introduction

American Indian and Alaska Native (AI/AN) populations include people who main-tain tribal affiliation or community attachment with the original populations of North America, South America, and Central America. In the United States (USA), there are 567 AI/AN tribes that are federally recognized, more than 100 tribes that are state recognized, and some tribes that are neither state nor federally recognized (Office of Minority Health, 2018). As of 2012, there were an estimated 5.2 million people, or 2% of the total US population, classified as AI/AN alone or AI/AN in combination with one or more other races. Approximately 25% of AI/AN live on reservations or other trust lands. Of the approximately 75% of the AI/AN who live outside of tribal areas, 60% live in metropolitan areas (Office of Minority Health, 2018). Each of these tribal communities has unique cultural teachings, traditions, and languages.

Rates of diseases and other adverse health outcomes are higher in AI/AN than in other communities in the USA. Heart disease, cancer, and unintentional injuries are the leading causes of death among AI/AN (Centers for Disease Control & Prevention [CDC], 2012, 2013). Compared to Whites, American Indians/Alaska Natives have higher rates of emphysema, chronic bronchitis, and asthma (Barnes, Adams, & Powell-Griner, 2010). Furthermore, AI/AN men and women are twice as likely to be diagnosed with chronic liver disease than Whites (Office of Minority Health, 2013), and rates of unintentional injuries and deaths are 60% higher in AI/AN compared to Whites (West & Naumann, 2011). The literature also demonstrates major health issues for AI/AN with regard to several behavioral health conditions: substance abuse, post-traumatic stress, violence, and suicide (Gone & Trimble, 2012; Myhra

J. A. Baldwin (✉) · E. R. Eaves · B. G. Brown · K. Elwell · H. J. Williamson
Northern Arizona University, Flagstaff, AZ, USA
e-mail: Julie.baldwin@nau.edu

© Springer Nature Switzerland AG 2020
B. L. Levin, A. Hanson (eds.), *Foundations of Behavioral Health*,
https://doi.org/10.1007/978-3-030-18435-3_10

& Wieling, 2014a, 2014b; Office of Minority Health, 2018; Spillane, Greenfield, Venner, & Kahler, 2015; Yuan, Duran, Walters, Pearson, & Evans-Campbell, 2014).

The American Indian Service Utilization, Psychiatric Epidemiology, Risk and Protective Factors Project found the prevalence of DSM-IV disorders was 35.7% for women to nearly 50% for men (Beals et al., 2005). The most common disorder for women was post-traumatic stress disorder and for men, alcohol abuse and dependence. Significant levels of comorbidity were found among those with depressive and/or anxiety and substance use disorders (Beals et al., 2005).

To fully understand the behavioral health disparities experienced by AI/AN, it is critical to examine the context in which they occur. High prevalence of behavioral disorders in AI/AN communities is believed to be linked to a number of historical and environmental factors, such as historical trauma and contemporary discrimination, as well as current-day unemployment, academic failure, high-risk occupations, and lack of health insurance (Andrews, Guerrero, Wooten, & Lengnick-Hall, 2015; Centers for Disease Control & Prevention, 2013; Moghaddam, Momper, & Fong, 2013; Stanley, Harness, Swaim, & Beauvais, 2014).

Currently, one in four AI/AN live in poverty (Macartney, Bishaw, & Fontenot, 2013, February). Although AI/AN health-care services are supposed to be provided by the Indian Health Service (HIS) and some tribal health offices, these services are not adequate to cover the health needs. Over one-third of AI/AN have no health insurance coverage (Office of Clinical and Preventive Services, 2011). AI/AN are also underrepresented in the Medicaid expansion population (Andrews et al., 2015), which affects access to and utilization of health and behavioral health services.

Studies of both urban and rural AI/AN populations have documented poor health, limited health-care options, and limited services utilization (Adekoya, Truman, & Landen, 2015; Brave Heart et al., 2016; Castor et al., 2006; Genovesi, Hastings, Edgerton, & Olson, 2014; Gone & Trimble, 2012; Liao et al., 2011; Murphy et al., 2014; Reilley et al., 2014; Siordia, Bell, & Haileselassie, 2017; Towne Jr., Probst, Mitchell, & Chen, 2015). Barriers to services and utilization include distance to a care facility, transportation, stigma, lack of cultural sensitivity among health-care professionals, relocation, difficulty navigating health-care delivery systems, lack of awareness of available health resources, long waiting times for health care, difficulty adhering to medication, preference for traditional healers, and poor incentives in health promotion (Kim, Bryant, Goins, Worley, & Chiriboga, 2012; Moghaddam et al., 2013; Shah et al., 2014). Other factors also affect services delivery, including gaps in state-tribal collaborations (Croff, Rieckmann, & Spence, 2014; Gone & Trimble, 2012).

Despite these challenges, AI/AN people have demonstrated resiliency and self-determination over the centuries. In this chapter, we describe the current state of behavioral health for AI/AN and the contributing factors to these disparities. We feature some of the successes AI/AN communities have in addressing these issues.

This chapter is organized by first presenting the epidemiology of behavioral disorders in AI/AN, including mental disorders, alcohol/drug disorders, disabilities, and co-occurring disorders. We emphasize both risk and protective factors. We then highlight some of the successful behavioral health prevention and treatment strategies. We conclude by discussing implications for behavioral health for AI/AN including future directions for research, services, programs, and policy.

Mental Health and Psychological Distress

AI/AN populations are at a high risk for poor mental health outcomes. Among those 18 years of age and older, AI/AN are more likely to experience serious psychological distress in the past 30 days (5.4%) than their White or Black/African American counterparts (3.4% and 3.5%, respectively) (National Center for Health Statistics [NCHS], 2016, May). AI/AN populations are also 50% more likely to report hopelessness, worthlessness, and feelings of nervousness or restlessness all or most of the time compared to non-Hispanic whites and 80% more likely to report frequent sadness (NCHS, 2016). Some researchers claim that accurate data on depression among AI/AN elders is challenging because most AI/AN do not seek treatment for depression and are, therefore, "hidden" conditions (Garrett, Baldridge, Benson, Crowder, & Aldrich, 2015). Using extrapolations from other minority data, Garrett et al. (2015) project that AI/AN in 2050 will experience four times the rate of depression in those over 65 years of age and approximately four-and-a-half times the rate of dementia as they experienced in 2010.

In an analysis of gender and ethnic differences in the National Epidemiologic Survey on Alcohol and Related Conditions, Brave Heart et al. (2016) reported that most AI/AN men (70%) and women (63%) experienced at least one lifetime mental disorder and were more likely to have experienced mental disorders (substance use and mood and personality disorders) than their non-Hispanic White counterparts (Brave Heart et al., 2016). The authors argue that historical trauma (e.g., boarding school experience but more broadly genocide, ethnocide, and attempts to assimilate into majority culture) likely contributed to unresolved grief that led to depression and substance abuse (Brave Heart, 2003; Brave Heart et al., 2016).

Historical genocide and the boarding school system have contributed to contemporary traumatic experiences and "multi-generational distress" in AI/AN (Warne & Lajimodiere, 2015). For example, Myhra and Wieling (2014b) examined the impact of trauma on the psychological well-being across two generations of AI/AN. Participants of both generations reported trauma from childhood, including substance abuse and neglect, sexual or physical abuse, family violence, loss, and death. Both generations reported past and current discrimination and racism, and attributed their elders' difficulties (such as substance abuse) to boarding school experiences. Soto, Baezconde-Garbanati, Schwartz, and Unger (2015) found that historical trauma was a risk factor for commercial tobacco use, both directly and through several mediating factors, such as cultural activities and ethnic identity. The impact of substance abuse complicates the effects of historical trauma, often amplifying negative impacts and putting users at increased risk of experiencing or inflicting trauma (Ehlers, Gizer, Gilder, Ellingson, & Yehuda, 2013).

In interviews with AI/AN elders, Grayshield, Rutherford, Salazar, Mihecoby, and Luna (2015) explored the effects of historical trauma. The elders described historical trauma in both individual and community levels: the disrespect and destruction of the land and its people, boarding school abuses, and internalization of oppression (low self-worth and negative messages about self). They believed that the current impact of this history included alcoholism, substance abuse, food abuse (Western foods lead to Western diseases), and a negative impact of technology. They also reported a loss of culture and language, community discord and violence, anger, and depression (Grayshield et al., 2015).

Other psychological stressors included poverty, poor housing, or homelessness; lack of opportunities on reservation (compared to urban environments); and neighborhood safety. Parents reported more difficulties with mental health than their adult children, which the authors suggest is attributable to parents' efforts to protect their children (Myhra & Wieling, 2014a).

Evans-Campbell, Walters, Pearson, and Campbell (2012) found that two-spirit individuals (gay, bisexual, or transgender) who had attended boarding schools reported higher rates of alcohol use, illicit drug use, and suicidal ideations or attempts than those who had not attended boarding schools. Further, people with a parent or caregiver who attended boarding school were significantly more likely to experience suicidal ideations, generalized anxiety disorders, or post-traumatic stress disorders than others, suggesting that boarding school attendance impacts intergenerational health (Evans-Campbell et al., 2012). In other research with AI/AN individuals, even having a grandparent who attended boarding school was associated with increased risk of suicide (20.4% compared to 13.1%) (Bombay, Matheson, & Anisman, 2014).

Youth

American Indian/Alaska Native children experience high rates of victimization, poverty, mental disorders, and gang involvement that impact mental well-being. Conditions of poverty, loss of culture, and discrimination lead many AI/AN youth to be attracted to gang activity (Hautala, Sittner Hartshorn, & Whitbeck, 2016), which is linked to higher rates of substance abuse and violence (Whitbeck, Hoyt, Chen, & Stubben, 2002). High rates of alcohol use among AI/AN youth are often linked to historical trauma and the consequences of cultural loss at many levels (Brown, Dickerson, & D'Amico, 2016). Among AI/AN youth in substance abuse treatment, high rates of comorbid PTSD and alcoholism, as well as a history of trauma, are common (Ehlers et al., 2013). Further, substance use is one of the leading factors contributing to unintentional injuries and disabilities among AI youth (Centers for Disease Control & Prevention, 2003).

Social problems among AI/AN adolescents resulting from perceived discrimination and weak social ties, particularly in urban public school settings, can contribute to extreme alcohol and other drug consumption (Rees, Freng, & Winfree Jr., 2014;

Whitbeck, Hoyt, McMorris, Chen, & Stubben, 2001). Binge alcohol use among AI/AN adolescents is often linked to family problems and aggressive behavior, suicide, non-suicidal self-injury, and persistent problems in later life (Tingey et al., 2016). Children who witness or experience household dysfunction (domestic violence, substance abuse, criminal activity, and mental illness in the home), for example, are more likely to report poor mental health outcomes (Dickerson & Johnson, 2012; Warne & Lajimodiere, 2015). A higher risk for depression has been linked to how adolescents describe life events. Negative narratives about adverse life events (e.g., attribution of negative events to individual stupidity vs. bad luck) vs. positive (protective) narratives are styles developed as early as 8th grade and underscore the need for early intervention (Mileviciute, Trujillo, Gray, & Scott, 2013). Youth receiving mental health services in one urban clinic most frequently reported mood disorders (41.5%), adjustment disorder (35.4%), and PTSD or acute stress (23.1%). Researchers suggest these are linked to the pervasive effects of abuse, injustice, historical trauma, and the loss of cultural identity (Brave Heart, 2003; Dickerson & Johnson, 2012).

Multiple risk factors put AI/AN youth at risk for suicidal ideation. In a study of youths in the Midwestern USA, 9.5% reported suicidal thoughts (Yoder, Whitbeck, Hoyt, & LaFromboise, 2006). Substance use was most strongly correlated with suicidal thoughts, but other factors included being female, perceived discrimination, and negative life events such as family, economic, and school-related stressors (Yoder et al., 2006). Depression and poor family social support were also associated with suicidal thoughts (Manson, Beals, Dick, & Duclos, 1989). Zamora-Kapoor et al. (2016) found that social isolation, exposure to the suicide of a friend or family member, and being overweight were associated with suicidal ideation in both AI/AN and non-Hispanic whites. Barlow et al. (2012) found that 64% of youth from a Southwest tribe, particularly males, were intoxicated at the time of suicide and 75% of those who had attempted suicide were intoxicated at the time. Alcohol was the most commonly reported source of intoxication in suicidal acts, and peer pressure was also cited as a contributing factor.

Deviant peers appear to influence delinquency and substance use behaviors among AI/AN youth (Rees et al., 2014). AI/AN youth experience more disability-based harassment and gender-based harassment compared to youth from other racial or ethnic groups (Bucchianeri, Gower, McMorris, & Eisenberg, 2016). However, Tingey et al. (2016) report that strong ethnic identity, connection to cultural values, and positive family and peer influences are protective factors among AI/AN youth against substance use disorders (Mmari, Blum, & Teufel-Shone, 2010).

Gender, Sexual Orientation, and Violence

American Indian women are more likely to be victims of violent crime than women of other ethnicities (Walters & Simoni, 2002) and to develop psychiatric symptoms due to trauma and their sequelae. Sexual violence against AI/AN women is especially deleterious. Based on the National Intimate Partner and Sexual Violence

Survey, 2011, the lifetime prevalence of rape in AI/AN women is 27.5%, with another 55% reporting other forms of sexual violence (Breiding et al., 2014). In AI/AN women aged 15–35 living on or near a reservation, exposure to trauma was associated with symptoms of PTSD, substance use, and risky sexual behavior. Those with high trauma exposure who met the criteria for PTSD were at greater risk for binge drinking and risky sexual behaviors that increased their risk for HIV (Pearson et al., 2015).

There is evidence that AI/ANs who identify as gay, bisexual, or transgendered ("two-spirit" individuals) experience disproportionately higher rates of both anti-Native and anti-gay discrimination and violence, particularly sexual violence in urban settings (Fieland, Walters, & Simoni, 2007; Lehavot, Walters, & Simoni, 2009). Two-spirit AI/AN women are at particular risk for substance abuse and mental health challenges such as PTSD due to their "multiple minority oppressed status" (Elm, Lewis, Walters, & Self, 2016, p. 352). Among two-spirit AI/AN, consequences of emotional trauma were exacerbated by boarding school attendance (Evans-Campbell et al., 2012).

Both AI/AN females and males experience high rates of intimate partner violence, usually before the age of 25. Among Native women, 51.7% reported physical violence, and 63.8% reported psychological aggression in intimate relationships (Breiding et al., 2014).

In a study of 18- to 45-year-old women at an IHS hospital, intimate partner violence was strongly associated with subsequent mood disorder (Stockman, Hayashi, & Campbell, 2015). Although 43% of Native men reported physical violence in their relationships, reports of psychological aggression were less frequent than in most other ethnicities (Breiding et al., 2014).

Veterans

Both rural and urban AI/AN veterans experience poor mental health from combat experience, most commonly depression and mood and other anxiety disorders (Westermeyer & Canive, 2013), and more lifetime PTSD than their white counterparts (Beals et al., 2002; Westermeyer & Canive, 2013). Among AI/ANs who served in the military, almost half report some type of disability associated with their service and identified their substance use problems as resulting from military service (Harada, Villa, Reifel, & Bayhylle, 2005). In a nationally representative sample of US veterans, Smith, Goldstein, and Grant (2016) found a higher prevalence of lifetime PTSD in AI/ANs (24.1%) than among Blacks (11%) or Whites (5.97%). In addition, AI/ANs are overrepresented among veterans who are homeless (making up 1.6% of veterans but 19% of the homeless veteran population) and experience higher rates of hospitalization for alcohol dependence than any other veteran group (Kasprow & Rosenheck, 1998).

Difficulty navigating the complex system of the Veterans Administration exacerbates stress in veterans and their families (Kaufman et al., 2016). This is particularly true on reservation lands that lack culturally competent care and transportation to access services (AlMasarweh & Ward, 2016).

Suicide

Suicide is one of the most serious outcomes of severe mental distress in AI/AN. In 2014, the second highest US rate of suicide was among AI/AN males (16.4 per 100,000) (NCHS, 2016). The highest rates of suicide in Native men occurred among those 15–24 years and 25–44 years (23.5 and 26.2 per 100,000, respectively). Native women completed suicide at lower rates than their male counter parts (5.5 per 100,000 overall), but those between 15 and 24 years of age were almost twice as likely to complete suicide as non-Hispanic whites of the same age (NCHS, 2016). Two-spirit women who attended boarding school were six times more likely to report suicidal thoughts than those who did not attend boarding school and almost nine times more likely to attempt suicide (Evans-Campbell et al., 2012).

Veteran suicide is increasing for all groups, especially for AI/AN. In addition to a lack of connectedness and sense of burden on family (if the veteran lived), Chiurliza, Michaels, and Joiner (2016) found higher rates of suicide risk in AI/AN compared to other ethnicities through consideration of an "acquired capability for suicide (i.e., a diminished fear of death and increased pain tolerance)" (p. 3), a quality that should be considered in suicide prevention at all levels of military service.

Substance Use in AI/AN Communities

AI/ANs have the highest rates of substance abuse of any racial/ethnic group in the USA, with rates of alcoholism and illicit drug use two to five times higher than the general population (Ehlers, Liang, & Gizer, 2012; Currie, Wild, Schopflocher, Laing, & Veugelers, 2013; Steen, 2015). Substance use is a principle causal factor in continued poor health outcomes in AI/AN communities. The IHS views the consequences of substance abuse as the root of the most urgent health problems in AI/AN communities (Ehlers et al., 2012).

AI/AN youth use tobacco, alcohol, and illicit substances at higher rates than adolescents of any other racial/ethnic group (Steen, 2015). Use is often initiated at younger ages compared to substance use debut in other groups (Brown et al., 2016; Whitesell et al., 2014). Stanley et al. (2014) found high prevalence rates for almost every substance, particularly marijuana, binge alcohol use, and OxyContin, among AI/AN as young as 8th grade. Dickerson and Johnson (2012) found that alcohol and marijuana were the most common substances used among a cohort of AI/AN youth. However, AI/AN youth also report relatively high rates of amphetamine/stimulant use, narcotic pain medication use, cocaine, tobacco, inhalants, hallucinogens, stimulant prescription medications, and over-the-counter medications (Barlow et al., 2010; Dickerson & Johnson, 2012).

Gender differences in substance use among AI/ANs vary by region and urban versus rural location. There is some evidence that substance abuse, such as methamphetamine and opioid analgesic use, is more prevalent among AI/AN women than men (Forcehimes et al., 2011). One study conducted in Los Angeles County found more AI/AN women seeking treatment for methamphetamine use than men (Spear, Crevecoeur, Rawson, & Clark, 2007); however, other research has found methamphetamine use to be more common among men (Iritani, Hallfors, & Bauer, 2007). AI/AN men have some of the highest substance use rates of any racial or ethnic group (O'Connell, Novins, Beals, & Spicer, 2005; Whitesell, Beals, Crow, Mitchell, & Novins, 2012). High rates of alcohol use among AI/AN men lead to intergenerational issues such as difficulty establishing positive fatherhood roles (Neault et al., 2012).

AI/AN women have one of the highest rates of drug-related mortality of any racial/ethnic group (up to 44 per 100,000 in 45–54 age category) (Walters & Simoni, 2002). In a study of female students attending tribal colleges, Schultz (2016) found that most women (62%) had used drugs at least once during their lifetime. In an urban sample, two-spirit individuals (gay, bisexual, or transgendered) were more likely to report being victimized or engaging in high-risk behaviors as a result of substance use (Simoni, Walters, Balsam, & Meyers, 2006). Two-spirit individuals also reported higher rates of mental health service utilization, higher rates of alcohol use, and higher rates of illicit drug use than other participants (Balsam, Huang, Fieland, Simoni, & Walters, 2004).

Although substance abuse is a major problem facing many AI/AN communities, there are major regional differences in substance abuse and related disorders between, for example, Southwest and Great Plains communities (Etz, Arroyo, Crump, Rosa, & Scott, 2012; Volkow & Warren, 2012). To understand substance abuse in both current and historical context, nuances and contextual factors influencing substance use in varied AI/AN populations must be considered (Etz et al., 2012). Although many cultural, social, economic, and contextual factors contribute to high rates of substance use, many strengths and sources of resilience among AI/AN communities, such as strong cultural traditions, family support, and cultural pride, also contribute to abstinence and to mitigating the effects of substance abuse (LaFromboise, Hoyt, Oliver, & Whitbeck, 2006).

Alcohol Use

Alcohol use is extremely prevalent in AI/AN communities, with lifetime prevalence of 96% for men and 92% for women by the time they finish 12th grade (Walters & Simoni, 2002). AI/AN have the highest rates of admission for substance use disorders in general, and they are more likely to report alcohol as the primary substance used than any other racial or ethnic group (Greenfield & Venner, 2012). Mortality resulting from alcohol use is much higher among AI/ANs than non-AI/ANs (Evans-Campbell et al., 2012), although mortality also varies considerably by region, with some of the highest rates in the Northern Plains and lowest in the Eastern USA (Landen, Roeber, Naimi, Nielsen, & Sewell, 2014). AI/AN people who use alcohol face an elevated risk of both mental and physical health consequences, including physical and sexual violence, accidents from intoxicated driving, and chronic health issues (Landen et al., 2014; Whitesell et al., 2012; Yuan et al., 2010).

Research suggests that AI/ANs display higher rates of abstinence from alcohol than the general population (Cunningham, Solomon, & Muramoto, 2016); however, adults who do engage in alcohol use often engage in heavier or binge use (O'Connell et al., 2005; Whitesell et al., 2012). Reservation-based populations exhibit greater abstinence than urban AI/AN populations, perhaps in part because many reservations prohibit the use and sale of alcohol within their borders (Landen et al., 2014; Walters, Simoni, & Evans-Campbell, 2002).

Considerable efforts to uncover genetic predispositions to alcoholism among AI/ANs have been unsuccessful, suggesting that social factors are largely responsible for elevated rates (Ehlers et al., 2012). Alcohol was not introduced into AI/AN communities until European colonization, and thus there are strong negative associations with its use. In qualitative interviews with AI/AN people, Spicer (2001) found that both drinkers and non-drinkers described alcohol use as incompatible with AI/AN worldviews and morality. AI/AN communities, however, report several dilemmas related to the embeddedness of alcohol use in many aspects of current social and cultural life (Yuan et al., 2010). Quintero (2001) argues that looking uncritically at AI/AN patterns of alcohol use without considering historical and contemporary contexts of discrimination and disadvantage faced by AI/AN peoples serves to reproduce colonialist images and perpetuates disadvantage among AI/AN people through the preservation of negative stereotypes.

Tobacco Use

According to the US Centers for Disease Control and Prevention (CDC), between 2005 and 2013, AI/AN people used tobacco at higher rates than all other US populations except individuals reporting multiple races (Jamal et al., 2014). Smoking is also more common among males and among people living in poverty (Jamal et al., 2014). AI/AN youth have the highest rates of commercial tobacco use in the USA (Unger, Soto, & Baezconde-Garbanati, 2006), and early tobacco use is often associated with stress or exposure to trauma and negative peer influences (Whitesell et al., 2014). AI/AN smokers are consistently more likely to drink heavily than non-smokers (Ryan, Cooke, & Leatherdale, 2016), and although tobacco use varies considerably by region, related health consequences tend to be disproportionately higher in AI/AN communities (Whitesell et al., 2012).

Illicit Drug Use

AI/AN communities have high rates of use for a range of illicit substances, including stimulants (Gilder, Gizer, Lau, & Ehlers, 2014), inhalants (Stockman et al., 2015), prescription medications (Katzman et al., 2016; Momper, Delva, Tauiliili, Mueller-Williams, & Goral, 2013; Wu, Pilowsky, & Patkar, 2008), and increasingly methamphetamines (Brown, 2010; Forcehimes et al., 2011).

Use of opioid analgesics for non-medical reasons is higher among AI/ANs than among Caucasians (6.2% and 5.6%, respectively) (Katzman et al., 2016). AI/AN people experience higher rates of accidental overdose as a result of opioid use (15.7% vs 14.7%) (Hirchak & Murphy, 2017). Among AI/AN adolescents, past year hospitalization or multiple arrests, as well as low family income and being treated for psychological problems, are associated with increased use of non-prescribed opioids (Wu et al., 2008).

Use of methamphetamines (MA) has been increasing in AI/AN communities (Forcehimes et al., 2011). Rural and reservation-dwelling AI/AN communities have experienced rates of stimulant dependence as high as 33%. Rural areas, including many American Indian reservations, are particularly attractive for MA production due to geographic isolation, poverty, and sparse law enforcement (Glover-Kerkvliet, 2009). Health disparities and vulnerability of AI/AN communities have been compounded by the MA crisis, with a broad range of health risks from dental and skin disorders to accidental poisoning of children, increases in crime, domestic violence, and child neglect/abuse (Glover-Kerkvliet, 2009; Spear et al., 2007).

Multi-Substance Use Disorders

Multi-substance use disorder impacts AI/AN communities disproportionately and those using multiple substances with alcohol experience symptoms of alcohol-related problems at higher rates than those who use alcohol alone (Gilder, Stouffer, Lau, & Ehlers, 2016). Use of multiple drugs in combination with alcohol use has been associated with increases in the rates of DSM-3R alcohol dependence disorders (Kunitz, 2008). In a study of Alaska Natives, the majority of alcohol users also used other substances, with the most common being marijuana, followed by cocaine and opiates (Malcolm, Hesselbrock, & Segal, 2006). Those who experience multi-substance use disorders often initiate drug and alcohol use at earlier ages and experience academic failure and other social difficulties (Gilder et al., 2016).

Disability and Substance Use

National estimates of disability status in 2014 found that 1 in 5 US adults have some type of disability. Among US adults, AI/ANs have the highest prevalence of experiencing any disability (35.5%) compared to all other racial and ethnic groups. AI/

ANs also have the highest prevalence of cognitive disability (19.4%), mobility disability (19.7%), vision disability (9%), self-care disability (6.3%), and independent living disability (12.3%) compared to all other racial/ethnic groups (Okoro, Hollis, Cyrus, & Griffin-Blake, 2018).

The prevalence of fetal alcohol syndrome is highest among AI/AN children as a result of higher alcohol use among AI/AN women (Fox et al., 2015). High rates of alcohol and tobacco use during pregnancy among AI/AN mothers (3 times and 1.5 times the national rate, respectively) also contribute to high rates of infant mortality in AI/AN populations (Walters et al., 2002).

Among AI/ANs with disabilities, drug use increases as disability severity increases (Grant et al., 2016). AI/AN males and females with disabilities have the highest prevalence of smoking as compared to other race/ethnic groups with disabilities. Lower education levels among AI/AN adults with disabilities contribute to increased nicotine use (Courtney-Long, Romano, Carroll, & Fox, 2017). Also, AI/AN males with disabilities are more likely to binge drink or engage in heavy drinking (Okoro et al., 2007). AI/ANs with traumatic brain injuries (TBI) are more likely to experience substance use disorders (Nelson, Rhoades, Noonan, & Manson, 2007).

Prevention, Intervention, and Treatment

Successful prevention, intervention, and treatment of behavioral health concerns in AI/AN populations are constrained by several barriers to services delivery. Difficulty of diagnosing mental health conditions, lack of access to treatment services, funding limitations, and stigma toward mental health impose barriers to appropriate treatment and care (Johnson & Cameron, 2001). One key barrier to designing and implementing effective treatment programs is that Western biomedical definitions of mental health and treatment are poorly aligned with AI/AN understandings of wellness and healing (Gone, 2008; Hartmann & Gone, 2012). Divergent models of health and illness pose barriers to providing adequate and culturally resonant treatment for mental health (Gone, 2016). Many AI/AN communities' understandings of mental health are incongruent with Western biomedical therapies (Office of the Surgeon General, 2001), and attempts to treat AI/AN patients from within biomedical paradigms are often perceived as colonialistic or even as "brainwashing" by AI/AN patients (Gone, 2016, p. 2).

Despite the reported prevalence of traumatic experience among AI/AN individuals, few seek treatment for trauma due to limited access to mental health services and fear of stigma and discrimination (United States Commission on Civil Rights, 2004). Gurley et al. (2001) found that although 75% of AI/AN veterans reported a mental health or substance abuse problem, PTSD, and alcohol abuse, fewer than 20% of these veterans sought mental health care and more commonly sought care for physical health concerns. Fears of stigma and discrimination when accessing mental health services present major barriers to improving behavioral health, particularly among AI/AN youth.

Research suggests that nearly half of AI/AN individuals diagnosed with mental illness seek treatment from traditional medical practitioners. Traditional medical services are often sought for the treatment of depression and anxiety. Walls, Johnson, Whitbeck, and Hoyt (2006) found that American Indian parents/caregivers strongly prefer traditional cultural services for mental health and substance abuse problems rather than formal behavioral health services and believe that these services are more effective. Increased anxiety, spiritual engagement, and past experiences with discrimination in health care were also associated with a preference for a traditional approach to care (Aronson, Johnson-Jennings, Kading, Smith, & Walls, 2016).

Other known barriers to care include geography, particularly access to services located in rural and remote locations, poverty, transportation, and an inadequate number of qualified treatment providers (Goodkind et al., 2010).

School-based prevention programs have become an increasingly popular means to enhance access to prevention services. These programs, which are located in tribal affiliated and public schools, have primarily focused on alcohol and drug prevention (Middlebrook, LeMaster, Beals, Novins, & Manson, 2001).

In order to assess whether existing prevention and treatment services are effectively meeting the mental health needs of individuals suffering from mental health conditions, there has been an increasing call for integrating evidence-based practices (EBPs) with these services. Behind the draw of EBP has been the desire to provide all individuals with quality care that has been scientifically validated to demonstrate effectiveness (Walker, Whitener, Trupin, & Migliarini, 2015). However, concerns have been raised that few studies have evaluated these programs using rigorous methods. Further, given the small size of the AI/AN population, AI/AN patients have been poorly represented in many studies. As a result, these studies fail to include large samples that would generate the reliability and validity characteristic of rigorous methods (Walker et al., 2015). Many AI/AN communities perceive EBP standards as incongruent with their values and a challenge to tribal sovereignty. Demonstrating the effectiveness of culturally adapted programs has been particularly challenging due to the limited representation of AI/AN communities in efficacy trials.

Ethnic Identity and Culturally Appropriate Approaches to Prevention and Healing

In recent years, scholars have turned to culturally adapted interventions to increase the effectiveness of prevention and treatment programs in diverse populations (Griner & Smith, 2006). Culturally adapted mental health interventions tailored to a specific ethnic population are up to four times more effective than traditional health interventions (Castro, Barrera, & Holleran Steiker, 2010). These interventions integrate key values, practices, and ideals within the community into intervention design and implementation. Griner and Smith (2006) found that interventions that use indigenous language are twice as effective as those conducted in English.

Often called culturally sensitive interventions (CSIs), these programs incorporate Native values, norms, beliefs, and practices into the design, implementation, and evaluation of the intervention. The underlying premise of CSIs is that intervention methods that align with the values, beliefs, practices, and norms of the target population increase access, promote engagement, and may be more effective (Jackson & Hodge, 2010). By defining health and wellness as balance within the individual and community, these interventions embrace a holistic perspective, integrating prevention and treatment strategies that promote both individual and community well-being. Many of these programs draw upon the knowledge and expertise of Native community members who play a key role in designing and administering the intervention (LaFromboise & Howard-Pitney, 1995).

Many substance abuse prevention programs foster participation in community service to reinforce key AI/AN values of family, service, respect, and spirituality. The National Indian Youth Leadership Project, deemed a model program by the Center for Substance Abuse Prevention, emphasizes community service while promoting skill development in the areas of problem-solving and wilderness education (Carter, Straits, & Hall, 2007).

To heal from the impact of historical trauma and increase mental well-being, AI/AN elders advocate for combatting negative narratives about self through increased awareness, education, and a return to culture and spiritual ways (Garrett et al., 2015). Elders also emphasize the importance of language, cultural identity, spirituality, tradition, and family support in building both individual and community resilience but call for changes in social, political, and economic resources to move communities forward (Reinschmidt, Attakai, Kahn, Whitewater, & Teufel-Shone, 2016). Families and communities that participate in the healing can regain strengths and positive qualities of being American Indian (Garrett et al., 2015).

Ethnic identity is especially significant for AI/AN youth and has had a positive influence on self-esteem and future optimism, which affects mental health. Higher self-esteem is associated with a decreased risk for depression, anxiety, and externalizing behaviors, such as fighting or breaking rules at school and home (Smokowski, Evans, Cotter, & Webber, 2014).

Participation in ceremonies and other traditional activities and supporting community cohesion, even in an urban environment, are critical to successful intervention (Hartmann & Gone, 2012). Programs that incorporate a balance of mind, body, spirit, and context (including community building and family support) have proved successful in helping adolescents overcome the impact of both historical and contemporary oppression in the urban setting and to make a successful transition to adulthood (Friesen et al., 2015).

Implications for Behavioral Health

Suggestions for future research to improve behavioral health among AI/AN include integrating prevention and treatment services, addressing the role of stress in mental health, embracing a holistic perspective for behavioral health, integrating Western biomedical and traditional AI/AN healing approaches, and acknowledging the role of historical social and cultural inequities that contribute to poor behavioral health outcomes (Goodkind et al., 2010). While Western biomedical approaches measure the success of substance abuse prevention with outcomes such as sobriety, traditional healing focuses on outcomes rooted in spiritual beliefs and practices, such as an individual's notion of spiritual connection and sense of belonging within the community. Spiritual ties to traditional Native American beliefs have been found to be particularly protective against suicide attempts (Garroutte, Goldberg, Beals, Herrell, & Manson, 2003).

Therefore, research should be based from Indigenous worldviews and perspectives using community-engaged approaches. Community members should be involved in the research from its conception to implementation to dissemination of results (Baldwin, Johnson, & Benally, 2009). Tribal, cultural, and linguistic diversity needs to be considered throughout all phases of the research process. Culturally appropriate evaluation tools need to be validated and used to determine effectiveness of programs (Caldwell et al., 2005). Finally, we need to build capacity for community members to design and oversee research projects in their own communities. More funding should be directed to train Native students and community members in behavioral health services research.

Services

Many would argue that to see reductions in behavioral health disparities among AI/AN, there must be a "genuine transformation of systems of care" (Goodkind et al., 2010, p. 391). System factors might include finding ways to reimburse healers for care, supporting behavioral health systems to address historical trauma and contemporary stressors, and creating alternative licensing and credentialing for AI/AN service providers. An excellent example is provided by the Alaska Native Tribal Health Consortium that has developed and implemented a Behavioral Health Aide Program (Goodkind et al., 2010). The program trains and certifies behavioral health workers to address mental health and substance abuse in Alaska Native villages and has met with significant success. There is also a need for providers to be trained in behavioral health cultural competency to first understand their own culture and how it impacts their practice (Gone, 2007). Finally, LaFromboise et al. (2006) argue that Western therapeutic approaches are too individually focused and discredit the benefits of traditional Native healing.

Programs

Increasingly, AI/AN communities are seeking culturally appropriate strategies to address the high rates of substance dependence, trauma, and violence that they are facing (Hartmann & Gone, 2012). The diverse worldviews of AI/AN communities often do not fit neatly into Western biomedical paradigms, leading to underutilization of biomedical treatment among AI/ANs even in urban areas (Hartmann & Gone, 2012). In a review of the use of AI/AN traditional healing in urban communities, Hartmann and Gone (2012) reported that participation in traditional healing activities led to stronger ethnocultural identity as well as community support, political empowerment, and resilience strategies for AI/AN communities. Walls, Whitbeck, and Armenta (2016) caution, however, that while indigenous spirituality was associated with poorer psychological outcomes, the effect was attenuated by controlling for moderating factors such as perceived discrimination and historical losses.

Emphasis on AI/AN culture and wellness ideals is a means of preventing substance abuse in AI/AN populations (Brown et al., 2016). Numerous treatment and prevention programs based on Native worldviews have demonstrated success, such as talking circles, family-based interventions, criminal sentences that incorporate traditional practices, and traditional ceremonies such as sweat lodge and drumming ceremonies (Greenfield & Venner, 2012; The National Congress of American Indians, 2006, November).

Strong cultural traditions, family and clan networks, and cultural beliefs surrounding abstinence in AI/AN communities serve as protective and resilience promoting factors (Barlow et al., 2012). Prevention and treatment programs should emphasize family values and tribal cohesion to reduce the sense of isolation and cultural disconnection reported by many AI/AN drinkers (Yuan et al., 2010). Also, research suggests that substance abuse prevention programs must target youth at early ages and account for the impacts of stress and exposure to traumatic events (Whitesell et al., 2014). Culturally relevant programs that incorporate mental health and substance abuse treatment can benefit both rural reservation-based and urban American Indian communities (Currie et al., 2013; Dickerson & Johnson, 2012).

Policy

Finally, it is important to discuss the policy implications associated with the behavioral health needs of AI/AN communities. Behavioral health services can be accessed through a variety of sources including private insurance, Medicaid, Indian Health Services, state and local funds, discretionary grants from state and federal resources, and Tribal funds (Office of Clinical and Preventive Services, 2011). Each of these funding options comes with its own policy implications, as each will be overseen by a variety of governmental groups including local, state, tribal, and federal governing bodies.

Tribal governments operate as sovereign nations and have power of authority over programs and services related to the health, safety, and welfare of their citizens similar to state governments (National Conference of State Legislatures, 2016). It is recommended that intergovernmental agreements including partnerships between state and tribal governments occur when planning for resources (National Conference of State Legislatures, 2016). Ongoing collaboration between federal, tribal, and state programs with a focus on cultural practices, traditional approaches, and community-healing will support sustainable policy solutions and mutual respect between partners (National Association of State Mental Health Program Directors, 2015; Office of Clinical and Preventive Services, 2011).

Tribal representatives should be involved in developing policy in the early stages of policy conceptualization (Willging et al., 2012). Using a CBPR approach to facilitate discussions regarding policy changes can facilitate trust and also commitment to implement proposed policy reforms (Blanchard, Petherick, & Basara, 2015). Any policy-based initiatives to reform behavioral health services should include enough flexibility to provide culturally sound services. Policies supporting behavioral health services can also emerge from efforts to implement culturally relevant evidence-based programs (EBPs). For example, the Suquamish community adapted EBPs to establish a mental health program titled *Healthy and Whole*. Based on the successes of the *Healthy and Whole* program, the Suquamish Tribal Council developed policies to promote sustainability of the program (Kinsey & Reed, 2015).

At the federal level, the Substance Abuse and Mental Health Services Administration (2017, December 21) acknowledges the importance and necessity for tribal consultation in all of their efforts to support trust, respect, and shared responsibility. In 2007, they developed a SAMSHA-Specific Tribal Consultation Policy (TCP) which outlines their consultation processes. The Substance Abuse and Mental Health Services Administration also provides technical assistance resources for working with Tribal groups and has several funding opportunities focused on behavioral health issues specific to AI/AN groups (SAMHSA, 2017, December 21). The 2010 Patient Protection and Affordable Care Act (ACA) included the Indian Health Care Improvement Reauthorization and Extension Act (IHCIA) in which Title VII called for a comprehensive behavioral health service initiatives in Indian Country (Office of Clinical and Preventive Services, 2011). Policies supporting integration of primary care and behavioral health support a holistic approach to care which aligns with traditional tribal healing practices (Office of Clinical and Preventive Services, 2011).

At the local, state, and tribal levels, there are also opportunities to reform policies to support more culturally relevant care. Policy efforts supported by local tribal groups resulted in the Arizona Medicaid program received approval for their Section 1115 Waiver in which Medicaid will now reimburse for Tribal-based Traditional Healing Services (Arizona Health Care Cost Containment System, 2016). Local and tribal groups can also work with IHS to establish a community health representative (CHR) work force through their local IHS offices (Old Elk, 2016, October, 31). Community health representatives are members of local tribal communities who know the local culture, can serve as advocates, and can also provide needed culturally sound behavioral health services.

In conclusion, while the AI/AN communities experience higher rates of a variety of behavioral health conditions than other US populations, there are opportunities through culturally relevant and collaborative research, services, programs, and policy efforts to improve behavioral health outcomes among AI/AN communities. Promising approaches include a focus on Native world views, community assets, cultural identity, and resiliency.

References

Adekoya, N., Truman, B., & Landen, M. (2015). Incidence of notifiable diseases among American Indians/Alaska Natives – United States, 2007-2011. *MMWR: Morbidity and Mortality Weekly Report, 64*(1), 16–19.

AlMasarweh, L., & Ward, C. (2016). Barriers to health care access and utilization: A study of Native American women veterans in two Montana reservations. *Research in the Sociology of Health Care, 34*, 33–60. [Special social groups, social factors and disparities in health and health care]. https://doi.org/10.1108/S0275-495920160000034003

Andrews, C. M., Guerrero, E. G., Wooten, N. R., & Lengnick-Hall, R. (2015). The Medicaid expansion gap and racial and ethnic minorities with substance use disorders. *American Journal of Public Health, 105*(*Suppl 3*), S452–S454. https://doi.org/10.2105/ajph.2015.302560

Arizona Health Care Cost Containment System. (2016). *Arizona's section 1115 waiver process.* [Web page]. Phoenix, AZ: Arizona Health Care Cost Containment System. https://www.aza-hcccs.gov/shared/FiveYear.html

Aronson, B. D., Johnson-Jennings, M., Kading, M. L., Smith, R. C., & Walls, M. L. (2016). Mental health service and provider preference among American Indians with type 2 diabetes. *American Indian and Alaska Native Mental Health Research, 23*(1), 1–23. https://doi.org/10.5820/aian.2301.2016.1

Baldwin, J. A., Johnson, J. L., & Benally, C. C. (2009). Building partnerships between indigenous communities and universities: lessons learned in HIV/AIDS and substance abuse prevention research. *American Journal of Public Health, 99*(*Suppl 1*), S77–S82. https://doi.org/10.2105/ajph.2008.134585

Balsam, K. F., Huang, B., Fieland, K. C., Simoni, J. M., & Walters, K. L. (2004). Culture, trauma, and wellness: A comparison of heterosexual and lesbian, gay, bisexual, and two-spirit Native Americans. *Cultural Diversity & Ethnic Minority Psychology, 10*(3), 287–301. https://doi.org/10.1037/1099-9809.10.3.287

Barlow, A., Mullany, B. C., Neault, N., Davis, Y., Billy, T., Hastings, R., ... Walkup, J. T. (2010). Examining correlates of methamphetamine and other drug use in pregnant American Indian adolescents. *American Indian and Alaska Native Mental Health Research, 17*(1), 1–24.

Barlow, A., Tingey, L., Cwik, M., Goklish, N., Larzelere-Hinton, F., Lee, A., ... Walkup, J. T. (2012). Understanding the relationship between substance use and self-injury in American Indian youth. *American Journal of Drug and Alcohol Abuse, 38*(5), 403–408. https://doi.org/10.3109/00952990.2012.696757

Barnes, P. M., Adams, P. F., & Powell-Griner, E. (2010). Health characteristics of the American Indian or Alaska Native adult population: United States, 2004-2008. *National Health Statistics Reports*(20), 1–22.

Beals, J., Manson, S. M., Shore, J. H., Friedman, M., Ashcraft, M., Fairbank, J. A., & Schlenger, W. E. (2002). The prevalence of posttraumatic stress disorder among American Indian Vietnam veterans: disparities and context. *Journal of Traumatic Stress, 15*(2), 89–97. https://doi.org/10.1023/a:1014894506325

Beals, J., Manson, S. M., Whitesell, N. R., Spicer, P., Novins, D. K., & Mitchell, C. M. (2005). Prevalence of DSM-IV disorders and attendant help-seeking in 2 American Indian reservation populations. *Archives of General Psychiatry, 62*(1), 99–108. https://doi.org/10.1001/archpsyc.62.1.99

Blanchard, J. W., Petherick, J. T., & Basara, H. (2015). Stakeholder engagement: a model for tobacco policy planning in Oklahoma Tribal communities. *American Journal of Preventive Medicine, 48*(1 Suppl 1), S44–S46. https://doi.org/10.1016/j.amepre.2014.09.025

Bombay, A., Matheson, K., & Anisman, H. (2014). The intergenerational effects of Indian Residential Schools: implications for the concept of historical trauma. *Transcultural Psychiatry, 51*(3), 320–338. https://doi.org/10.1177/1363461513503380

Brave Heart, M. Y. (2003). The historical trauma response among natives and its relationship with substance abuse: A Lakota illustration. *Journal of Psychoactive Drugs, 35*(1), 7–13. https://doi.org/10.1080/02791072.2003.10399988

Brave Heart, M. Y., Lewis-Fernandez, R., Beals, J., Hasin, D. S., Sugaya, L., Wang, S., ... Blanco, C. (2016). Psychiatric disorders and mental health treatment in American Indians and Alaska Natives: Results of the National Epidemiologic Survey on Alcohol and Related Conditions. *Social Psychiatry and Psychiatric Epidemiology, 51*(7), 1033–1046. https://doi.org/10.1007/s00127-016-1225-4

Breiding, M. J., Smith, S. G., Basile, K. C., Walters, M. L., Chen, J., & Merrick, M. T. (2014). Prevalence and characteristics of sexual violence, stalking, and intimate partner violence victimization – national intimate partner and sexual violence survey, United States, 2011. *MMWR: Surveillance Summaries, 63*(8), 1–18.

Brown, R. A. (2010). Crystal methamphetamine use among American Indian and White youth in Appalachia: Social context, masculinity, and desistance. *Addiction Research & Theory, 18*(3), 250–269. https://doi.org/10.3109/16066350902802319

Brown, R. A., Dickerson, D. L., & D'Amico, E. J. (2016). Cultural identity among urban American Indian/Alaska Native youth: Implications for alcohol and drug use. *Prevention Science, 17*(7), 852–861. https://doi.org/10.1007/s11121-016-0680-1

Bucchianeri, M. M., Gower, A. L., McMorris, B. J., & Eisenberg, M. E. (2016). Youth experiences with multiple types of prejudice-based harassment. *Journal of Adolescence, 51*, 68–75. https://doi.org/10.1016/j.adolescence.2016.05.012

Caldwell, J. Y., Davis, J. D., Du Bois, B., Echo-Hawk, H., Erickson, J. S., Coins, R. T., ... Stone, J. B. (2005). Culturally competent research with American Indians and Alaska Natives: Findings and recommendations of the First Symposium of the Work Group on American Indian Research and Program Evaluation Methodology. *American Indian and Alaska Native Mental Health Research, 12*(1), 1–21. https://doi.org/10.5820/aian.1201.2005.1

Carter, S., Straits, K. J., & Hall, M. (2007). Project Venture: Evaluation of an experiential, culturally based approach to substance abuse prevention with American Indian youth. *The Journal of Experiential Education, 29*(3), 397–400. https://doi.org/10.1177/105382590702900315

Castor, M. L., Smyser, M. S., Taualii, M. M., Park, A. N., Lawson, S. A., & Forquera, R. A. (2006). A nationwide population-based study identifying health disparities between American Indians/Alaska Natives and the general populations living in select urban counties. *American Journal of Public Health, 96*(8), 1478–1484. https://doi.org/10.2105/ajph.2004.053942

Castro, F. G., Barrera, M., & Holleran Steiker, L. K. (2010). Issues and challenges in the design of culturally adapted evidence-based interventions. *Annual Review of Clinical Psychology, 6*(1), 213–239. https://doi.org/10.1146/annurev-clinpsy-033109-132032

Centers for Disease Control & Prevention. (2003). Tobacco, alcohol, and other drug use among high school students in Bureau of Indian Affairs-funded schools – United States, 2001. *MMWR: Morbidity and Mortality Weekly Report, 52*(44), 1070–1072.

Centers for Disease Control & Prevention. (2012). Vital signs: Unintentional injury deaths among persons aged 0-19 years – United States, 2000-2009. *MMWR: Morbidity and Mortality Weekly Report, 61*, 270–276.

Centers for Disease Control & Prevention. (2013). CDC health disparities and inequalities report: United States, 2013. *MMWR: Supplements, 62*(3), 1–2. https://www.cdc.gov/mmwr/pdf/other/su6203.pdf

Chiurliza, B., Michaels, M. S., & Joiner, T. E. (2016). Acquired capability for suicide among individuals with American Indian/Alaska Native backgrounds within the military. *American*

Indian and Alaska Native Mental Health Research, 23(4), 1–15. https://doi.org/10.5820/aian. 2304.2016.1

Courtney-Long, E. A., Romano, S. D., Carroll, D. D., & Fox, M. H. (2017). Socioeconomic factors at the intersection of race and ethnicity influencing health risks for people with disabilities. *Journal of Racial and Ethnic Health Disparities, 4*(2), 213–222. https://doi.org/10.1007/s40615-016-0220-5

Croff, R. L., Rieckmann, T. R., & Spence, J. D. (2014). Provider and state perspectives on implementing cultural-based models of care for American Indian and Alaska native patients with substance use disorders. *Journal of Behavioral Health Services and Research, 41*(1), 64–79. https://doi.org/10.1007/s11414-013-9322-6

Cunningham, J. K., Solomon, T. A., & Muramoto, M. L. (2016). Alcohol use among Native Americans compared to whites: Examining the veracity of the 'Native American elevated alcohol consumption' belief. *Drug and Alcohol Dependence, 160*, 65–75. https://doi.org/10.1016/j.drugalcdep.2015.12.015

Currie, C. L., Wild, T. C., Schopflocher, D. P., Laing, L., & Veugelers, P. (2013). Illicit and prescription drug problems among urban Aboriginal adults in Canada: The role of traditional culture in protection and resilience. *Social Science and Medicine, 88*, 1–9. https://doi.org/10.1016/j.socscimed.2013.03.032

Dickerson, D. L., & Johnson, C. L. (2012). Mental health and substance abuse characteristics among a clinical sample of urban American Indian/Alaska Native youths in a large California Metropolitan area: A descriptive study. *Community Mental Health Journal, 48*(1), 56–62. https://doi.org/10.1007/s10597-010-9368-3

Ehlers, C. L., Gizer, I. R., Gilder, D. A., Ellingson, J. M., & Yehuda, R. (2013). Measuring historical trauma in an American Indian community sample: Contributions of substance dependence, affective disorder, conduct disorder and PTSD. *Drug and Alcohol Dependence, 133*(1), 180–187. https://doi.org/10.1016/j.drugalcdep.2013.05.011

Ehlers, C. L., Liang, T., & Gizer, I. R. (2012). ADH and ALDH polymorphisms and alcohol dependence in Mexican and Native Americans. *American Journal of Drug and Alcohol Abuse, 38*(5), 389–394. https://doi.org/10.3109/00952990.2012.694526

Elm, J. H., Lewis, J. P., Walters, K. L., & Self, J. M. (2016). "I'm in this world for a reason": Resilience and recovery among American Indian and Alaska Native two-spirit women. *Journal of Lesbian Studies, 20*(3-4), 352–371. https://doi.org/10.1080/10894160.2016.1152813

Etz, K. E., Arroyo, J. A., Crump, A. D., Rosa, C. L., & Scott, M. S. (2012). Advancing American Indian and Alaska Native substance abuse research: Current science and future directions. *American Journal of Drug and Alcohol Abuse, 38*(5), 372–375. https://doi.org/10.3109/00952990.2012.712173

Evans-Campbell, T., Walters, K. L., Pearson, C. R., & Campbell, C. D. (2012). Indian boarding school experience, substance use, and mental health among urban two-spirit American Indian/Alaska natives. *American Journal of Drug and Alcohol Abuse, 38*(5), 421–427. https://doi.org/10.3109/00952990.2012.701358

Fieland, K. C., Walters, K. L., & Simoni, J. M. (2007). Determinants of health among two-spirit American Indians and Alaska Natives. In H. Meyer & M. E. Northridge (Eds.), *The health of sexual minorities: Public health perspectives on lesbian, gay, bisexual, and transgender populations* (pp. 268–300). New York, NY: Springer.

Forcehimes, A. A., Venner, K. L., Bogenschutz, M. P., Foley, K., Davis, M. P., Houck, J. M., … Begaye, P. (2011). American Indian methamphetamine and other drug use in the Southwestern United States. *Cultural Diversity & Ethnic Minority Psychology, 17*(4), 366–376. https://doi.org/10.1037/a0025431

Fox, D. J., Pettygrove, S., Cunniff, C., O'Leary, L. A., Gilboa, S. M., Bertrand, J., … Meaney, F. J. (2015). Fetal alcohol syndrome among children aged 7-9 years – Arizona, Colorado, and New York, 2010. *MMWR: Morbidity and Mortality Weekly Report, 64*(3), 54–57.

Friesen, B. J., Cross, T. L., Jivanjee, P., Thirstrup, A., Bandurraga, A., Gowen, L. K., & Rountree, J. (2015). Meeting the transition needs of urban American Indian/Alaska Native youth through culturally based services. *The Journal of Behavioral Health Services & Research, 42*(2), 191–205. https://doi.org/10.1007/s11414-014-9447-2

Garrett, M. D., Baldridge, D., Benson, W., Crowder, J., & Aldrich, N. (2015). Mental health disorders among an invisible minority: Depression and dementia among American Indian and Alaska Native elders. *The Gerontologist, 55*(2), 227–236. https://doi.org/10.1093/geront/gnu181

Garroutte, E. M., Goldberg, J., Beals, J., Herrell, R., & Manson, S. M. (2003). Spirituality and attempted suicide among American Indians. *Social Science and Medicine, 56*(7), 1571–1579.

Genovesi, A. L., Hastings, B., Edgerton, E. A., & Olson, L. M. (2014). Pediatric emergency care capabilities of Indian Health Service emergency medical service agencies serving American Indians/Alaska Natives in rural and frontier areas. *Rural and Remote Health, 14*(2), 2688.

Gilder, D. A., Gizer, I. R., Lau, P., & Ehlers, C. L. (2014). Item response theory analyses of DSM-IV and DSM-5 stimulant use disorder criteria in an American Indian community sample. *Drug and Alcohol Dependence, 135*, 29–36. https://doi.org/10.1016/j.drugalcdep.2013.10.010

Gilder, D. A., Stouffer, G. M., Lau, P., & Ehlers, C. L. (2016). Clinical characteristics of alcohol combined with other substance use disorders in an American Indian community sample. *Drug and Alcohol Dependence, 161*, 222–229. https://doi.org/10.1016/j.drugalcdep.2016.02.006

Glover-Kerkvliet, J. (2009). The methamphetamine crisis in American Indian and Native Alaskan communities. *Inquiries, 1*(12), 1/1.

Gone, J. P. (2007). 'We never was happy living like a Whiteman': Mental health disparities and the postcolonial predicament in American Indian communities. *American Journal of Community Psychology, 40*(3-4), 290–300. https://doi.org/10.1007/s10464-007-9136-x

Gone, J. P. (2008). 'So I can be like a Whiteman': The cultural psychology of space and place in American Indian mental health. *Culture & Psychology, 14*(3), 369–399. https://doi.org/10.1177/1354067X08092639

Gone, J. P. (2016). Alternative knowledges and the future of community psychology: Provocations from an American Indian healing tradition. *American Journal of Community Psychology, 58*(3–4), 314–321. https://doi.org/10.1002/ajcp.12046

Gone, J. P., & Trimble, J. E. (2012). American Indian and Alaska native mental health: Diverse perspectives on enduring disparities. *Annual Review of Clinical Psychology, 8*, 31–60. https://doi.org/10.1146/annurev-clinpsy-032511-143127

Goodkind, J. R., Ross-Toledo, K., John, S., Hall, J. L., Ross, L., Freeland, L., … Lee, C. (2010). Promoting healing and restoring trust: Policy recommendations for improving behavioral health care for American Indian/Alaska Native adolescents. *American Journal of Community Psychology, 46*(3–4), 386–394. https://doi.org/10.1007/s10464-010-9347-4

Grant, B. F., Saha, T. D., Ruan, W. J., Goldstein, R. B., Chou, S. P., Jung, J., … Hasin, D. S. (2016). Epidemiology of DSM-5 drug use disorder: Results from the National Epidemiologic Survey on Alcohol and Related Conditions-III. *JAMA Psychiatry, 73*(1), 39–47. https://doi.org/10.1001/jamapsychiatry.2015.2132

Grayshield, L., Rutherford, J. J., Salazar, S. B., Mihecoby, A. L., & Luna, L. L. (2015). Understanding and healing historical trauma: The perspectives of Native American elders. *Journal of Mental Health Counseling, 37*(4), 295–307. https://doi.org/10.17744/mehc.37.4.02

Greenfield, B. L., & Venner, K. L. (2012). Review of substance use disorder treatment research in Indian country: Future directions to strive toward health equity. *American Journal of Drug and Alcohol Abuse, 38*(5), 483–492. https://doi.org/10.3109/00952990.2012.702170

Griner, D., & Smith, T. B. (2006). Culturally adapted mental health intervention: A meta-analytic review. *Psychotherapy, 43*(4), 531–548. https://doi.org/10.1037/0033-3204.43.4.531

Gurley, D., Novins, D. K., Jones, M. C., Beals, J., Shore, J. H., & Manson, S. M. (2001). Comparative use of biomedical services and traditional healing options by American Indian veterans. *Psychiatric Services, 52*(1), 68–74. https://doi.org/10.1176/appi.ps.52.1.68

Harada, N. D., Villa, V. M., Reifel, N., & Bayhylle, R. (2005). Exploring veteran identity and health services use among Native American veterans. *Military Medicine, 170*(9), 782–786.

Hartmann, W. E., & Gone, J. P. (2012). Incorporating traditional healing into an urban American Indian health organization: A case study of community member perspectives. *Journal of Counseling Psychology, 59*(4), 542–554. https://doi.org/10.1037/a0029067

Hautala, D. S., Sittner Hartshorn, K. J., & Whitbeck, L. B. (2016). Prospective childhood risk factors for gang involvement among north american indigenous adolescents. *Youth Violence and Juvenile Justice, 14*(4), 390–410. https://doi.org/10.1177/1541204015585173

Hirchak, K. A., & Murphy, S. M. (2017). Assessing differences in the availability of opioid addiction therapy options: Rural versus urban and American Indian reservation versus nonreservation. *The Journal of Rural Health, 33*(1), 102–109. https://doi.org/10.1111/jrh.12178

Iritani, B. J., Hallfors, D. D., & Bauer, D. J. (2007). Crystal methamphetamine use among young adults in the USA. *Addiction, 102*(7), 1102–1113. https://doi.org/10.1111/j.1360-0443.2007.01847.x

Jackson, K. F., & Hodge, D. R. (2010). Native American youth and culturally sensitive interventions: A systematic review. *Research on Social Work Practice, 20*(3), 260–270. https://doi.org/10.1177/1049731509347862

Jamal, A., Agaku, I. T., O'Connor, E., King, B. A., Kenemer, J. B., & Neff, L. (2014). Current cigarette smoking among adults – United States, 2005-2013. *MMWR: Morbidity and Mortality Weekly Report, 63*(47), 1108–1112.

Johnson, J. L., & Cameron, M. C. (2001). Barriers to providing effective mental health services to American Indians. *Mental Health Services Research, 3*(4), 215–223.

Kasprow, W. J., & Rosenheck, R. (1998). Substance use and psychiatric problems of homeless Native American veterans. *Psychiatric Services, 49*(3), 345–350. https://doi.org/10.1176/ps.49.3.345

Katzman, J. G., Fore, C., Bhatt, S., Greenberg, N., Griffin Salvador, J., Comerci, G. C., … Karol, S. (2016). Evaluation of American Indian health service training in pain management and opioid substance use disorder. *American Journal of Public Health, 106*(8), 1427–1429. https://doi.org/10.2105/ajph.2016.303193

Kaufman, C. E., Kaufman, L. J., Shangreau, C., Dailey, N., Blair, B., & Shore, J. (2016). American Indian veterans and VA services in three tribes. *American Indian and Alaska Native Mental Health Research, 23*(2), 64–83. https://doi.org/10.5820/aian.2302.2016.64

Kim, G., Bryant, A. N., Goins, R. T., Worley, C. B., & Chiriboga, D. A. (2012). Disparities in health status and health care access and use among older American Indians and Alaska Natives and non-Hispanic Whites in California. *Journal of Aging and Health, 24*(5), 799–811. https://doi.org/10.1177/0898264312444309

Kinsey, K., & Reed, P. G. (2015). Linking Native American tribal policy to practice in mental health care. *Nursing Science Quarterly, 28*(1), 82–87. https://doi.org/10.1177/0894318414558616

Kunitz, S. J. (2008). Risk factors for polydrug use in a Native American population. *Substance Use and Misuse, 43*(3-4), 331–339. https://doi.org/10.1080/10826080701202783

LaFromboise, T. D., & Howard-Pitney, B. (1995). The Zuni life skills development curriculum: Description and evaluation of a suicide prevention program. *Journal of Counseling Psychology, 42*(4), 479–486. https://doi.org/10.1037/0022-0167.42.4.479

LaFromboise, T. D., Hoyt, D. R., Oliver, L., & Whitbeck, L. B. (2006). Family, community, and school influences on resilience among American Indian adolescents in the upper Midwest. *Journal of Community Psychology, 34*(2), 193–209. https://doi.org/10.1002/jcop.20090

Landen, M., Roeber, J., Naimi, T., Nielsen, L., & Sewell, M. (2014). Alcohol-attributable mortality among American Indians and Alaska Natives in the United States, 1999-2009. *American Journal of Public Health, 104*(Suppl 3), S343–S349. https://doi.org/10.2105/ajph.2013.301648

Lehavot, K., Walters, K. L., & Simoni, J. M. (2009). Abuse, mastery, and health among lesbian, bisexual, and two-spirit American Indian and Alaska Native women. *Cultural Diversity & Ethnic Minority Psychology, 15*(3), 275–284. https://doi.org/10.1037/a0013458

Liao, Y., Bang, D., Cosgrove, S., Dulin, R., Harris, Z., Taylor, A., … Giles, W. (2011). Surveillance of health status in minority communities: Racial and Ethnic Approaches to Community Health

Across the U.S. (REACH U.S.) Risk Factor Survey, United States, 2009. *MMWR: Surveillance Summaries, 60*(6), 1–44.

Macartney, S., Bishaw, A., & Fontenot, K. (2013, February). *Poverty rates for selected detailed race and Hispanic groups by state and place: 2007-2011* (American Community Survey Briefs, ACSBR/11-17). Washington, DC: U. S. Census Bureau. https://www2.census.gov/library/publications/2013/acs/acsbr11-17.pdf

Malcolm, B. P., Hesselbrock, M. N., & Segal, B. (2006). Multiple substance dependence and course of alcoholism among Alaska native men and women. *Substance Use and Misuse, 41*(5), 729–741. https://doi.org/10.1080/10826080500391803

Manson, S. M., Beals, J., Dick, R. W., & Duclos, C. (1989). Risk factors for suicide among Indian adolescents at a boarding school. *Public Health Reports, 104*(6), 609–614.

Middlebrook, D. L., LeMaster, P. L., Beals, J., Novins, D. K., & Manson, S. M. (2001). Suicide prevention in American Indian and Alaska Native communities: A critical review of programs. *Suicide and Life-Threatening Behavior, 31*(Suppl), 132–149.

Mileviciute, I., Trujillo, J., Gray, M., & Scott, W. D. (2013). The role of explanatory style and negative life events in depression: A cross-sectional study with youth from a North American plains reservation. *American Indian and Alaska Native Mental Health Research, 20*(3), 42–58. https://doi.org/10.5820/aian.2003.2013.42

Mmari, K. N., Blum, R. W., & Teufel-Shone, N. (2010). What increases risk and protection for delinquent behaviors among American Indian youth?: Findings from three tribal communities. *Youth & Society, 41*(3), 382–413. https://doi.org/10.1177/0044118X09333645

Moghaddam, J. F., Momper, S. L., & Fong, T. (2013). Discrimination and participation in traditional healing for American Indians and Alaska Natives. *Journal of Community Health, 38*(6), 1115–1123. https://doi.org/10.1007/s10900-013-9721-x

Momper, S. L., Delva, J., Tauiliili, D., Mueller-Williams, A. C., & Goral, P. (2013). OxyContin use on a rural midwest American Indian reservation: Demographic correlates and reasons for using. *American Journal of Public Health, 103*(11), 1997–1999. https://doi.org/10.2105/ajph.2013.301372

Murphy, T., Pokhrel, P., Worthington, A., Billie, H., Sewell, M., & Bill, N. (2014). Unintentional injury mortality among American Indians and Alaska Natives in the United States, 1990-2009. *American Journal of Public Health, 104*(Suppl 3), S470–S480. https://doi.org/10.2105/ajph.2013.301854

Myhra, L. L., & Wieling, E. (2014a). Intergenerational patterns of substance abuse among urban American Indian families. *Journal of Ethnicity in Substance Abuse, 13*(1), 1–22. https://doi.org/10.1080/15332640.2013.847391

Myhra, L. L., & Wieling, E. (2014b). Psychological trauma among American Indian families: A two-generation study. *Journal of Loss and Trauma, 19*(4), 289–313. https://doi.org/10.1080/15325024.2013.771561

National Association of State Mental Health Program Directors. (2015). *Partnering with tribal governments to meet the mental health needs of American Indian/Alaska Native consumers: Assessment #4.* Alexandria, VA: National Association of State Mental Health Program Directors. https://www.nasmhpd.org/sites/default/files/Assessment%20%234_Partnering%20with%20Tribal%20Governments%20to%20Meet%20the%20Mental%20Health%20Needs%20of%20American%20Indian_Alaska%20Native%20Consumers.pdf

National Center for Health Statistics. (2016, May). *Health, United States, 2015: with special feature on racial and ethnic health disparities* (DHHS Publication No. 2016-1232). Washington, DC: National Center for Health Statistics. http://www.cdc.gov/nchs/data/hus/hus15.pdf

National Conference of State Legislatures. (2016). *Separation of powers-state tribal relations and interstate compacts.* [Web page]. Washington, DC: National Conference of State Legislatures. http://www.ncsl.org/research/about-state-legislatures/separation-of-powers-tribal-interstate-relations.aspx

Neault, N., Mullany, B., Powers, J., Coho-Mescal, V., Parker, S., Walkup, J., & Barlow, A. (2012). Fatherhood roles and drug use among young American Indian men. *American Journal of Drug and Alcohol Abuse, 38*(5), 395–402. https://doi.org/10.3109/00952990.2012.703735

Nelson, L. A., Rhoades, D. A., Noonan, C., & Manson, S. M. (2007). Traumatic brain injury and mental health among two American Indian populations. *Journal of Head Trauma Rehabilitation, 22*(2), 105–112. https://doi.org/10.1097/01.HTR.0000265098.52306.a9

O'Connell, J. M., Novins, D. K., Beals, J., & Spicer, P. (2005). Disparities in patterns of alcohol use among reservation-based and geographically dispersed American Indian populations. *Alcoholism, Clinical and Experimental Research, 29*(1), 107–116.

Office of Clinical and Preventive Services. (2011). *American Indian/Alaska Native behavioral health briefing book.* Rockville, MD: U. S. Department of Health and Human Services, Indian Health Service, Division of Behavioral Health. https://www.ihs.gov/newsroom/includes/themes/newihstheme/display_objects/documents/2011_Letters/AIANBHBriefingBook.pdf

Office of Minority Health. (2013). *Chronic liver disease and American Indians/Alaska Natives.* [Web page]. Washington, DC: U. S. Department of Health and Human Services. https://minorityhealth.hhs.gov/omh/browse.aspx?lvl=4&lvlid=32

Office of Minority Health. (2018). *Profile: American Indian/Alaska Native* [Web page]. Washington, DC: U. S. Department of Health and Human Services. https://minorityhealth.hhs.gov/omh/browse.aspx?lvl=3&lvlid=62

Office of the Surgeon General. (2001). *Mental health: Culture, race, and ethnicity: A supplement to Mental health, a report of the Surgeon General.* https://www.ncbi.nlm.nih.gov/pubmed/20669516

Okoro, C. A., Denny, C. H., McGuire, L. C., Balluz, L. S., Goins, R. T., & Mokdad, A. H. (2007). Disability among older American Indians and Alaska Natives: Disparities in prevalence, health-risk behaviors, obesity, and chronic conditions. *Ethnicity and Disease, 17*(4), 686–692.

Okoro, C. A., Hollis, N. D., Cyrus, A. C., & Griffin-Blake, S. (2018). Prevalence of disabilities and health care access by disability status and type among adults – United States, 2016. *MMWR: Morbidity and Mortality Weekly Report, 67*(32), 882–887. https://doi.org/10.15585/mmwr.mm6732a3

Old Elk, G. (2016, October, 31). *CHRs embody the local community.* [Web page]. Washington, DC: Indian Health Service. https://www.ihs.gov/newsroom/index.cfm/ihs-blog/october2016/chrs-embody-the-local-community/

Pearson, C. R., Kaysen, D., Belcourt, A., Stappenbeck, C. A., Zhou, C., Smartlowit-Briggs, L., & Whitefoot, P. (2015). Post-traumatic stress disorder and HIV risk behaviors among rural American Indian/Alaska Native women. *American Indian and Alaska Native Mental Health Research, 22*(3), 1–20. https://doi.org/10.5820/aian.2203.2015.1

Quintero, G. (2001). Making the Indian: Colonial knowledge, alcohol, and Native Americans. *American Indian Culture and Research Journal, 25*(4), 57–71. https://doi.org/10.17953/aicr.25.4.d7703373656686m4

Rees, C., Freng, A., & Winfree, L. T., Jr. (2014). The Native American adolescent: Social network structure and perceptions of alcohol induced social problems. *Journal of Youth and Adolescence, 43*(3), 405–425. https://doi.org/10.1007/s10964-013-0018-2

Reilley, B., Bloss, E., Byrd, K. K., Iralu, J., Neel, L., & Cheek, J. (2014). Death rates from human immunodeficiency virus and tuberculosis among American Indians/Alaska Natives in the United States, 1990-2009. *American Journal of Public Health, 104*(Suppl 3), S453–S459. https://doi.org/10.2105/ajph.2013.301746

Reinschmidt, K. M., Attakai, A., Kahn, C. B., Whitewater, S., & Teufel-Shone, N. (2016). Shaping a stories of resilience model from urban American Indian elders' narratives of historical trauma and resilience. *American Indian and Alaska Native Mental Health Research, 23*(4), 63–85. https://doi.org/10.5820/aian.2304.2016.63

Ryan, C. J., Cooke, M., & Leatherdale, S. T. (2016). Factors associated with heavy drinking among off-reserve First Nations and Metis youth and adults: Evidence from the 2012 Canadian Aboriginal Peoples Survey. *Preventive Medicine, 87*, 95–102. https://doi.org/10.1016/j.ypmed.2016.02.008

Schultz, K. (2016). *Native women, intimate partner violence, and drug use and consequences: Prevalence and associations among tribal college and university students.* (PhD Dissertation), University of Washington, Seattle, WA. Retrieved from https://digital.lib.washington.edu/researchworks/bitstream/handle/1773/37241/Schultz_washington_0250E_16388.pdf?sequence=1&isAllowed=y

Shah, V. O., Ghahate, D. M., Bobelu, J., Sandy, P., Newman, S., Helitzer, D. L., … Zager, P. (2014). Identifying barriers to healthcare to reduce health disparity in Zuni Indians using focus group conducted by community health workers. *Clinical and Translational Science, 7*(1), 6–11. https://doi.org/10.1111/cts.12127

Simoni, J. M., Walters, K. L., Balsam, K. F., & Meyers, S. B. (2006). Victimization, substance use, and HIV risk behaviors among gay/bisexual/two-spirit and heterosexual American Indian Men in New York City. *American Journal of Public Health, 96*(12), 2240–2245. https://doi.org/10.2105/ajph.2004.054056

Siordia, C., Bell, R. A., & Haileselassie, S. L. (2017). Prevalence and risk for negative disability outcomes between American Indians-Alaskan Natives and other race-ethnic groups in the Southwestern United States. *Journal of Racial and Ethnic Health Disparities, 4*(2), 195–200. https://doi.org/10.1007/s40615-016-0218-z

Smith, S. M., Goldstein, R. B., & Grant, B. F. (2016). The association between post-traumatic stress disorder and lifetime DSM-5 psychiatric disorders among veterans: Data from the National Epidemiologic Survey on Alcohol and Related Conditions-III (NESARC-III). *Journal of Psychiatric Research, 82*, 16–22. https://doi.org/10.1016/j.jpsychires.2016.06.022

Smokowski, P. R., Evans, C. B., Cotter, K. L., & Webber, K. C. (2014). Ethnic identity and mental health in American Indian youth: Examining mediation pathways through self-esteem, and future optimism. *Journal of Youth and Adolescence, 43*(3), 343–355. https://doi.org/10.1007/s10964-013-9992-7

Soto, C., Baezconde-Garbanati, L., Schwartz, S. J., & Unger, J. B. (2015). Stressful life events, ethnic identity, historical trauma, and participation in cultural activities: Associations with smoking behaviors among American Indian adolescents in California. *Addictive Behaviors, 50*, 64–69. https://doi.org/10.1016/j.addbeh.2015.06.005

Spear, S., Crevecoeur, D. A., Rawson, R. A., & Clark, R. (2007). The rise in methamphetamine use among American Indians in Los Angeles County. *American Indian and Alaska Native Mental Health Research, 14*(2), 1–15.

Spicer, P. (2001). Culture and the restoration of self among former American Indian drinkers. *Social Science and Medicine, 53*(2), 227–240.

Spillane, N. S., Greenfield, B., Venner, K., & Kahler, C. W. (2015). Alcohol use among reserve-dwelling adult First Nation members: Use, problems, and intention to change drinking behavior. *Addictive Behaviors, 41*, 232–237. https://doi.org/10.1016/j.addbeh.2014.10.015

Stanley, L. R., Harness, S. D., Swaim, R. C., & Beauvais, F. (2014). Rates of substance use of American Indian students in 8th, 10th, and 12th grades living on or near reservations: update, 2009-2012. *Public Health Reports, 129*(2), 156–163. https://doi.org/10.1177/003335491412900209

Steen, N. (2015). Resiliency and recovery: Factor analysis of youth indigenous in United States. *Asian Journal of Indigenous Studies, 1*(1), 1–13.

Stockman, J. K., Hayashi, H., & Campbell, J. C. (2015). Intimate partner violence and its health impact on ethnic minority women, including minorities and impoverished groups. *Journal of Women's Health, 24*(1), 62–79. https://doi.org/10.1089/jwh.2014.4879

Substance Abuse and Mental Health Services Administration. (2017, December 21). *SAMSHA's efforts*. [Web page]. Rockville, MD: Substance Abuse and Mental Health Services Administration. http://www.samhsa.gov/tribal-affairs/samhsas-efforts

The National Congress of American Indians. (2006). *Methamphetamine in Indian Country: An American problem uniquely affecting Indian country*. Washington, DC: U.S. Department of Justice. https://www.justice.gov/archive/tribal/docs/fv_tjs/session_1/session1_presentations/Meth_Overview.pdf

Tingey, L., Cwik, M. F., Rosenstock, S., Goklish, N., Larzelere-Hinton, F., Lee, A., … Barlow, A. (2016). Risk and protective factors for heavy binge alcohol use among American Indian adolescents utilizing emergency health services. *American Journal of Drug and Alcohol Abuse, 42*(6), 715–725. https://doi.org/10.1080/00952990.2016.1181762

Towne, S. D., Jr., Probst, J. C., Mitchell, J., & Chen, Z. (2015). Poorer quality outcomes of medicare-certified home health care in areas with high levels of Native American/Alaska native residents. *Journal of Aging and Health, 27*(8), 1339–1357. https://doi.org/10.1177/0898264315583051

Unger, J. B., Soto, C., & Baezconde-Garbanati, L. (2006). Perceptions of ceremonial and noncer-emonial uses of tobacco by American-Indian adolescents in California. *Journal of Adolescent Health, 38*(4), 443.e449–443.e416. https://doi.org/10.1016/j.jadohealth.2005.02.002

United States Commission on Civil Rights. (2004). *Broken promises: Evaluating the Native American health care system.* Washington, DC: United States Commission on Civil Rights. https://www.sprc.org/resources-programs/broken-promises-evaluating-native-american-health-care-system

Volkow, N. D., & Warren, K. R. (2012). Advancing American Indian/Alaska Native substance abuse research. *American Journal of Drug and Alcohol Abuse, 38*(5), 371. https://doi.org/10.3109/00952990.2012.712174

Walker, S. C., Whitener, R., Trupin, E. W., & Migliarini, N. (2015). American Indian perspectives on evidence-based practice implementation: Results from a statewide Tribal Mental Health Gathering. *Administration and Policy in Mental Health, 42*(1), 29–39. https://doi.org/10.1007/s10488-013-0530-4

Walls, M. L., Johnson, K. D., Whitbeck, L. B., & Hoyt, D. R. (2006). Mental health and substance abuse services preferences among American Indian people of the northern Midwest. *Community Mental Health Journal, 42*(6), 521–535. https://doi.org/10.1007/s10597-006-9054-7

Walls, M. L., Whitbeck, L., & Armenta, B. (2016). A cautionary tale: Examining the interplay of culturally specific risk and resilience factors in indigenous communities. *Clinical Psychological Science, 4*(4), 732–743. https://doi.org/10.1177/2167702616645795

Walters, K. L., & Simoni, J. M. (2002). Reconceptualizing native women's health: an "indigenist" stress-coping model. *American Journal of Public Health, 92*(4), 520–524. https://www.ncbi.nlm.nih.gov/pmc/articles/PMC1447108/pdf/0920520.pdf

Walters, K. L., Simoni, J. M., & Evans-Campbell, T. (2002). Substance use among American Indians and Alaska natives: Incorporating culture in an "indigenist" stress-coping paradigm. *Public Health Reports, 117*(*Suppl 1*), S104–S117.

Warne, D., & Lajimodiere, D. (2015). American Indian health disparities: Psychosocial influences. *Social and Personality Compass, 9*(10), 567–569.

West, B. A., & Naumann, R. B. (2011). Motor vehicle-related deaths – United States, 2003-2007. *MMWR: Supplements, 60*(1), 52–55.

Westermeyer, J., & Canive, J. (2013). Posttraumatic stress disorder and its comorbidities among American Indian veterans. *Community Mental Health Journal, 49*(6), 704–708. https://doi.org/10.1007/s10597-012-9565-3

Whitbeck, L. B., Hoyt, D. R., Chen, X., & Stubben, J. D. (2002). Predictors of gang involvement among American Indian adolescents. *Journal of Gang Research, 10*(1), 11–26.

Whitbeck, L. B., Hoyt, D. R., McMorris, B. J., Chen, X., & Stubben, J. D. (2001). Perceived dis-crimination and early substance abuse among American Indian children. *Journal of Health and Social Behavior, 42*(4), 405–424.

Whitesell, N. R., Asdigian, N. L., Kaufman, C. E., Big Crow, C., Shangreau, C., Keane, E. M., ... Mitchell, C. M. (2014). Trajectories of substance use among young American Indian adoles-cents: Patterns and predictors. *Journal of Youth and Adolescence, 43*(3), 437–453. https://doi.org/10.1007/s10964-013-0026-2

Whitesell, N. R., Beals, J., Crow, C. B., Mitchell, C. M., & Novins, D. K. (2012). Epidemiology and etiology of substance use among American Indians and Alaska Natives: Risk, protection, and implications for prevention. *American Journal of Drug and Alcohol Abuse, 38*(5), 376–382. https://doi.org/10.3109/00952990.2012.694527

Willging, C. E., Goodkind, J., Lamphere, L., Saul, G., Fluder, S., & Seanez, P. (2012). The impact of state behavioral health reform on Native American individuals, families, and communities. *Qualitative Health Research, 22*(7), 880–896. https://doi.org/10.1177/1049732312440329

Wu, L. T., Pilowsky, D. J., & Patkar, A. A. (2008). Non-prescribed use of pain relievers among adolescents in the United States. *Drug and Alcohol Dependence, 94*(1–3), 1–11. https://doi.org/10.1016/j.drugalcdep.2007.09.023

Yoder, K. A., Whitbeck, L. B., Hoyt, D. R., & LaFromboise, T. (2006). Suicidal ideation among American Indian youths. *Archives of Suicide Research, 10*(2), 177–190. https://doi.org/10.1080/13811110600558240

Yuan, N. P., Duran, B. M., Walters, K. L., Pearson, C. R., & Evans-Campbell, T. A. (2014). Alcohol misuse and associations with childhood maltreatment and out-of-home placement among urban two-spirit American Indian and Alaska Native people. *International Journal of Environmental Research and Public Health, 11*(10), 10461–10479. https://doi.org/10.3390/ijerph111010461

Yuan, N. P., Eaves, E. R., Koss, M. P., Polacca, M., Bletzer, K., & Goldman, D. (2010). "Alcohol is something that been with us like a common cold": Community perceptions of American Indian drinking. *Substance Use and Misuse, 45*(12), 1909–1929. https://doi.org/10.3109/10826081003682115

Zamora-Kapoor, A., Nelson, L. A., Barbosa-Leiker, C., Comtois, K. A., Walker, L. R., & Buchwald, D. S. (2016). Suicidal ideation in American Indian/Alaska Native and White adolescents: The role of social isolation, exposure to suicide, and overweight. *American Indian and Alaska Native Mental Health Research, 23*(4), 86–100. https://doi.org/10.5820/aian.2304.2016.86

Older Adults

Donna Cohen and Andrew Krajewski

Introduction

Behavioral health care for a rapidly aging population is and will continue to be a national and global public health priority because mental health problems are the single greatest cause of health disability (Steel et al., 2014; Whiteford et al., 2013). The swift growth and increasing biopsychosocial heterogeneity of the older population in the United States (USA) and the rest of the world have been a bittersweet success. More people are living longer and in better health than ever before in most countries. However, advancing age carries an increasing risk for multiple physical and behavioral health problems, chronic conditions, functional impairments and excess disability, frailty, and a changed quality of life. All of these adverse circumstances not only affect the psychosocial and economic health and well-being of individuals with behavioral health problems but also their families and the communities in which they live.

Geriatric behavioral health policy cannot be understood in isolation from health, social, economic, and welfare policies (Cohen & Eisdorfer, 2011). Aging is a developmental process mediated by biopsychosocial-environmental factors that interact to influence health or disease, functional effectiveness or disability, and resilience or vulnerability. The emergence of illness, including mental illness, in later life usually reflects the consequences of genetics, accumulated trauma, exposure to toxins, health and lifestyle behaviors, environmental factors, and a variety of stressors. Physical health and behavioral health are intimately interrelated

D. Cohen (✉)
Department of Child and Family Studies, College of Behavioral and Community Sciences, University of South Florida, Tampa, FL, USA
e-mail: cohen@usf.edu

A. Krajewski
Department of Sociology and Criminology, College of the Liberal Arts, Pennsylvania State University, State College, PA, USA

© Springer Nature Switzerland AG 2020
B. L. Levin, A. Hanson (eds.), *Foundations of Behavioral Health*,
https://doi.org/10.1007/978-3-030-18435-3_11

with one another (Weiss, Haber, Horowitz, Stuart, & Wolfe, 2009), and it is estimated that currently at least 50% of all diseases are affected by behavioral factors, e.g., poor nutrition and exercise patterns, substance abuse, lack of adherence to prescribed medications, and sexual activities (Institute of Medicine, 2001; Johnson, Hayes, Brown, Hoo, & Ethier, 2014).

Aging is also a sociopolitical experience that affects every person, family, and community as well as every component of a society's infrastructure. Thus, a healthy society must develop policies that create and sustain behavioral and physical health, vitality, economic security, and meaningful productivity for people of all ages.

This chapter has four objectives:

1. To review demographic changes in the unprecedented growth of an aging society.
2. To identify the prevalence and impact of geriatric behavioral health challenges.
3. To examine the history of public policies that have shaped geriatric behavioral health policies in the USA.
4. To examine geriatric behavioral health policies within the broader context of public policies.

The Demographic Landscape of an Aging Society

Persons aged 65 years and older in the USA will almost double from 48 million (14.1% of the population) in 2015 to 88 million in 2050 (Ortman & Velkoff, 2014; Population Reference Bureau, 2016). The world population aged 65 and older will more than double to 1.6 billion (22% of the world's population) from 2015 to 2050 (He, Goodkind, & Kowal, 2016). The oldest-old, persons aged 85 and older, who are at the highest risk for certain disorders and conditions, will continue to grow more rapidly than any other age group, from 2% in 2000 (four million persons) to 5% in 2050 (19 million persons) (United Nations Department of Economic and Social Affairs Population Division, 2015).

Demographic heterogeneity as well as the rapid expansion of an aging population has important implications for developing responsive policies and practices. In spite of greater prosperity, health, vitality, and well-being, there are significant gender, racial, ethnic, and economic disparities that merit attention to the needs of a culturally diverse older population as well as their family caregivers (Ortman & Velkoff, 2014). Women account for 58% of the population aged 65 and older and 75% of the population aged 85 and older. This gender inequality is relevant for several reasons. Older women experience and express illnesses differently than men. In addition, they are more vulnerable due to marital status, living arrangements, economic insecurity, and inadequacies in our knowledge of women's health. Older women are less likely than older men to be married and are more likely to live alone, circumstances that can affect an individual's well-being, economically and emotionally, and leave women without a spouse caregiver (Ortman & Velkoff, 2014).

Of the 35 million persons aged 65 and older living in the USA, 16% (5.6 million) are members of ethnic and racial minority groups, and 11% (1.2 million) are foreign-born (Ortman & Velkoff, 2014). In 2000, non-Hispanic whites made up 84% of the population aged 65 and older: 8% were non-Hispanic Black, 6% were Hispanic, 2% were Asian and Pacific Islander, and less than 1% were American Indians and Alaskan Natives. However, by 2050, the non-Hispanic white older population will decline from 84% to 64%, with the Hispanic population increasing to 16%, the Black population increasing to 12%, and Asian and Pacific Islanders as well as American Indians and Alaskan Natives growing to 8% of the older population. The fastest growth will occur in the older Hispanic population, from two million in 2000 to more than 13 million in 2050, and they will outnumber the older Black population by 2028 (Ortman & Velkoff, 2014). Thus, the increasing racial and ethnic diversity in the USA will require greater knowledge about differences in health and illness behaviors, help-seeking, patterns of family caregiving, as well as the need for greater flexibility in the organization and delivery of mental health services.

Behavioral Health Care Challenges of an Aging Society

There are many indications that behavioral health problems affect a significant proportion of older adults in the USA. A total of 5.2 million older Americans have Alzheimer's disease and related dementias, and that number is estimated to triple to 14–16 million by 2050 (Alzheimer's Association, 2016). Between 5.6 and 8 million older people (14–20%) have a diagnosable behavioral health condition, including mood disorders, anxiety disorders, substance abuse disorders, and other disorders (e.g., personality disorders, sleep disorders). That number is expected to double by 2030 (Eden, Maslow, Le, & Blazer, 2012). Within this population, it is estimated that 3–8% of individuals have a serious mental disorder (e.g., schizophrenia, bipolar disorder, or chronic depression). In addition to the prevalence of both alcohol and medication misuse, about 15% of community-residing older persons have symptoms of depression (Blazer, 2003), and every 68 min, an older person kills themselves (Drapeau & McIntosh, 2015).

In spite of the high prevalence of behavioral health conditions in the older population now and as projected in the future, there is a serious shortage of trained geriatric behavioral health manpower, appropriate clinical services, and tailored psychosocial interventions that coordinate with medical and social service providers (Bartels, Pepin, & Gill, 2014; Cohen & Eisdorfer, 2011). In spite of an urgent need for professionals with expertise in geriatric mental health care, there are currently only 1800 geriatric psychiatrists in the USA, and that number will decrease in the foreseeable future, amounting to only 1 geriatric psychiatrist for every 6000 older adults with a behavioral disorder (Bartels & Naslund, 2013). Unfortunately, the pattern of a severe shortfall in providers is the same for other clinicians in geriatric psychology, nursing, social work, and counseling.

The unmet needs for mental health care are a serious problem, with a substantial proportion of the affected population at risk for ongoing poor physical and mental health outcomes and unnecessary disability (Bartels et al., 2014). Two-thirds of older persons with a mental disorder do not receive needed services, and although they are more willing to pursue mental health care than in the past, the outcome is distressing (Bartels et al., 2014). Only 48% of older persons who received psychiatric help were considered to have received minimally adequate care, and of the large majority who received mental health care in the general medical sector, only 13% received adequate care (Bartels et al., 2014). Since the majority of Americans, especially older Americans, use primary care physicians as their de facto mental health-care providers, these data reflect the inadequacy of current practice patterns.

Many characteristics of clinical providers and health-care system operations contribute to the poor quality of care throughout the continuum of acute and long-term care. Provider factors include the following: ageism and therapeutic nihilism; lack of knowledge about psychosocial needs, functional effectiveness, diagnostic protocols, and effective treatments; and low referral rates from primary care physicians to mental health specialists. A number of barriers are created by the organization and financing of health-care services. These include the lack of available and accessible mental health services, the lack of integration of mental health care with other medical services, limited reimbursement in long-term care settings, limited coverage for specific treatment, and perceptions by many third-party payers that care of mental health problems is open-ended, leading to high costs.

The lack of adequate treatment for the range of behavioral disorders has a significant adverse impact on older adults, their family caregivers, and the greater society. Older persons are at risk for decreased functional effectiveness and increased disability, continuing poor physical and behavioral health, a decreased quality of life, and increased mortality. Family members living with the increasing burden of caregiving demands have higher rates of depression and poorer health status. These factors all contribute to dramatic increased health-care costs. Mental health conditions are among the most costly of eight health conditions in older adults (IOM, 2008), and for those who are beneficiaries of both Medicare and Medicaid, mental health conditions increase costs two to three times (Bartels et al., 2003).

A review of historical and contemporary public health policies can provide a perspective about why the behavioral health needs of older adults are underserved. The present system of geriatric behavioral health care is not working, and it will not even begin to meet the future needs of a rapidly growing population of older people (Jeste et al., 1999; National Association of Mental Health Planning and Advisory Councils, 2007). The sad irony is these system failures are occurring in the USA, which has the highest per capita health-care expenditures in the world for older people as well as the largest research investments in developing geriatric behavioral health interventions (Bartels et al., 2014).

Historical Review of US Public Policy on Geriatric Behavioral Health Research, Policy, and Practice

The social and economic needs of an aging population emerged as a federal public policy agenda in the 1930s, followed by a public policy agenda for health care in the 1960s. The 1930 Census reported there were 6,634,000 people aged 65 years and older (5.49% of the total population) (US Census Bureau, 1931). A series of actions by the executive and legislative branches of government led to the passage of the Social Security Act in 1935 during President Roosevelt's administration to help sustain the economic and social welfare of families with older relatives. Recognition of the impact of a growing aging population led President Truman to charge the Federal Security Administration to hold a national conference on aging to evaluate the shifting age demographics. Several other national conferences after that laid the groundwork for the first designated White House Conference on Aging (WHCoA) held in 1961. Six WHCoAs, spanning 65 years, led to a number of key national policies and programs that have had an impact on geriatric behavioral health care.

Health care was the major focus of the 1961 WHCoA, which led to legislation establishing Medicare and Medicaid in 1965 under President Johnson (Tibbitts, 1960). However, long-term care largely was overlooked, and reimbursement for mental health care, other than inpatient psychiatric care and psychological testing, was limited relative to physical medical care services. The Older Americans Act, also was passed in 1965, creating the Federal Administration on Aging, an advisory body to the US Secretary of Health and Human Services.

The spotlight of the 1971 WHCoA, held during President Nixon's administration, was on economic security, but several recommendations targeted the need to fund research and training initiatives (WHCoA, 1971). Significant outcomes of the Conference included the establishment of the National Institute on Aging in 1974 and the creation of the Center for the Study of Mental Health and Aging within the National Institute of Mental Health. Other major developments included a national nutrition program for older adults as well as the creation of the Federal Council on Aging and the Senate Special Committee on Aging (WHCoA, 1971).

The 1981 WHCoA was planned under President Carter's administration and implemented under President Reagan (Cowell, 1981). Social security and long-term care were signal areas of concentration. Based on the Conference recommendations, the federal Omnibus Reconciliation Act, passed in 1987, mandated that mental health services be provided in long-term care facilities. The 1981 Conference also produced other mental health recommendations that were implemented over the years. The cap on outpatient mental health services under Medicare Part B increased (repealed 8 years later under the Omnibus Reconciliation Act of 1989). Modifications to Medicare allowed psychologists and clinical social workers to be reimbursed for specific services. However, parity between somatic health care and mental health care was not achieved at that time. Mental health-care services continued to be reimbursed at 50% in contrast to 80% for other medical care. It would not be until 2008 that parity was achieved. The passage of the 2008 Paul Wellstone and Pete

Domenici Mental Health Parity and Addiction Equity Act mandated insurance parity for companies of fifty or more employees beginning in 2010.

During the 1980s, there was increased interest at the federal level. New legislation expanded reimbursement for home health care, occupational therapy, and specific therapies in long-term care institutions and increased funds for mental health research and research on Alzheimer's disease. In addition to an interagency task force on Alzheimer's disease, additional funding created Clinical Research Centers for Geriatric Mental Health and Geriatric Mental Health Training Awards. The Department of Veterans Affairs (VA) recommended new programs for the integration of behavioral and primary health care and more clinical geriatric research and demonstration programs at medical centers for older adult populations.

The 1995 WHCoA convened under President Clinton focused on supporting and reforming existing social and health programs, including Medicare, Medicaid, and the Older Americans Act (Blancato, 1994). Although the Conference did not endorse any new initiatives, a commitment was voiced to support the field of geriatric mental health and target future national policy focused on an aging population.

Four major developments occurred in the 1990s. Funding for research on Alzheimer's disease grew. In 1991, representatives of several organizations formed the National Coalition on Mental Health and Aging with a mission to advocate for policy reform (National Coalition on Mental Health and Aging, 2018).

Another milestone was the 1999 Surgeon General's report on mental health identifying the prevalence and impact of disability due to mental illness among older Americans now and in the future (Office of the Surgeon General, 1999). Finally, the 1999 Olmstead decision of the US Supreme Court determined that institutionalizing individuals with disabilities as well as mental illnesses, who could live in the community with supports, is discrimination that violates the Americans with Disabilities Act (Bartels, Miles, Dums, & Levine, 2003).

The 2005 WHCoA, convened under President George W. Bush, passed many resolutions, and among the top ten priorities was the need to improve the recognition, detection, and treatment of mental illness, especially depression among older Americans. Mental health issues were also the focus of other resolutions regarding Medicare and Medicaid, geriatric manpower, and long-term care reform (Gloth 3rd., 2007).

The 2015 WHCoA, held in Washington under President Obama's administration, was the first to use social media to transform the activities of the conference into opportunities for national and international participation. The overall theme was healthy aging for people of all ages, and there were four priority concentration areas: (1) healthy aging, (2) retirement security, (3) long-term services and supports, and (4) elder justice (WHCoA, 2015). The Healthy Aging Section included discussions and recommendations to optimize cognitive health and increase research on the dementias as well as the need for programs and resources to support the expansion of research, training, and practices to maximize behavioral health (WHCoA, 2015).

An Integrated Behavioral Health and Social Policy Framework

Future behavioral health-care policies need to continue to consider the many biopsychosocial and environmental factors that interact to promote behavioral health and maximize vitality and quality of life. Cohen and Eisdorfer (2011) suggest there are three main assumptions regarding integrated geriatric behavioral health policy reform. First, later life should be a time to feel secure regardless of the level of dependency and need for care. Second, later life should be a time, for those who choose, to remain actively engaged in family and community life. Third, any policy (or lack thereof) that diminishes the independence of older adults damages their health and quality of life by increasing marginalization and eventual deterioration and dependency. Working from these assumptions, they created the SAFE HAVENS framework with ten core themes: (1) Security, (2) Alternatives, (3) Functionality, (4) Engagement, (5) Health, (6) Abilities, (7) Values, (8) Environment, (9) New information, and (10) Simplicity.

Security

The many axes of security, financial, physical, emotional, and psychosocial create a foundation for behavioral health in older people, and some of the major policy issues that enhance security include retirement benefits, Social Security, Medicare, and other health-care benefits. Although social policies are economically based and executed, they must be steered by beliefs that older people are valuable and merit a secure future. Since the generativity of older generations has supported their families and communities, they not only deserve respect for these contributions but also opportunities to continue contributing in meaningful ways. This country has a moral responsibility to maintain an investment in the older population because programs that benefit older people also help their families and the greater community.

Social Security and Medicare, funded by Federal tax revenues from the workforce, are not solely entitlement programs for older people. They are designed to help families and younger people in the community. Social Security was conceived to save families from economic hardship because parents and older family members were living longer. Likewise, Medicare was intended to assist families with the costs of acute health care for aging relatives. However, continued federal financing of these programs has been an ongoing challenge given the rapid aging of the population, a decreasing ratio of workers to retirees, and other factors.

Medicare has been a successful policy providing health insurance for the older population as well as blind and disabled populations. It has eased the burden of health-care payments for millions of middle-aged Americans, who would otherwise be paying for the care of parents and grandparents as well as their children. It improved access to health care and therefore the health and quality of life of older persons. Medicare also allowed family members in the workforce to support their children's development and education and also pay for housing, transportation, health care, and other expenses which might have otherwise been consumed by the health-care costs of parents and grandparents. Although Medicare has weaknesses including restrictions in long-term care, rising overall costs, and fraudulent abuse, the basic principle of investing in Medicare remains a sound one.

Economic insecurity is a growing worry, especially among older women, given the projected future shortfall in Social Security financing and the changing structure and availability of pension plans. The soundness of Social Security is contingent on two major factors: (1) the ratio of workers to retirees and (2) level of taxation. Current projections indicate that over time, there will be a shortfall of available funds for the growing population of retirees who in turn are supported by fewer workers paying into the program. At the same time, private pension programs are disappearing, as major corporations are defaulting or scaling down employee pensions to maintain profits. Thus, older persons, even those who had done everything possible to plan and save for retirement, are facing the risk of financial insecurity.

There are several options to reform Social Security to protect today's older population as well as those who will age into Social Security in future years. These include, but are not limited to, the following: (1) raising the full retirement age, (2) increasing or eliminating the payroll earnings cap, (3) reducing benefits for high-income earners, (4) increasing the payroll tax rates, and (5) establishing parallel Federal investment programs. Increasing the retirement age by 2 or 3 years and/or increasing the level of taxable employee earnings to a higher cap would go a long way to resolve economic disparities. However, there are pros and cons to reform options, and it is essential that Social Security not be politicized. Reform will only occur with public education and involvement advocating a bipartisan review of national pension reform.

Alternatives

The rapidly growing population of older adults is characterized by increasing heterogeneity, i.e., they are less alike than any other age group on all biological, psychological, behavioral, and social variables. Scientific advances coupled with the successes of Medicare have contributed to a healthier, more active population, and successive generations of older people have become more diversified. Therefore, it is inappropriate to create policies based on beliefs that with advancing age, people are all sick and dependent, lose their cognitive abilities, and/or are less capable in work-related tasks and responsibilities.

Policy reform needs to focus on increasing opportunities for older people to participate in meaningful roles instead of promoting barriers that force individuals to retire and become marginalized. The ability to make meaningful choices and perceive alternatives in later life enhances mental and physical well-being, and policies must encourage alternatives by removing barriers and/or providing incentives to facilitate engagement. Provision of reimbursement for personal assistive devices and maximizing functioning through architectural design should enhance barrier freedom in transportation options, home design, workplace sites, and public environments (e.g., hospitals, libraries, malls, courthouses). The older adult population has the largest amount of discretionary income, which should be attractive to many industries to develop a wide range of products, from clothing to travel, to enhance lifestyle and bolster the economy. There are a wide range of attractive products for the senior lifestyle.

Functionality

Functionality is a core concept in geriatric health and behavioral health care, and caring for individuals impaired or disabled by illness, frailty, and injuries is often more challenging than curing or managing a disease. Since many geriatric diseases are chronic, the clinician's role is to optimize functioning by integrating behavioral, social, and pharmacological strategies to maximize performance and minimize the occurrence of acute crises.

Not only can rehabilitation and assistive devices improve many age- or illness-related impairments, these technologies can address opportunities for lifestyle enhancement. Functionality is the outcome of preventive screening and incorporating health promotion/risk prevention behaviors into personal lifestyles. Education about depression, nutrition, obesity, and other health maintenance strategies as well as establishing new behaviors, such as physical and cognitive exercise, enhance functional capacity.

Medicare and private insurance policies now cover screening and prevention strategies in health and mental health. Medicare Part B covers, at no cost to beneficiaries, a one-time "Welcome to Medicare" preventive visit, which includes a review of risk factors for depression, an annual screening for depression in primary care settings, and a yearly "Wellness Visit" to review changes in mental health. The Affordable Care Act, since 2014, required all non-grandfathered health plans to cover a range of preventative services at no cost, including screenings for depression and alcohol misuse.

Engagement

One of the most significant policy challenges is to provide meaningful roles for older adults in contemporary society and find ways to support them. Just as it is possible to use many approaches to reduce barriers to mobility and enhance functional effectiveness, it is necessary to maximize older people's engagement in meaningful pursuits and reduce or eliminate barriers to participation.

Engagement has many different meanings: to engage in work or an occupation, to engage to with others to accomplish mutual goals, to initiate or carry out activities, to enter into a loyal relationship with someone, to interact with other individuals, and to participate in long-term projects and activities. Thus, engagement is manifest in many ways, including but not limited to supporting older people to work or volunteer, encouraging contributional roles within the family and community, helping older persons remain active in physical and social activities that provide personal pleasure and a sense of meaningful participation, appreciating the value of intimate relationships and friendships in later life, and developing policies that will continue to engage the growing aging population.

Individuals may also be engaged in a range of personally satisfying creative artistic activities as well as political and social causes. Vital involvement, life satisfaction, and personal achievement are potent interventions to combat loneliness, inactivity, and social isolation. Many older people find meaning in family, parenting, and grandparenting relationships as well as in work and volunteer roles in the community. However, there are more broad-based concerns in the development of policies that encourage engagement. As life expectancy continues to increase, a number of challenging questions emerge: What is the "shelf life" of an individual? What mechanisms are needed to maximize independence and interdependence as well as successful aging within sociopolitical structures? What is the range of stakeholders responsible for developing and implementing policy changes?

These questions are not theoretical issues. Among the most powerful predictors of emotional well-being in later life are the availability of a confidante and meaningful social relationships and supports. Not having a relationship(s) that facilitates engagement is anomie or disconnectedness, characterized by isolation and loneliness, especially among the very old. Disconnectedness has a profound negative impact on mental and physical health, security, and quality of life. Durkheim referred to anomie as a cause of suicide (Johnson, 1965), and older persons, especially older white males, have high suicide rates (Ivey-Stephenson, Crosby, Jack, Haileyesus, & Kresnow-Sedacca, 2017).

Societal responsibility for facilitating the engagement of older adults goes hand in hand with individual responsibility to be active, productive, and engaged. Policies that support mechanisms to provide help and assist others are powerful forces that encourage and sustain productive social interactions and productivity. There are many sources of help, including, but not limited to, family, friends, educational institutions, professionals, community groups, business, and governmental agencies. Those who are old, frail, and vulnerable also require a range of affordable and accessible medical as well as home- and community-based services in addition to family and psychosocial support.

Health

Four issues are critical in the development of geriatric health and behavioral health policy: (1) availability, (2) accessibility, (3) affordability, and (4) appropriateness of health care.

Availability refers to two issues: (1) having enough trained geriatric behavioral health professionals and (2) having a knowledge base for clinical guidelines and tools to diagnose, treat, manage, and prevent diseases. The current and projected numbers of behavioral health professionals are woefully inadequate as discussed earlier, making this the single greatest barrier to suitable care. Thus, policies targeting increased training programs for medical students, residents, clinical graduate students, and postdoctoral fellows, as well as practitioners, must be a priority. Although more older people are living longer in good health, the burden of chronic illnesses, including the increasing prevalence of comorbidity and the increased dependency on medications and other expensive procedures, such as imaging and dialysis, is costly. From a policy perspective, identifying ways to increase the speed of translation of research results from bench to bedside is essential. Just as important is the responsibility to monitor the safety of new clinical interventions such as drugs and devices once they have been approved and are on the market. At the moment, there are no clear policies about the ongoing surveillance of medication effects as well as "natural" products not subject to FDA regulation.

Accessibility and affordability are closely related issues. Accessibility refers to the ease of obtaining care, and affordability refers to the ability to pay for care. The ability to find quality health care and behavioral health care that is affordable and accessible and also deals with the functional needs of older adults remains a challenge. In order to work toward these objectives, the structure and financing of the health-care delivery system need to be reformed. Relatively independent and uncoordinated generalist and specialist physicians deliver most of the health care in this country, despite the recognition that the availability of non-medical supportive services can decrease the burden of health-care management, reduce acuity, enhance function, and prevent institutionalization. Policies to encourage the coupling of health and supportive services as well as to increase geriatric health-care manpower, woefully insufficient at this time, are critical to improve accessible and affordable care. The critical need to boost the numbers of health-care professionals in geriatrics was among the top ten recommendations of the 2005 White House Conference on Aging (Gloth 3rd., 2007) and a 2008 IOM report (Institute of Medicine Committee on the Future Health Care Workforce for Older Americans, 2008).

Although behavioral health and physical health are interrelated, the systems of delivering and financing care are very different (Unutzer & Park, 2012). Mental health has a powerful impact on health-care costs, in large measure, because mental illnesses are so prevalent, are frequently undetected, and dramatically affect physical health and functional effectiveness (Mojtabai, 2011; Unutzer & Park, 2012). Studies repeatedly show that the cost of health care is significantly impacted by mental health problems, and depression and anxiety disorders significantly increase the cost of a patient's general medical or surgical care (Kleine-Budde et al., 2013; Mihalopoulos & Vos, 2013).

Since health behaviors mediate an individual's risk many for different illnesses and consequently influence health-care costs, health-care reform must consider reinforcing appropriate health promotion and risk reduction health and behavioral health behaviors. A related policy consideration lies in the personal vs. societal responsibility to pay for health care for those who smoke, fail to control their blood pressure by failure to adhere to medications or diet, refuse to exercise, abuse drugs, or refuse rehabilitation or counseling. Health programs should be available without cost to individuals with these behavioral problems who want help, and incentives such as reduced out-of-pocket payments or better insurance rates should be considered for those who practice healthy lifestyles.

A central issue in health and behavioral health policy is the best ways to craft a three-way partnership between people, providers, and third-party payers to provide quality care, minimize medical errors, and contain costs. This not only includes a partnership for the provision and payment of acute medical care and long-term care services but also preventative screening and interventions (e.g., cholesterol, blood pressure, malnutrition, obesity, bone density screening) as well as vaccinations for conditions such as pneumonia and influenza. Health maintenance behavior programs not only need to be implemented for patients but also family members who are frequently critical partners in the treatment/management plans.

A number of other important policy issues need to be addressed:

- Reimbursement should be provided for health professionals, including physician assistants, nurse practitioners, and psychiatric nurse practitioners, who play a crucial role in health.
- Electronic health records (HER) need to be implemented. EHRs focus on the total health of the patient and are designed to share information with all clinicians involved in the patient's care. EHRs track data over time, identify when patients are due for preventive screenings or checkups, monitor how patients are doing on various procedures, and monitor and improve overall quality of care within the practice.
- More health-care and human services professionals trained in geriatric care are urgent.
- Family caregiver supports and services should be inclusive of children and adolescent caregivers as well as adults.
- Initiatives that provide many health-care and social services in the same location are needed to provide "one stop shopping."
- Resident-centered geriatric care and psychosocial interventions are priorities to improve long-term care.

Ability

The ability domain refers to the productive capacities and performance of older persons. Since the language used in policy communicates underlying values as well as specific content, the concept of ability needs to be emphasized in policy statements. In the absence of serious, crippling health problems, older adults can be productive, able, and generative members of society. The concept of "use it or lose it" underscores the premise that older adults have capabilities and skills that can be enhanced by physical and cognitive exercises as well as active participation in social or creative activities.

Predicting competencies requires that performance be measured according to specific criteria. The standards for evaluating performance on tasks such as driving a car, flying an airplane, sitting as a judge, performing surgery, or performing other workplace roles are very different, but performance benchmarks can be defined, measured, and evaluated. Unfortunately, negative biases and unfounded beliefs about older people often presume age-related declining abilities without testing them. As a consequence, policies emerge that diminish or curtail the ability to perform various roles and responsibilities, such as mandatory retirement ages. Although older adults with cognitive, sensory, and physical impairments may be limited in their ability to perform certain activities, these should be addressed on a case-by-case basis. Individual performance criteria should be used instead of chronological age. Age-based mandatory retirement in the corporate sector, state judges, and other occupations, age of entry cut-offs for law enforcement and other public safety occupations, and the age 60 rule for retirement of commercial airline pilots are prime examples of occupational requirements that presume but do not evaluate job-related abilities.

Values

Policies need to acknowledge older people as valuable members of society, not reinforce a devaluation because of age. The essence of the concept of value is that it shifts the model of eldercare from a charitable concept to an investment concept. It is an investment in every individual and society to promote dignity and quality of life in the care of older adults, indeed people of all ages. Educating individuals to adopt moral values about the importance of caring for others leads to new ways of thinking about investing in those who are frail and sick.

Social and health policies need to be formulated to address issues that create access to meaningful pursuits, improves vitality, enhances quality of life, and ultimately promotes behavioral health. For example, the development of community programs to allow older persons to train and participate in voluntary work as well as paid employment should be a priority. Policies restricting the participation of older adults in the workplace need to be carefully justified.

Values, however, are not synonymous with paid employment. There are many generative roles for older adults to invest time and/or money to help others in the family as well as the greater community. Furthermore, older persons can become models of revitalization and inspiration to others when they pursue personal creative activities, such as art, music, writing, drama, or sports.

Environment

Older adults generally prefer to continue to live at home, even when frailty and medical conditions threaten mobility, self-care, and safety. "Aging in Place" is used to describe a broad policy goal to enable older persons to remain in their homes or a familiar community of their choice as long as possible with services and assistance as needs change (Cutchin, 2003). Although many psychosocial, family, and political factors affect how well older adults can age in place, financial circumstances probably have the greatest impact. Those who rent apartments, houses, or trailers may not have the option to remain at home or in familiar communities when properties are sold, and finding affordable, desirable housing may be difficult. Even individuals who own their homes may face diminishing financial resources to pay the mortgage, taxes, maintenance, insurance, and other housing expenses.

Aging in place is seen as desirable, but this will not be possible unless states have policies that provide support for needed services. These policies need to address the availability of community referral sources and home- and community-based services, accessible health care, coordination among health and aging networks, public transportation, caregiver support services, and affordable and available housing, including home repair services.

New Information

The rapid expansion of information, access to information, and utilization/integration of information are a challenge for all age groups, and individuals who are not able to access and deal with information become less well informed and able to function in our rapidly changing society. Policies that support educational and training programs, sustain cognitive capacities, and help older adults develop new skills to prevent obsolescence are critical, and to do this, a public-private sector partnership of many different stakeholders needs to become involved in extending educational opportunities to the older population. Abundant research has established the value of lifespan learning for enhancing cognitive skills. Computer literacy is now well within the capacity of many older adults, and access to the information on the Internet has become a valuable instrument for decision-making about virtually all aspects of life, including health care.

Continuing education of health and human service professionals is a serious issue for policy formulation as well. Professional associations concerned with aging and mental health provide training programs about the latest research and clinical practice advances. Evidenced-based practice has become the gold standard for clinical care, including behavioral health and social programs. This approach recognizes the importance of using results confirmed by multiple studies to inform clinicians and patients about empirical standards of care and available choices.

From a policy perspective, evidence-based practice is becoming more accepted as the basis for developing social and mental health programs. Evidence-based practice standards are evolving for the treatment of older adults, but the research is limited at this time to a few areas, including community outreach mental health services and homecare mental health services.

Simplicity

The many governmental and non-governmental programs and services for older people and their family caregivers are a confusing quagmire for consumers. The full range of available social and health programs for the older population should be integrated and seamless. Just as having multiple physicians with poor communication patterns adversely affects health care, so do multiple private and governmental agencies become a barrier to quality care. Many of these agencies and health-care settings have different sets of qualifications for the populations served, records are rarely shared between professionals, and older people themselves may not communicate information to staff across the many settings they access. The unfortunate consequence may be if they are turned away in one setting, they may not be aware of other options for assistance.

Orchestrating and simplifying the process of caring are the most problematic challenges faced by the clinical community. Behavioral health clinicians frequently need to become involved to help patients negotiate the system. Policy reform should include assurances of funding for multi-agency collaboration and the availability of service managers to help patients and families find the right care.

New Directions in Behavioral Health Care for Older Adults

New health-care policy programs are fueling changes in the behavioral health care of all Americans, including older people. The Patient Protection and Affordable Care Act (ACA), signed into law by President Obama in 2010 but with most provisions going into effect in 2014, has resulted in some basic changes in health-care delivery. Most of the ACA does not explicitly address geriatric mental health, but some reforms have major implications for costly patients, including older adults with behavioral health disorders who account for a disproportionate portion of health-care costs, e.g., Medicare and dually eligible (Medicare and Medicaid) patients (Bartels, Gill, & Naslund, 2015).

The ACA expands the provisions of the 2008 Mental Health Parity and Addiction Equity Act, requiring insurers to provide the equivalent level of coverage for mental health and substance abuse treatment as provided for other medical/surgical services. Specific components of the ACA relevant to geriatric mental health include nine major components. These include "accountable care organizations (ACOs), patient-centered medical homes (PCMHs), Medicaid-financed specialty health homes, hospital readmission and health care transition initiatives, a Medicare annual wellness visit, quality standards, support for the use of health information technology and telehealth, the Independence at Home and the 1915(i) State Plan Home and Community-Based Services program, as well as the Centers for Medicare Services' Medicare-Medicaid Coordination Office, the Center for Medicare and Medicaid Innovation, and the Patient-Centered Outcomes Research Institute" (Bartels et al., 2015, p. 304).

Accountable Care Organizations

ACOs are groups of providers that are accountable for the cost and quality of health care delivered to a patient population based on prescribed performance and payment criteria. A new type of ACO, Totally Accountable Care Organizations, integrates physical health and behavioral health as well as social and public health and long-term care services based on an overall payment structure with financial incentives to reduce costs. These programs provide opportunities to integrate a full range of management and preventative care options to manage high-cost older patients who use more behavioral health services.

Patient-Centered Medical Homes

PCMHs deliver a coordinated and comprehensive range of health-care services at lower per capita costs targeting the distinctive needs of individual patients. They are ideally suited to provide accessible and extensive physical and behavioral health care for older persons with multiple chronic health problems, including major depression. This model originated in the 1960s as a program to care for children with complex chronic illnesses.

Medicaid-Financed Specialty Health Home

This model coordinates comprehensive physical and mental health care at a single site for Medicaid patients with complex and/or multiple chronic conditions. Most Medicaid patients are not older persons. However, 17% of Medicaid beneficiaries are dually eligible under Medicare and Medicare, more than 9% are low-income older adults, and 10% of newly eligible individuals are between the ages of 55 and 64 years (Centers for Medicare & Medicaid Services, 2018).

Hospital Readmission and Health-Care Transitions

Several ACA programs focus on successfully transitioning patients from hospitals to community settings and decreasing hospital readmission rates. These include a pilot program creating working partnerships between hospitals and post-acute providers, a pilot program utilizing payment bundling to hospitals for the total care of patients, and a community-based care transition initiative that delivers at least one transitional care intervention to Medicare patients. A number of studies have reported the effectiveness of transitional initiatives in improving care and reducing readmissions to hospitals in adults, and a few have examined the effect on frail older adults. However, there is scant research on the impact of transitional care for older adults with behavioral health conditions, who usually have other chronic health problems and are at high risk for nursing home admission.

The Annual Medicare Wellness Visit

The ACA pays for time-intensive annual wellness visits, at no cost to Medicare beneficiaries (Bartels et al., 2015). The wellness visits include a health professional's review of a patient's history, a patient's questionnaire about health risks, physical and functional health assessments, individualized health advice, and follow-up. Follow-up may include diagnostic tests, referrals to specialists, and/or setting goals for health promotion and risk prevention behaviors.

The visit only includes screens for two behavioral health areas: a depression screen using the Patient Health Questionnaire (PHQ-9) and a cognitive assessment based on family member reports using an evidence-based, cognitive-screening instrument. However, other aspects of the visits that may be relevant for behavioral health include screening for tobacco dependence and obesity as well as counseling for managing weight and smoking cessation.

Quality Standards and Incentives

Health plans must submit annual reports reporting specific measures of health-care delivery, including health outcomes and quality indicators. The intent of these reports is to decrease/avoid unnecessary emergency room visits and hospital readmissions. Quality measures include the care experiences of patients and caregivers, care coordination, patient safety, health promotion/disease prevention, and management of complicated high-cost conditions. Some health plans provide incentives to encourage patient participation in health promotion activities, such as physical fitness or smoking cessation programs.

The ACA includes two quality benchmarks for behavioral health: (1) the scores on the screens for depression and cognitive impairment included in the Medicare annual wellness visit and (2) quality measures of integrated mental health-care programming provided in patient-centered medical homes (Bartels et al., 2015). It also specifies more structured requirements for psychiatric hospitals to follow and report outcomes, which if not submitted results in a payment penalty. Finally, a pilot Medicare program is testing the effectiveness of providing positive incentives for hospitals that achieve specific performance standards.

Information Health Technology and Telehealth

One of the expectations for the ACA is that a number of health-care providers will adopt mobile, online, and remote health-care information technologies for diagnosis and treatment, symptom monitoring, and health-care administration.

Independence at Home Demonstration

The Independence At Home (IAH) demonstration project from the Center for Medicare and Medicaid Innovation tests the delivery of primary care services at home for individuals with complex, chronic clinical care conditions (Moon, Hollin, Nicholas, Schoen, & Davis, 2015). The IAH program was extended for another 2 years in February 2018 raising the number of participating beneficiaries to 15,000.

1915(i) State Plan Home and Community-Based Services Program

This program delivers health care to Medicare beneficiaries with chronic health conditions using home-based primary care teams and provides both acute and long-term medical services on a needs basis (Centers for Medicare & Medicaid Services, 2014). Under Section 1915(i), states may provide a range of services to special populations, such as older persons with behavioral health conditions. These services include clinic care, case management, psychosocial rehabilitation, behavioral support, and health monitoring and promotion (Centers for Medicare & Medicaid Services, 2014).

Center for Medicare and Medicaid Services (CMS) Coordination Office, Center for Medicare and Medicaid Innovation (CMMI), and Patient-Centered Outcomes Research Institute (PCORI)

The CMS Coordination Office coordinates Medicare and Medicaid benefits between the federal government and states for dually eligible individuals, many of whom are older adults with mental health problems. CMMI tests service delivery and payment models to ensure quality of care and minimize expenditures. PCORI develops better standards of evidence for quality of care to improve decision-making for health-care professionals and patients. Both the CMMI and PCORI solicit and fund a number of projects that focus on integrating physical and behavioral health care for vulnerable populations that include older adults with behavioral health conditions.

Implications for Behavioral Health

Dedicated and concerted advocacy by public and private stakeholders will be essential to pave the way to provide optimal care for the population of older adults with behavioral health challenges who will double by 2030, unfortunately at the same time as the number of trained geriatric behavioral health professionals decreases (Eden et al., 2012). The IOM report underscored the necessity to train and support a sufficient cadre of practitioners to provide integrated diagnosis and treatment of geriatric mental health conditions across the broad spectrum of primary care, acute and long-term care, social services, and home- and community-based care settings (Eden et al., 2012). Sadly, no government agencies have been charged with the specific responsibility to focus on the mental health-care needs older adults, and despite the IOM's charge that SAMHSA prioritize geriatric mental health, SAMHSA's 2015–2018 strategic plan did not identify older adults as a priority and did not specify programmatic initiatives for geriatric mental health services (SAMHSA, 2014, 2017).

The ACA does not specifically focus on the needs of number of older adults with behavioral health needs, but a number of the provisions discussed provide opportunities for improving care. However, the battle will be an uphill one to meet the needs of this high-risk population who go unrecognized.

References

Alzheimer's Association. (2016). *2016 Alzheimer's disease facts and figures*. Chicago, IL: Author. https://www.alz.org/documents_custom/2016-facts-and-figures.pdf

Bartels, S. J., Dums, A. R., Oxman, T. E., Schneider, L. S., Arean, P. A., Alexopoulos, G. S., & Jeste, D. V. (2003). Evidence-based practices in geriatric mental health care: An overview of systematic reviews and meta-analyses. *The Psychiatric Clinics of North America, 26*(4), 971–990, x-xi.

Bartels, S. J., Gill, L., & Naslund, J. A. (2015). The Affordable Care Act, accountable care organizations, and mental health care for older adults: Implications and opportunities. *Harvard Review of Psychiatry, 23*(5), 304–319. https://doi.org/10.1097/hrp.0000000000000086

Bartels, S. J., Miles, K. M., Dums, A. R., & Levine, K. J. (2003). Are nursing homes appropriate for older adults with severe mental illness? Conflicting consumer and clinician views and implications for the Olmstead decision. *Journal of the American Geriatrics Society, 51*(11), 1571–1579. https://doi.org/10.1046/j.1532-5415.2003.51508.x

Bartels, S. J., & Naslund, J. A. (2013). The underside of the silver tsunami: Older adults and mental health care. *The New England Journal of Medicine, 368*(6), 493–496. https://doi.org/10.1056/NEJMp1211456

Bartels, S. J., Pepin, R., & Gill, L. E. (2014). The paradox of scarcity in a land of plenty: Meeting the needs of older adults with mental health and substance use disorders. *Generations, 38*(3), 6–13. https://www.ncbi.nlm.nih.gov/pmc/articles/PMC4316367/pdf/nihms656697.pdf

Blancato, R. B. (1994). The 1995 White House Conference on Aging. *Journal of Aging & Social Policy, 6*(1–2), xiii–xxvi. https://doi.org/10.1300/J031v06n01_a

Blazer, D. G. (2003). Depression in late life: Review and commentary. *The Journals of Gerontology. Series A, Biological Sciences and Medical Sciences, 58*(3), 249–265.

Centers for Medicare & Medicaid Services. (2014). Medicaid program; state plan home and community-based services, 5-year period for waivers, provider payment reassignment, and home and community-based setting requirements for Community First Choice and home and community-based services (HCBS) waivers. Final rule. *Federal Register, 79*(11), 2947–3039.

Centers for Medicare & Medicaid Services. (2018). *Seniors & Medicare and Medicaid enrollees* [Web page]. Baltimore, MD: Author. https://www.medicaid.gov/medicaid/eligibility/medicaid-enrollees/index.html

Cohen, D., & Eisdorfer, C. (2011). *Integrated textbook of geriatric mental health*. Baltimore, MD: Johns Hopkins University Press.

Cowell, D. D. (1981). *White House Conference on Aging, 1981*. Abstracts of the Technical Committee Reports, Mini White House Conference Reports, and State White House Conference Reports. Washington, DC: White House Conference on Aging. http://files.eric.ed.gov/fulltext/ED215262.pdf

Cutchin, M. P. (2003). The process of mediated aging-in-place: A theoretically and empirically based model. *Social Science & Medicine, 57*(6), 1077–1090.

Drapeau, C. W., & McIntosh, J. L. (2015, January 22). *U.S.A. suicide: 2013 official final data.* Washington, DC: American Academy of Suicidology. http://www.suicidology.org/portals/14/docs/resources/factsheets/2013datapgsv2alt.pdf

Eden, J., Maslow, K., Le, M., & Blazer, D. G. (2012). *The mental health and substance use workforce for older adults: In whose hands?* Washington, DC: National Academies Press. http://www.ncbi.nlm.nih.gov/books/NBK201410/

Gloth, F. M., 3rd. (2007). The 2005 White House Conference on Aging: A new day for White House conferences on aging and food for the future. *Journal of the American Geriatrics Society, 55*(2), 305–307. https://doi.org/10.1111/j.1532-5415.2007.01051.x

He, W., Goodkind, D., & Kowal, P. (2016, March). *An aging world: 2015* (International Population Reports, P95/16-1). Washington, DC: U.S. Government Publishing Office. https://www.census.gov/content/dam/Census/library/publications/2016/demo/p95-16-1.pdf

Institute of Medicine. (2001). *Health and behavior: The interplay of biological, behavioral, and societal influences.* Washington, DC: National Academy Press.

Institute of Medicine Committee on the Future Health Care Workforce for Older Americans. (2008). *Retooling for an aging America: Building the health care workforce.* Washington, DC: National Academies Press.

Ivey-Stephenson, A. Z., Crosby, A. E., Jack, S. P. D., Haileyesus, T., & Kresnow-Sedacca, M. J. (2017). Suicide trends among and within urbanization levels by sex, race/ethnicity, age group, and mechanism of death – United States, 2001-2015. *Morbidity and Mortality Weekly Report. Surveillance Summaries, 66*(18), 1–16. https://doi.org/10.15585/mmwr.ss6618a1

Jeste, D. V., Alexopoulos, G. S., Bartels, S. J., Cummings, J. L., Gallo, J. J., Gottlieb, G. L., … Lebowitz, B. D. (1999). Consensus statement on the upcoming crisis in geriatric mental health: Research agenda for the next 2 decades. *Archives of General Psychiatry, 56*(9), 848–853. https://doi.org/10.1001/archpsyc.56.9.848

Johnson, B. D. (1965). Durkheim's one cause of suicide. *American Sociological Review, 30*(6), 875–886. https://doi.org/10.2307/2090966

Johnson, N. B., Hayes, L. D., Brown, K., Hoo, E. C., & Ethier, K. A. (2014). CDC National Health Report: Leading causes of morbidity and mortality and associated behavioral risk and protective factors – United States, 2005-2013. *MMWR Supplements, 63*(4), 3–27.

Kleine-Budde, K., Muller, R., Kawohl, W., Bramesfeld, A., Moock, J., & Rossler, W. (2013). The cost of depression: A cost analysis from a large database. *Journal of Affective Disorders, 147*(1–3), 137–143. https://doi.org/10.1016/j.jad.2012.10.024

Mihalopoulos, C., & Vos, T. (2013). Cost-effectiveness of preventive interventions for depressive disorders: An overview. *Expert Review of Pharmacoeconomics & Outcomes Research, 13*(2), 237–242. https://doi.org/10.1586/erp.13.5

Mojtabai, R. (2011). National trends in mental health disability, 1997-2009. *American Journal of Public Health, 101*(11), 2156–2163. https://doi.org/10.2105/ajph.2011.300258

Moon, M., Hollin, I. L., Nicholas, L. H., Schoen, C., & Davis, K. (2015). Serving older adults with complex care needs: A new benefit option for Medicare. *Issue Brief (Commonwealth Fund), 23*, 1–11.

National Association of Mental Health Planning and Advisory Councils. (2007). *Older adults and mental health: A time for reform.* Rockville, MD: Center for Mental Health Services, Substance Abuse and Mental Health Services Administration.

National Coalition on Mental Health and Aging. (2018). *History* [Web page]. s.l.: Author. http://www.ncmha.org/?page_id=52

Office of the Surgeon General. (1999). *Mental health: A report of the Surgeon General.* Rockville, MD: Department of Health and Human Services, U.S. Public Health Service.

Ortman, J. M., & Velkoff, V. A. (2014, May). *An aging nation: The older population in the United States: Population estimates and projections* (Current Population Reports, P25-1140). Washington, DC: U.S. Census Bureau. https://www.census.gov/prod/2014pubs/p25-1140.pdf

Population Reference Bureau. (2016). *2016 world population data sheet with a special focus on human needs and sustainable resources*. Washington, DC: Author. http://www.prb.org/pdf16/prb-wpds2016-web-2016.pdf

Steel, Z., Marnane, C., Iranpour, C., Chey, T., Jackson, J. W., Patel, V., & Silove, D. (2014). The global prevalence of common mental disorders: A systematic review and meta-analysis 1980-2013. *International Journal of Epidemiology, 43*(2), 476–493. https://doi.org/10.1093/ije/dyu038

Substance Abuse and Mental Health Services Administration. (2014). *Leading change 2.0: Advancing the behavioral health of the nation 2015–2018* (HHS Publication No. (PEP) 14-LEADCHANGE2). Rockville, MD: Author. http://store.samhsa.gov/shin/content//PEP14-LEADCHANGE2/PEP14-LEADCHANGE2.pdf

Substance Abuse and Mental Health Services Administration. (2017). *Get connected: Linking older adults with resources on medication, alcohol, and mental health* (HHS Pub. No. (SMA) 03-3824)). Rockville, MD: Author. https://store.samhsa.gov/shin/content/SMA03-3824/SMA03-3824.pdf

Tibbitts, C. (1960). The 1961 White House Conference on Aging: Its rationale, objectives, and procedures. *Journal of the American Geriatrics Society, 8*, 373–377.

U. S. Bureau of the Census. (1931). *Fifteenth census of the United States, 1930* (Vol. 1. Number and distribution of inhabitants). Washington, DC: U. S. Government Printing Office.

United Nations Department of Economic and Social Affairs Population Division. (2015). *World population ageing 2015*. New York, NY: Author. http://www.un.org/en/development/desa/population/publications/pdf/ageing/WPA2015_Report.pdf

Unutzer, J., & Park, M. (2012). Strategies to improve the management of depression in primary care. *Primary Care, 39*(2), 415–431. https://doi.org/10.1016/j.pop.2012.03.010

Weiss, S. J., Haber, J., Horowitz, J. A., Stuart, G. W., & Wolfe, B. (2009). The inextricable nature of mental and physical health: Implications for integrative care. *Journal of the American Psychiatric Nurses Association, 15*(6), 371–382. https://doi.org/10.1177/1078390309352513

White House Conference on Aging. (1971). *White House Conference on Aging: A report to the delegates from the conference sections and special concerns sessions, November 28–December 2*. Washington, DC: U.S. Government Printing Office. http://files.eric.ed.gov/fulltext/ED058541.pdf

White House Conference on Aging. (2015). *2015 White House Conference on Aging: Final report*. Washington, DC: Author. https://archive.whitehouseconferenceonaging.gov/2015-WHCOA-Final-Report.pdf

Whiteford, H. A., Degenhardt, L., Rehm, J., Baxter, A. J., Ferrari, A. J., Erskine, H. E., … Vos, T. (2013). Global burden of disease attributable to mental and substance use disorders: Findings from the Global Burden of Disease Study 2010. *Lancet, 382*(9904), 1575–1586. https://doi.org/10.1016/s0140-6736(13)61611-6

Behavioral Health Services for Persons with Intellectual and Developmental Disabilities

Marc J. Tassé, Elizabeth A. Perkins, Tammy Jorgensen Smith, and Richard Chapman

Overview of Intellectual and Developmental Disabilities

Intellectual and developmental disabilities (IDD) do not possess any protective factor against the onset of behavioral disorders. In fact, research has shown that persons with intellectual disability, autism spectrum disorder, and related developmental disabilities are more susceptible to certain behavioral disorders than persons in the general population. Due to an individual's intellectual disability and/or developmental disability, the correct identification and treatment do not always follow a standard and expected course. We also know that the presence of behavioral health issues increases the challenges of properly supporting these individuals to live successful lives at home, school, and work and in the community. In this chapter we will focus on intellectual and developmental disabilities as well as touch upon autism spectrum disorder.

The American Association on Intellectual and Developmental Disabilities (AAIDD; Schalock et al., 2010), an interdisciplinary professional society founded almost 140 years ago, and the American Psychiatric Association (APA, 2013) define intellectual disability as originating during the developmental period and being characterized by significant impairments in both intellectual functioning and adaptive behavior.

M. J. Tassé (✉)
The Ohio State University, Columbus, OH, USA
e-mail: Marc.tasse@osumc.edu

E. A. Perkins
Department of Child & Family Studies, College of Behavioral and Community Sciences, University of South Florida, Tampa, FL, USA

T. J. Smith
College of Behavioral and Community Sciences, University of South Florida, Tampa, FL, USA

R. Chapman
University of South Florida, Tampa, FL, USA

© Springer Nature Switzerland AG 2020
B. L. Levin, A. Hanson (eds.), *Foundations of Behavioral Health*,
https://doi.org/10.1007/978-3-030-18435-3_12

Significant impairments are defined as functioning that is approximately two standard deviations or more below the population mean, and limitations in adaptive behavior include skill deficits in the performance of conceptual, social, and/or practical skills.

The *Diagnostic and Statistical Manual for Mental Disorders* (DSM-5) (APA, 2013) defines autism spectrum disorder (ASD) as being characterized by impairments in two realms: (1) social use of communication (including interpersonal skills and reciprocity, back-and-forth communication, understanding non-verbal social cues, eye contact, use and recognition of body language, understanding gestures, recognizing different emotions embedded in facial expressions, etc.) and (2) restricted, repetitive, and stereotyped patterns of behavior and interests or activities, including stereotyped motor behaviors, echolalia, idiosyncratic phrases, insistence on sameness, and hypo- or hyper-reactivity to sensory input or other sensory aspects. The presence of social communication deficits and restricted, repetitive behaviors and interests manifest during the developmental period and result in significant impairments across multiple life areas.

Developmental disabilities also are an administrative category of individuals defined under the federal Developmental Disabilities Assistance and Bill of Rights Act of 2000 (DD Act; Public Law 106-402) and can include a variety of known conditions. Section 102(8) of the DD Act defines developmental disability as a severe, chronic disability that:

1. "Is attributable to a mental or physical impairment or combination of mental and physical impairments"
2. "Is manifested before the individual attains age 22"
3. "Is likely to continue indefinitely"
4. "Results in substantial functional limitations in three or more of the following areas of major life activity: self-care, receptive and expressive language, learning, mobility, self-direction, capacity for independent living, and economic self-sufficiency"
5. "Reflects the individual's need for a combination and sequence of special, interdisciplinary, or generic services, individualized supports, or other forms of assistance that are of lifelong or extended duration and are individually planned and coordinated" (DD Act; Pub. L. 106-402, §102.8, pp. 1683–1684).

In addition, the Act also addresses infants and children to age 9 who have substantial developmental delays or specific congenital or acquired conditions. These children may be considered to have a developmental disability without meeting three or more of the criteria described above in 1 through 5 if the individual, without services and supports, has a high probability of meeting those criteria later in life (DD Act; Pub. L. 106–402, §102.8, p. 1684).

Epidemiology

Some broader definitions of developmental disabilities are inclusive of conditions such as hearing loss, vision impairment, learning disability, and attention deficit/hyperactivity disorder, and, with such definitions, the prevalence rates are as high as

14% of the total population of children between the ages of 3 and 17 years (Boyle et al., 2011). For the purposes of this chapter, however, we will use the definition of developmental disability found in the DD Act of 2000.

According to Larson et al. (2001), developmental disability and intellectual disability are not perfectly overlapping conditions. In their study on the prevalence of DD and ID, 48% of individuals had a developmental disability but no co-occurring intellectual disability, 28% had a developmental disability and an intellectual disability, and the remaining 24% had an intellectual disability but no developmental disability (Larson et al., 2001).

The estimated prevalence of intellectual disability is theoretically between 2 and 3% of the general population. This estimate is based on our knowledge of the normal distribution of abilities in the general population and the expected proportion of individuals who would be approximately two standard deviations below the population mean (Tassé & Grover, 2013). However, because the condition is diagnosed when the individual's functioning in both intellectual functioning and adaptive behavior are significantly subaverage, the actual estimated prevalence falls to approximately 1% of the total population (APA, 2013). Since intellectual disability is a condition that is diagnosed based entirely on the individual's intellectual and adaptive functioning, its etiology can be almost anything and is often multifactorial, including prenatal, perinatal, and postnatal risk factors (see Table 1). It is estimated that 30–40% of all cases of intellectual disability have no known cause(s).

The prevalence of ASD has been on the rise for the past two decades, increasing almost 300% between 1996 and 2010 (Van Naarden Braun et al., 2015). Boys have consistently been at greater risk of having ASD than girls (i.e., 4:1). The Centers for Disease Control and Prevention (CDC) publishes regular estimates of the prevalence of ASD at approximately 2-year intervals. In 2014, the CDC reported the prevalence of ASD to be approximately 1 in 68, up from its previous 2012 published report of 1 in 88 (Autism and Developmental Disabilities Monitoring Network Surveillance Year 2010 Principal Investigators, 2012, 2014).

There is some debate within the field whether the extent to which these increases in prevalence might be a reflection of better case ascertainment and identification, possibly as a result of an increase in awareness and access to services, or whether these changes in prevalence rate are a result of a true increase in incidence. It should be noted that the most recent prevalence statistics published by the CDC in April 2016 indicated, for the first time in many years, no change in the prevalence of ASD, remaining at 1 in 68 (Christensen et al., 2016). Hence, autism spectrum disorder remains an important public health concern in the United States, with lifetime costs

Table 1 Risk factors

Prenatal	Genetic or chromosomal disorders, metabolic disorders, trauma or injury that impacts fetal development, infection/toxins
Perinatal	Anoxia, infection, other trauma
Postnatal	Sensory deprivation, nutritional deficiency, environmental toxins/poisons (e.g., lead, mercury, pesticides, etc.), trauma/infection, or brain injury

associated to ASD estimated at approximately $3.2 million per person. These costs are driven largely by behavioral therapies in childhood, extensive adult care, as well as large indirect societal costs due to lost productivity (Ganz, 2007).

Behavioral Health and IDD

People with IDD are susceptible to presenting all forms of behavioral health problems found in the DSM-5 (APA, 2013). Not only are they susceptible, but they are three to four times more likely than the general population to present with behavioral health problems (Fletcher, Loschen, Stavrakaki, & First, 2007). Among the more common comorbid behavioral health conditions in people with ID, not unlike in the general population, are conditions such as depression and anxiety disorder (Fletcher et al., 2007). Whereas individuals with ASD may also present with high frequencies of comorbidity of anxiety disorder and depressive disorders, children also may present frequently with oppositional defiant/conduct disorder and attention deficit/hyperactivity disorder (Simonoff et al., 2008).

Some evidence has supported the need to adapt the symptoms or signs characteristic of psychiatric disorders in people with intellectual and developmental disabilities. This led to the publication of the *Diagnostic Manuals—Intellectual Disability (DM-ID): A Textbook of Diagnosis of Mental Disorders in Persons with Intellectual Disability* (Fletcher et al., 2007), which adapted the diagnostic criteria of the DSM-IV-TR (APA, 2000) for persons with IDD. An adaptation of the DSM-5 (APA, 2013) was published in 2016 (Fletcher, Barnhill, & Cooper, 2016). In most cases, the diagnostic criteria are relatively the same for people with milder forms of ID, but differences in number count and type of signs and symptoms associated with various DSM diagnoses appear with more significant levels of impairment in cognitive functioning and expressive language.

Problem behavior is also a common concern among clinicians working with individuals with IDD. Siegel et al. (2014) reported the most common reasons for admission to a specialized in-patient unit for children with IDD were problem behaviors, such as aggression, self-injurious behavior, property destruction, and tantrums, which led to placement in this restrictive clinical setting. The presence of problem behavior in individuals with IDD is, in fact, the most often cited reason for exclusion from more inclusive settings or placement into a segregated classroom/ school, home, in-patient unit, and/or employment (Bruininks, Hill, & Morreau, 1988; Lakin & Stancliffe, 2005). Children with ASD are also six times more likely to be hospitalized in a psychiatric unit than children without ASD (Croen, Najjar, Ray, Lotspeich, & Bernal, 2006). Therefore, effective and coordinated intervention strategies are crucial to preventing and eliminating problem behaviors and increasing adaptive skills and overall quality of life in people with IDD.

Substance Abuse

There was a time when few individuals with IDD had opportunity to access illicit drugs and alcohol. With the movements of normalization, valorization of social role, and self-determination, as well as the reduction of coercive controls and restriction of individual rights and freedoms of persons with IDD, came the greater likelihood of individuals with IDD making bad choices that led to less desirable outcomes. The increased prevalence of substance abuse is one such example. While the prevalence of illicit drug and alcohol use in people with IDD is relatively low, their risk of having a substance-related problem is comparatively high (Carroll Chapman & Wu, 2012). The severity of the problem of substance abuse in people with IDD is exacerbated by the fact that few effective treatments available for people with IDD exist and people with IDD typically avoid or rapidly abandon treatment interventions for substance abuse (Frielink, Schuengel, Kroon, & Embregts, 2015).

Although individuals with IDD face a variety of barriers to achieve meaningful inclusion in the community, opportunities that support inclusion for individuals with IDD include customized employment strategies, the promotion of self-advocacy and self-determination for individuals with IDD, and strategies for successful support at the end-of-life.

Customized Employment

Customized employment (CE) is defined by the Workforce Innovation and Opportunity Act (WIOA, Pub. L. No. 113–128) as: "*competitive integrated employment*, for an individual with a significant disability, that is based on an individualized determination of the *strengths, needs, and interests of the individual* with a significant disability, *designed to meet the specific abilities of the individual* with a significant disability *and the business needs of the employer*, and carried out through flexible strategies" (USC 29 Chapter "Pharmacy Services in Behavioral Health", §705(35)(A), pp. 186–187, *italics by authors*). CE "utilizes an individualized approach to employment planning and job development—one person at a time… one employer at a time" (Office of Disability Employment Policy, ODEP, (2018), para. 1).

The CE process facilitates employment possibilities for job seekers with disabilities who, due to life complexities, have had difficulty obtaining employment through traditional vocational rehabilitation processes. It considers unique aspects of each person such as age, type of disability, functional capacities, disposition, and interaction style. The CE process also recognizes contextual factors including resources, living arrangements, geographical location, and services and supports that the person receives (Smith, Dillahunt-Aspillaga, & Kenney, 2017).

Why Customized Employment?

CE is a positive process that focuses on "real work in the real world" and involves:

- Painting an accurate picture of a job seeker through the discovery process;
- Utilizing a strength-based approach to identify talents, interests, abilities, and conditions in which the job seeker can be successful;
- Welcoming and empowering others, especially those closest to the job seeker, as active participants in the process through development of a person-centered team.
- Developing relationships with potential connectors and mentors in the community.

Negotiating employment opportunities that meet the needs of both the job seeker and the employer presents a number of challenges. To do so, to create "real work in the real world", the CE process consists of the six key elements: (1) the discovery process, (2) the vocational profile, (3) the customized employment planning meeting, (4) the visual resume, (5) customized job development and negotiation, and (6) accommodations and post-employment support.

Discovery

Discovery is a type of naturalistic assessment that uses qualitative methods to gather information useful in building a narrative snapshot of a job seeker to facilitate the identification of ideal working conditions (Callahan & Condon, 2007). Discovery is a vital part of the CE process because it promotes improved employment matching. The discovery process takes place in natural environments, such as the home, neighborhood, and community. It includes interviews, conversations, observations, and records reviews to get to know the job seeker and his or her interests, talents, and conditions for employment (e.g., environmental tolerances, social interaction skills, etc.).

Vocational Profile

The discovery process culminates in the development of a vocational profile that provides a descriptive picture of the job seeker. It is a robust, narrative report that provides a foundation for effectively negotiating personalized potential job opportunities with employers (Condon & Callahan, 2008). The profile is a living document that can be amended as new information is uncovered making it a particularly useful tool for students transitioning from school to the community and workforce. Profiles provide "an alternative format to traditional evaluation reports that compare persons with complexities to general standards and others" (Callahan, Shumpert, & Condon, 2011, p. 5).

Customized Employment Planning

The customized planning meeting includes the job seeker, family, friends, advocates, service providers, vocational rehabilitation (VR) counselors, and other stakeholders chosen by the job seeker. Ideally, it occurs within 2 weeks of the completion of the vocational profile. The purpose of the meeting is to develop a CE blueprint that bridges the gap between discovery and job placement. The information contained in the vocational profile is utilized to develop a specific plan of action for achieving a competitive, integrated employment outcome in a job that matches the individual's interests, talents, requirements, and conditions for employment.

Visual Resume

The visual resume is a sales tool to introduce the job seeker to potential employers. It is different from a typical resume in that it utilizes photos or video clips to demonstrate the job seeker completing tasks/skills essential to the position. This tool is very useful for individuals who may not be able to express their talents and abilities verbally as is traditionally done through the interviewing process. The visual resume may also be utilized to explain the concept of CE to an employer.

Customized Job Development and Negotiation

Customized employment includes negotiating employment opportunities with employers through the identification of unmet business needs that may be fulfilled by the talents of a job seeker. Typically, this process does not begin with a response to an advertisement for employees but rather through meeting with employers and touring businesses to identify mutually beneficial matches. Customized job development strategies include (1) job carving, the process of breaking jobs down into their key components and reassigning those pieces in more efficient or understandable way; (2) job sharing where two or more people share a position based on the strengths of each; and/or (3) job creation where a new job description is developed based on unmet needs of the employer (ODEP, 2018).

Accommodation and Post-Employment Support

Post-employment supports have been proven to be beneficial for people with disabilities who may encounter issues that they are not prepared to handle without assistance (Targett, Wehman, McKinley, & Young, 2004). Prior to vocational rehabilitation case closure, assistance should be provided in the development of natural supports and resources for targeting solutions to challenges prior to the loss of employment. In addition, employees and employers should be aware of the services available through the Job Accommodation Network (askjan.org) to aid in the identification and implementation of accommodations as required by the Americans with Disabilities Act.

An Example of Customized Employment

Individual	Allen has autism with limited speech. Through the discovery process, Allen is identified as having an interest in video games and a talent for organization and data entry
Setting	A local video store that sells new and used games has multiple employees who, when interviewed, state that they all prefer answering questions and selling games to stocking and organizing. While they are helping customers, games that have been ordered or bought for resale are typically set aside until there is time to enter the inventory into the computer and put it on the shelves. The sales floor quickly becomes disorganized due to movement of product by browsers. When a customer requests a particular game, the system does not show that it is in stock because it has not yet been entered into the computer, or the system does show it is in stock but the game cannot be located on the shelf because it is out of place. The employer indicates that, typically, employees are hired to perform all aspects of the job (selling, stocking, etc.)
Result	A customized approach allows the individual with autism to be hired to enter games into the computer, stock, and organize product. This leaves more time for other employees to sell and makes it much easier to access games that are in stock. In addition to an increase in sales, morale is increased because employees spend more time doing work that they enjoy. A win-win!

With the possibility of finding employment tailored to an individual's ability, persons with IDD become more independent and take on more responsibility for their lives, such as making decisions regarding work, housing, transportation, and health. Becoming more independent means they must learn to advocate for themselves.

The Self-Advocacy Movement for Individuals with IDD

The self-advocacy movement for individuals with intellectual and developmental disabilities is, in itself, a civil rights movement. The movement has its own unique values and beliefs that constitute self-advocacy. The related disability rights movement, also known as self-determination, places a strong emphasis on psychological independence and control over one's life (Conyers, 2003). The efforts to establish disability rights also may be seen as a political movement with a unique set of values, which include self-warmth and involvement in the political process (Putnam, 2005).

In the United States, the self-advocacy movement has a very vibrant history that dates back to the 1980s (Traustadóttir, 2006). Self-advocacy organizations were formed to help individuals with disabilities take control over their lives and to help individuals with disabilities have the right to leave institutions to live in the community and live in their communities (Traustadóttir, 2006).

Definition of Self-Advocacy

Self-Advocates Becoming Empowered (SABE), a national self-advocacy organization, defines self-advocacy as follows:

> Self-advocacy is about independent groups of people with disabilities working together for justice by helping each other take charge of our lives and fight discrimination. It teaches us how to make decisions and choices that affect our lives so we can be more independent. It also teaches us about our rights, but along with learning about our rights we learn responsibilities. The way we learn about advocating for ourselves is by supporting each other and helping each other gain confidence in ourselves so we can speak out for what we believe.(Hayden & Nelis, 2002, as cited in Caldwell, Aaron, & Rizzolo, 2011, p. 1)

Other alliances, such as the Florida Self-Advocacy Alliance (FSAA), have developed similar lists of values. The FSAA focuses on seven values: (1) moving forward, (2) expressing choices, (3) being independent, (4) knowing when to ask for help, (5) not being afraid to ask for help, (6) believing in oneself, and (7) letting go (Chapman & Jenkins, 2011).

The self-advocacy movement was based on the foundation of two models defining disabilities: (1) the medical and (2) the social models (Pledger, 2003). The medical model, also known as the biomedical model of disability, sees individuals with disabilities as having limitations that affect their ability to function and that need to be "fixed." Since the medical model views individuals with disabilities as having medical problems, the medical professional is the expert who can "fix" their problems. The social model of disability views disability as a culture that is affected by social oppression (Magasi, 2008) and has been used successfully for political activism. The "social model" does not view disability as a limitation that needs to be treated by a medical professional but rather promotes the concept of disability pride (Magasi, 2008).

Disability pride is seen as a rejection of the medical model of disability and recognizes disability as a vibrant culture (Magasi, 2008) and part of a unique cultural identity. Over 155 people participated in a study of a group of disability rights activists from the Americans Disabled for Assistance Programs Today (ADAPT) movement. Participants reported having a great sense of pride about being an individual with a disability, and they indicated that they would not want to be "cured" of their disability (Hahn & Beaulaurier, 2001).

Self-Advocacy as a Federal Priority

Self-advocacy is a major priority for the Federal government. Guidelines for federally funded State Councils on Developmental Disabilities are written into 42 US Code §15,025, and these Councils have a primary responsibility of supporting self-advocacy for individuals with DD (Caldwell et al., 2011). The Administration on Intellectual and Developmental Disabilities (AIDD), an agency within the Federal government, has taken a new interest in supporting self-advocates who have IDD. The AIDD sponsored two self-advocacy summits to (1) examine how the Federal government can support self-advocates throughout the country and (2) to note the issues and challenges that self-advocates face (Caldwell et al., 2011). The report features four areas challenging self-advocates around the country. These four areas are (1) barriers to self-advocacy, such as transportation; (2) public perception of individuals with developmental disabilities, mainly the continued use of such outdated language as mentally retarded; (3) support of self-advocates; and (4) the establishment of a technical assistance center to support the self-advocacy movement (Caldwell et al., 2011).

There are a number of national organizations involved in the self-advocacy movement; however, three are of particular note: (1) Self-Advocates Becoming Empowered (SABE), (2) ADAPT, and (3) Autistic Self-Advocacy Network (ASAN).

Self-Advocates Becoming Empowered (SABE) is a self-advocacy organization comprised of individuals with developmental disabilities. Founded in 1993, SABE was the initial self-advocacy organization for individuals with developmental disabilities (Ward & Meyer, 1999). The mission of the organization is to "ensure that people with disabilities are treated as equals and that they are given the same decisions, choices, rights, responsibilities, and chances to speak up to empower themselves; opportunities to make new friends; and to learn from their mistakes" (SABE, 2011). A major focus of the organization is advocating for the deinstitutionalization of individuals with developmental disabilities.

ADAPT, considered the radical component of the self-advocacy movement, seeks to promote change on behalf of individuals with disabilities by utilizing civil disobedience. One of the oldest self-advocacy organizations, ADAPT (then American Disabled for Accessible Public Transit) began its national campaign for lifts on buses and access to public transit for people with disabilities in 1983. It played a major role in gaining passage of the Americans with Disabilities Act (ADA), focusing on requirements relating to accessible transit, and the perception of the ADA as civil rights law. Describing itself as "a national grass-roots community that organizes disability rights activists to engage in nonviolent direct action, including civil disobedience, to assure the civil and human rights of people with disabilities to live in freedom" (ADAPT, 2018), APAPT advocated for the Disability Integration Act (2017). The Act would require changes to policies of public entities and long-term service and supports insurance providers to increase resources and supports for persons with disabilities to live independently within their communities.

The Autistic Self-Advocacy Network (ASAN), a national self-advocacy organization for individuals with ASD, advances the principles of the disability rights movement with regard to ASD. ASAN believes that the goal of autism advocacy should be to facilitate a world in which people with ASD enjoy the same access, rights, and opportunities as all other citizens. ASAN works to empower people with ASD across the globe to take control of their lives and the future of their common communities. The Network seeks to organize the community of persons with ASD to ensure their voices are heard in national conversations. Their slogan is "Nothing About Us, Without Us!" (ASAN: Autistic Self-Advocate Network, 2018).

With the increased emphases on self-advocacy and longer life-spans for persons with IDD, there is growing concern, from social and public policy perspectives, on how persons with IDD can age successfully with appropriate community and residential supports.

Aging with an Intellectual and Developmental Disability

The need to research the diverse processes of aging, whether social, physical, psychological, or biological, led to the discipline of gerontology (i.e., the study of aging) and geriatrics (i.e., medical care of older adults). In general terms, gerontology generally refers to those who are 65+ years of age. As the population aged 65+ rapidly increases, so will the demand rise for practitioners who serve the aging population. In the United States, we are in the midst of the aging of the baby boomer generation (i.e., people born during 1946–1964). Every day over 10,000 Baby Boomers reach age 65, increasing the current percentage of the US population of older adults from 13% to 18% by 2030 (Cohn & Taylor, 2010). This demographic change is well known to those in the fields of geropsychology and geropsychiatry who specialize in the study, prevention, and treatment of mental disorders in old age (see Chapter "Older Adults" in this volume for additional information on older adults and behavioral health).

The majority of individuals with IDD now have a similar life expectancy (LE) to that of the general population. Historically, the gap had been far greater, but in recent decades, the gap has closed quite dramatically. For example, between 1983 and 1997, LE rose an astonishing 24 years for people with Down syndrome, eight times the rate of increase for the general population in that same period (Yang, Rasmussen, & Friedman, 2002). Comparatively speaking, people with IDD are a relatively small segment of the aging population, with 641,860 people aged 60 years in 2000, a figure that is expected to double to 1.2 million by 2030 (Heller, Stafford, Davis, Sedlezky, & Gaylord, 2010).

Nevertheless, there is a significant proportion of aging individuals with IDD who need lifelong supports or will be accessing support services when their family caregivers can no longer provide such care. Unfortunately few professionals are ready to meet the challenges that arise in providing appropriate supports for aging people with IDD, even though their numbers are rapidly rising (Perkins & Moran,

2010). According to the National Association for the Dually Diagnosed (NADD, 2016), 30–35% of people with IDD have behavioral health problems. Therefore, 1/3 of aging people with IDD are likely to have lifelong behavioral health issues (e.g. depression, anxiety) or develop new ones. The remainder of this section will draw attention to three topics that are often overlooked areas of practice that behavioral health practitioners can provide invaluable supports to people aging people with IDD: Alzheimer's disease; coping with loss, grief, and death; and preparation for end-of-life.

Alzheimer's Disease and IDD

Justifiably, Alzheimer's disease is a major public health and behavioral health concern, prompting the passage of the National Alzheimer's Project Act in 2011 (Pub. L. 111-375). This legislation provides for a coordinated national strategy and essential framework to combat what the Alzheimer's Association describes as "one of America's most feared and costly diseases" (Alzheimer's Association, 2016). Currently 5.4 million Americans have Alzheimer's disease, which is projected to almost triple to 13.8 million persons by 2050, if efforts to prevent or cure the disease are not successful (Alzheimer's Association, 2016).

The National Task Group on Intellectual Disabilities and Dementia Practices (NTG) was formed to examine and report on the needs of adults with ID and dementia. After the National Alzheimer's Project Act was passed, the NTG advocated for and tracked progress on the implementation of the national plan with specific emphasis on inclusion of people with intellectual disabilities (Bishop et al., 2015). The NTG, a nationwide collaboration of researchers, clinicians, and long-term care providers, has produced a range of practice guidelines, screening tools, education and training curricula (see www.AADMD.org/NTG for further information).

People with Down syndrome are at an increased risk of developing Alzheimer's disease. Onset occurs at a much earlier age, between 40 and 49 years, compared with 72 years in the general population. Duration is 5–8 years compared with 7–20 years in the general population (Head, Powell, Gold, & Schmitt, 2012; Head, Silverman, Patterson, & Lott, 2012). Though not all conditions associated with IDD present with any greater risk of developing Alzheimer's disease than the general population, one unfortunate ramification of increased longevity of all people with IDD is there are many more individuals reaching ages when the prevalence of developing Alzheimer's disease increases. Also, a number of potential risk factors differentially impact people with IDD, including more limited cognitive reserve, greater propensity for significant head injuries, obesity, and poor cardiovascular health (NTG, 2012).

Though Alzheimer's disease has no known cure, pharmacological and environmental treatments can slow the disease's progression and improve quality of life. An early diagnosis is crucial to maximize treatment effects. Unfortunately, this can be very difficult because the onset of the disease can be harder to detect in those with pre-existing intellectual disability. Furthermore, commonly used screening instruments are not normed or appropriate for people with intellectual disability. As such, the NTG-Early Detection Screen for Dementia is highly recommended, as it can help identify people with dementia-like symptoms whose behaviors are from other causes (e.g., medication interactions, depression, thyroid disorders), and the screen can be easily incorporated into an annual wellness check (NTG, 2016). It is crucial to establish a baseline of functioning to discern what may be a new potentially dementia-related symptom or behavior and what is the established idiosyncratic behavior for a particular individual. Compiling a detailed history can be more problematic in people with IDD, especially those who live in residential group homes, due to gaps in caregivers' knowledge.

Diagnostic overshadowing (Reiss & Szyszko, 1983) is a particular challenge, whereby behavioral health professionals attribute signs and symptoms to the intellectual disability and not to the manifestation of a behavioral health condition. Indeed, for some individuals who are non-verbal, new or novel behaviors may be their attempt to communicate the changes and confusion that they are experiencing with their cognitive functioning. Conversely, some can do so very eloquently. "My Thinker's Not Working," an aptly named title of a report from NTG (2012), is actually a quote from an individual with IDD who was describing the effects of Alzheimer's disease.

Careful probing and observation by professionals and caregivers may assist the communication of symptoms of forgetfulness and the differential impact on spatial, short, and long-term memory. All general protocols for Alzheimer's disease management, psychosocial, behavioral, environmental, and pharmaceutical are equally applicable to people with IDD, but for more specific guidance refer to Moran, Rafii, Keller, Singh, and Janicki (2013).

Coping with Loss, Grief, and Death

An inevitable part of life is experiencing loss, and with increasing age, one is more likely to do so. It is a part of the human experience, and as such, people with IDD should be fully supported to express their feelings when losses occur. Aside from all the usual situations that can result in a sense of loss (e.g., changes of job, moving home, death of a loved one, the ending of significant intimate relationships and friendships, development of chronic health issues, etc.), it is important to consider other events and changes that may trigger a sense of loss with people with IDD.

The vast majority of people with IDD will live with their parents and other family caregivers for their entire life. Gains in longevity have resulted in many people with IDD now outliving their parents and potentially siblings, too. The death of family caregivers may also coincide with a move out of the family home into a completely new environment (e.g., to a group home). Such changes can be extremely abrupt and very traumatic.

Another scenario that arises for those who live in group homes and other residential settings is the loss/retirement of a formal support worker with whom the individual with IDD was particularly close and does not understand why someone who was a daily presence in their lives is now only seen occasionally, if at all. Similarly, a noted issue is the high turnover of direct support professionals, leading to instability and constant change in the staff that people with IDD may form close attachments. Professionals should be alert to the variety of potential and perhaps innocuous causes of loss that may trigger a grief reaction and be sensitive to the relative impact it may have upon the individual.

When people with IDD experience grief, they will have the same range of physical, emotional, and behavioral reactions. However, the degree to which the person understands the traumatic loss and the reasons behind the loss, coupled with their ability to express and/or communicate their feelings, can all impact how a loss is processed and grieved. Furthermore, a person may experience a death of a loved one but has never really conceptualized or had the opportunity to learn about the finality of death. Interestingly, Lipe-Goodson and Goebel's work (1983) suggested that the understanding of death is not as dependent on intellectual disability and more so on chronological age, emphasizing the importance of experiential learning. Thus, any type of loss experienced across the lifespan is an opportunity to increase understanding about loss. Such understanding can be further cemented by having discussions of former friends/relatives who have died, or favorite pets. Inclusion of people with IDD at funeral/memorial services is also very important, in saying goodbye and collectively grieving with others.

People with IDD may manifest their grief in different ways, including having an unwarranted sense of guilt or displacement of their sense of anger on others, especially in those with limited understanding to why an event has occurred (Doka, 2010). Another issue is *disenfranchised grief*, when an individual experiences a loss but that loss is not mourned, socially supported, or worse still even acknowledged (Doka, 2002). Unfortunately, people with IDD often experience disenfranchised grief from inappropriate and inadequate response from family or professional caregivers who have had little training or guidance on how to support people with IDD in their grief (Lavin, 2002).

Another issue is that professionals, friends, or family may feel that people with IDD need to be protected and may shield them from open discussion regarding death, disclosure of a particular event, and attendance at funerals (Lavin, 2002). Such overprotectiveness actually denies the right of the individual to learn how to cope with the loss and can lead to an increased sense of isolation, confusion, and anxiety. Generally, it should be remembered that constant reassurance and extra time may be needed to establish a therapeutic relationship when a person with IDD receives grief counseling. When a death is imminent, or occurs, the individual with IDD should have the same opportunities to be physically present and involved with the dying/dead person as any other would (Doka, 2010). Unfortunately, though many people with IDD may need additional support to cope with the death/significant loss, few may actually receive it, as professionals are generally unaware and uneducated about their unique issues. Fortunately, there is a growing interest to address this shortcoming. The Hospice Foundation of America's (2013) self-study course, "Supporting Individuals with IDD through Serious Illness, Grief, and Loss," is one such example.

Preparation for the End-of-Life

Thinking about our own mortality and preparing for our death and beyond is something we universally acknowledge as something we should do, but increasing age does increase the probability that we would formalize such plans. Even so, according to a survey conducted by the AARP Research Group (2000), in those aged 50+, 60% have a will, 23% have a living trust, and 45% have a durable power of attorney, but only 17% have all three! Another study found that in those 18 years and older, 60% want their end-of-life wishes to be respected, yet only a third of them had completed advance directives (Pollack, Morhaim, & Williams, 2010). Against the apparent reluctance for end-of-life planning for people with no intellectual/cognitive difficulties, one can imagine the task can seem even more onerous for people with IDD, their family caregivers, and professionals who support them. However, Kingsbury (2010) advocates that advanced care planning for health/ end-of-life wishes can and should be incorporated into regular person-centered-planning practices.

One of the major tenets of person-centered planning is to empower individuals to have control over their own lives and make choices that reflect their own needs. Person-centered planning gives the advantage of having a structured process to identify cultural, spiritual, and family rituals that may not be known and can be updated and modified as circumstances may dictate or with changes in someone's expressed wishes (Kingsbury, 2010). Also it is recommended to start these conversations sooner rather than later, although approaching general decision-making issues first, before the more poignant end-of-life planning is advisable (Kingsbury, 2010). For example, begin with general topics such as potential organ donation, versus personal wishes for interment. For further guidance, resources, such as *People Planning Ahead: Communicating Healthcare and End-of-Life Wishes* (Kingsbury, 2009), provide an invaluable framework for professionals engaged in this area.

Traditionally, many people with IDD have had all major decisions in their life made by legal guardians, but there is a growing movement that advocates for "Supported Decision-Making," whereby people use trusted family/friends and professionals, so they can make decisions without the need for "overly broad and restrictive guardianships" (Blanck & Martinis, 2015). The right to make one's own decisions on critical aspects of one's health, choices for treatment, and ultimately death are some of the most fundamental decisions we make. Friedman and Helm (2010) rightly describe end-of-life choices as being one of the most compelling issues that require clarification and insight. Such importance is not diminished in any way whatsoever by having an intellectual disability; quite the reverse, it is even more critical that such decisions, and wishes, are correctly identified, respected, and implemented.

Implications for Behavioral Health

Working with persons with IDD can be challenging, due to the burden of disease attributed to co-occurring intellectual/developmental disabilities and mental illnesses (Einfeld, Ellis, & Emerson, 2011). However, in the United States, approximately one-third (32.9%) of the total number of individuals with IDD served by state developmental disability agencies have mental illnesses (MI), one-third (32.9%) have some combination of IDD and MI, and 22.7% needed support to manage self-injurious behavior, 38.8% for disruptive behavior, and 25.1% for destructive behavior (Human Services Research Institute & National Association of State Directors of Developmental Disabilities Services, 2013). Clearly, individuals with IDD and co-occurring MI require a flexible array of services to help them effectively reside in their communities. Services and funding models need to be designed to promote the necessary flexibility and services infrastructure persons with IDD and MI need based on the individual.

Behavioral health professionals must be prepared to competently provide treatment to individuals with disabilities. According to the self-advocacy movement, the medical model is not an acceptable treatment framework for individuals with disabilities. Many of those who are involved in the self-advocacy movement believe that having a disability is an extraordinary gift. Behavioral health professionals must be able to recognize this and to help individuals with disabilities become empowered.

Behavioral health professionals also need to recognize individuals with disabilities as a unique culture rather than a population that should be pathologized and treated with special care. It is important for professionals to embrace this vibrant culture and become aware of the disability rights movement and how it affects the counseling relationship. Empowerment is a critical responsibility of behavioral health professionals. Behavioral healthcare professionals need to work with individuals with disabilities and be willing to get involved in the self-advocacy movement.

As we close this chapter, we would like to reiterate the importance of being able to "age in place," in local communities, with person-centered services, developing workforce competencies, receiving integrated and effective services provision, and helping to develop and implement proven models of care and treatment for people with IDD and behavioral health disorders.

References

AARP Research Group. (2000). *Where there is a will... Legal documents among the 50+ population: Findings from an AARP survey*. Washington, DC: AARP. http://assets.aarp.org/rgcenter/econ/will.pdf

ADAPT. (2018). *Welcome to ADAPT* [Web page]. Philadelphia PA: National ADAPT. https://adapt.org/

Alzheimer's Association. (2016). *2016 Alzheimer's disease facts and figures*. Chicago, IL: Author. https://www.alz.org/documents_custom/2016-facts-and-figures.pdf

American Psychiatric Association. (2000). *Diagnostic and statistical manual of mental disorders: DSM-IV-TR*. Washington, DC: American Psychiatric Association.

American Psychiatric Association. (2013). *Diagnostic and statistical manual of mental disorders: DSM-5*. Arlington, VA: Author.

ASAN: Autistic Self-Advocate Network. (2018). *About* [Web page]. Washington, DC: ASAN. http://autisticadvocacy.org/about-asan/

Autism and Developmental Disabilities Monitoring Network Surveillance Year 2010 Principal Investigators. (2012). Prevalence of autism spectrum disorders – Autism and Developmental Disabilities Monitoring Network, 14 sites, United States, 2008. *MMWR: Surveillance Summaries, 61*(3), 1–19.

Autism and Developmental Disabilities Monitoring Network Surveillance Year 2010 Principal Investigators. (2014). Prevalence of autism spectrum disorder among children aged 8 years – autism and developmental disabilities monitoring network, 11 sites, United States, 2010. *MMWR: Surveillance Summaries, 63*(2), 1–21.

Bishop, K. M., Hogan, M., Janicki, M. P., Keller, S. M., Lucchino, R., Mughal, D. T., … Wolfson, S. (2015). Guidelines for dementia-related health advocacy for adults with intellectual disability and dementia: National Task Group on Intellectual Disabilities and Dementia Practices. *Intellectual and Developmental Disabilities, 53*(1), 2–29. https://doi.org/10.1352/1934-9556-53.1.2

Blanck, P., & Martinis, J. G. (2015). "The right to make choices": The national resource center for supported decision-making. *Inclusion, 3*(1), 24–33. https://doi.org/10.1352/2326-6988-3.1.24

Boyle, C. A., Boulet, S., Schieve, L. A., Cohen, R. A., Blumberg, S. J., Yeargin-Allsopp, M., … Kogan, M. D. (2011). Trends in the prevalence of developmental disabilities in US children, 1997-2008. *Pediatrics, 127*(6), 1034–1042. https://doi.org/10.1542/peds.2010-2989

Bruininks, R., Hill, B. K., & Morreau, L. E. (1988). Prevalence and implications of maladaptive behaviors and dual diagnosis in residential and other service programs. In J. A. Stark, F. J. Menolascino, M. H. Albarelli, V. C. Gray, & National Strategies Conference on Mental Illness in the Mentally Retarded (Eds.), *Mental retardation and mental health: Classification, diagnosis, treatment, services* (pp. 1–29). New York, NY: Springer.

Caldwell, J., Aaron, K. K., & Rizzolo, M. K. (2011, September). *Envisioning the future: Allies in self advocacy: Final report*. Washington, DC: The University of Illinois at Chicago, Institute on Disability and Human Development. https://nccdd.org/images/Public_Policy/Public_Policy_Topics/Full_Self-Advocacy_Summit_Report.pdf

Callahan, M., & Condon, E. (2007). Discovery: The foundation of job development. In C. Griffin, D. Hammis, & T. Geary (Eds.), *The job developer's handbook: Practical tactics for customized employment* (pp. 23–35). Baltimore, MD: Paul H. Brookes Publishing.

Callahan, M., Shumpert, N., & Condon, E. (2011). *Profiles: Capturing the information of discovery*. Gautier, MS: Marc Gold & Associates.

Carroll Chapman, S. L., & Wu, L. T. (2012). Substance abuse among individuals with intellectual disabilities. *Research in Developmental Disabilities, 33*(4), 1147–1156. https://doi.org/10.1016/j.ridd.2012.02.009

Chapman, R. A., & Jenkins, A. (2011). *The values of the self advocacy movement*. Tampa, FL: The Florida Self Advocacy Alliance.

Christensen, D. L., Baio, J., Van Naarden Braun, K., Bilder, D., Charles, J., Constantino, J. N., … Yeargin-Allsopp, M. (2016). Prevalence and characteristics of autism spectrum disorder among children aged 8 years–autism and developmental disabilities monitoring network, 11 sites, United States, 2012. *MMWR: Surveillance Summaries, 65*(3), 1–23. https://doi.org/10.15585/mmwr.ss6503a1

Cohn, D. V., & Taylor, P. (2010, December 20). *Baby boomers approach 65 – glumly*. Washington, DC: Pew Research Center Social & Demographic Trends. http://www.pewsocialtrends.org/2010/12/20/baby-boomers-approach-65-glumly/

Condon, E., & Callahan, M. (2008). Individualized career planning for students with significant support needs utilizing the discovery and vocational profile process, cross-agency collaborative funding and social security work incentives. *Journal of Vocational Rehabilitation, 28*(2), 85–96.

Conyers, L. M. (2003). Disability culture: A cultural model of disability. *Rehabilitation Education, 17*(3), 139–154.

Croen, L. A., Najjar, D. V., Ray, G. T., Lotspeich, L., & Bernal, P. (2006). A comparison of health care utilization and costs of children with and without autism spectrum disorders in a large group-model health plan. *Pediatrics, 118*(4), e1203–e1211. https://doi.org/10.1542/peds.2006-0127

Developmental Disabilities Assistance and Bill of Rights Act, Pub. L. No. 106–402. (2000). https://www.gpo.gov/fdsys/pkg/PLAW-106publ402/html/PLAW-106publ402.htm

Disability Integration Act, S.910, 115th Congress. (2017). https://www.congress.gov/bill/115th-congress/senate-bill/910

Doka, K. J. (2002). *Disenfranchised grief: New directions, challenges, and strategies for practice.* Champaign, IL: Research Press.

Doka, K. J. (2010). In S. L. Friedman & D. T. Helm (Eds.), *End-of-life care for children and adults with intellectual and developmental disabilities* (pp. 261–271). Washington, DC: American Association on Intellectual and Developmental Disabilities.

Einfeld, S. L., Ellis, L. A., & Emerson, E. (2011). Comorbidity of intellectual disability and mental disorder in children and adolescents: A systematic review. *Journal of Intellectual and Developmental Disability, 36*(2), 137–143. https://doi.org/10.1080/13668250.2011.572548

Fletcher, R. J., Barnhill, J., & Cooper, S.-A. (2016). *DM-ID-2: Diagnostic manual, intellectual disability: A textbook of diagnosis of mental disorders in persons with intellectual disability.* Kingston, NY: NADD Press: National Association for the Dually Diagnosed.

Fletcher, R. J., Loschen, E., Stavrakaki, C., & First, M. (2007). *Diagnostic manual-intellectual disability: A textbook of diagnosis of mental disorders in persons with intellectual disability.* Kingston, NY: NADD Press.

Friedman, S. L., & Helm, D. T. (2010). *End-of-life care for children and adults with intellectual and developmental disabilities.* Washington, DC: American Association on Intellectual and Developmental Disabilities.

Frielink, N., Schuengel, C., Kroon, A., & Embregts, P. J. C. M. (2015). Pretreatment for substance-abusing people with intellectual disabilities: Intervening on autonomous motivation for treatment entry. *Journal of Intellectual Disability Research, 59*(12), 1168–1182. https://doi.org/10.1111/jir.12221

Ganz, M. L. (2007). The lifetime distribution of the incremental societal costs of autism. *Archives of Pediatrics and Adolescent Medicine, 161*(4), 343–349. https://doi.org/10.1001/archpedi.161.4.343

Hahn, H., & Beaulaurier, R. L. (2001). Attitudes toward disabilities: A research note on activists with disabilities. *Journal of Disability Policy Studies, 12*(1), 40–46. https://doi.org/10.1177/104420730101200105

Hayden, M., & Nelis, T. (2002). Self-advocacy. In P. C. Baker, M. D. Croser, & R. L. Schalock (Eds.), *Embarking on a new century: Mental retardation at the end of the 20th century* (pp. 221–233). Washington, DC: American Association on Mental Retardation (AAMR).

Head, E., Powell, D., Gold, B. T., & Schmitt, F. A. (2012). Alzheimer's disease in down syndrome. *European Journal of Neurodegenerative Disease, 1*(3), 353–364.

Head, E., Silverman, W., Patterson, D., & Lott, I. T. (2012). Aging and down syndrome. *Current Gerontology and Geriatrics Research, 2012*, 412536. https://doi.org/10.1155/2012/412536

Heller, T., Stafford, P., Davis, L. A., Sedlezky, L., & Gaylord, V. (2010). People with intellectual and developmental disabilities growing old: An overview. *Impact: Feature Issue on Aging and People with Intellectual and Developmental Disabilities, 23*(1), 2–3. https://ici.umn.edu/products/impact/231/231.pdf

Hospice Foundation of America. (2013). *Supporting individuals with IDD through serious illness, grief, and loss* [Web page]. Washington, DC: Author. https://register.hospicefoundation.org/products/supporting-individuals-with-idd-self-study-dvd

Human Services Research Institute, & National Association of State Directors of Developmental Disabilities Services. (2013). *National Core Indicators Adult Consumer Survey 2011–12 final report.* Cambridge, MA: Authors. http://www.nationalcoreindicators.org/upload/core-indicators/CS_2011-12_Final_Report.pdf

Kingsbury, L. A. C. (2009). *People planning ahead: A guide to communicating healthcare and end of life wishes.* Washington, DC: American Association on Intellectual and Developmental Disabilities.

Kingsbury, L. A. C. (2010). Use of person-centered planning for end-of-life decision making. In S. L. Friedman & D. T. Helm (Eds.), *End-of-life care for children and adults with intellectual and developmental disabilities* (pp. 275–289). Washington, DC: American Association on Intellectual and Developmental Disabilities.

Lakin, K. C., & Stancliffe, R. (2005). *Costs and outcomes of community services for people with intellectual disabilities*. Baltimore, MD: P.H. Brookes Pub. Co.

Larson, S. A., Lakin, K. C., Anderson, L., Kwak, N., Lee, J. H., & Anderson, D. (2001). Prevalence of mental retardation and developmental disabilities: Estimates from the 1994/1995 National Health Interview Survey Disability Supplements. *American Journal of Mental Retardation, 106*(3), 231–252.

Lavin, C. (2002). Disenfranchised grief and individuals with developmental disabilities. In K. J. Doka (Ed.), *Disenfranchised grief: New directions, challenges, and strategies for practice* (pp. 307–322). Champaign, IL: Research Press.

Lipe-Goodson, P. S., & Goebel, B. L. (1983). Perception of age and death in mentally retarded adults. *Mental Retardation, 21*(2), 68–75.

Magasi, S. (2008). Infusing disability studies into the rehabilitation sciences. *Topics in Stroke Rehabilitation, 15*(3), 283–287. https://doi.org/10.1310/tsr1503-283

Moran, J. A., Rafii, M. S., Keller, S. M., Singh, B. K., & Janicki, M. P. (2013). The National Task Group on Intellectual Disabilities and Dementia Practices consensus recommendations for the evaluation and management of dementia in adults with intellectual disabilities. *Mayo Clinic Proceedings, 88*(8), 831–840. https://doi.org/10.1016/j.mayocp.2013.04.024

National Association for the Dually Diagnosed. (2016). *Information on dual diagnosis* [Web page]. Kingston, NY: Author. http://thenadd.org/resources/information-on-dual-diagnosis-2/

National Task Group on Intellectual Disabilities and Dementia Practices. (2012). *My thinker's not working: A national strategy for enabling adults with intellectual disabilities affected by dementia to remain in their community and receive quality supports*. Chicago, IL: University of Illinois at Chicago, Department of Disability and Human Development, Rehabilitation Research and Training Center on Aging with Developmental Disabilities-Lifespan Health and Function. http://aadmd.org/sites/default/files/NTG_Thinker_Report.pdf

National Task Group on Intellectual Disabilities and Dementia Practices. (2016). *NTG-EDSD screening instrument* [Web page]. Hamden, CT: Author. http://aadmd.org/ntg/screening

Office of Disability Employment Policy. (2018). *What is customized employment?* [Web page]. Washington, DC: U.S. Department of Labor. https://www.dol.gov/odep/categories/workforce/CustomizedEmployment/what/index.htm

Perkins, E. A., & Moran, J. A. (2010). Aging adults with intellectual disabilities. *JAMA, 304*(1), 91–92. https://doi.org/10.1001/jama.2010.906

Pledger, C. (2003). Discourse on disability and rehabilitation issues. Opportunities for psychology. *American Psychologist, 58*(4), 279–284.

Pollack, K. M., Morhaim, D., & Williams, M. A. (2010). The public's perspectives on advance directives: Implications for state legislative and regulatory policy. *Health Policy, 96*(1), 57–63. https://doi.org/10.1016/j.healthpol.2010.01.004

Putnam, M. (2005). Conceptualizing disability: Developing a framework for political disability identity. *Journal of Disability Policy Studies, 16*(3), 188–198. https://doi.org/10.1177/104420 73050160030601

Reiss, S., & Szyszko, J. (1983). Diagnostic overshadowing and professional experience with mentally retarded persons. *American Journal of Mental Deficiency, 87*(4), 396–402. http://search.ebscohost.com/login.aspx?direct=true&db=psyh&AN=1983-10672-001&site=ehost-live

Schalock, R. L., Borthwick-Duffy, S. A., Bradley, V. J., Buntinx, W. H. E., Coulter, D. L., Craig, E. M., … Developmental, D. (2010). *Intellectual disability: Definition, classification, and systems of supports* (11th ed.). Washington, DC: American Association on Intellectual and Developmental Disabilities.

Self-Advocates Becoming Empowered. (2011). *Welcome to SABE!* [Web page]. Author [SABE]. http://www.sabeusa.org

Siegel, M., Milligan, B., Chemelski, B., Payne, D., Ellsworth, B., Harmon, J., … Smith, K. A. (2014). Specialized inpatient psychiatry for serious behavioral disturbance in autism and intellectual disability. *Journal of Autism and Developmental Disorders, 44*(12), 3026–3032. https://doi.org/10.1007/s10803-014-2157-z

Simonoff, E., Pickles, A., Charman, T., Chandler, S., Loucas, T., & Baird, G. (2008). Psychiatric disorders in children with autism spectrum disorders: Prevalence, comorbidity, and associated factors in a population-derived sample. *Journal of the American Academy of Child and Adolescent Psychiatry, 47*(8), 921–929. https://doi.org/10.1097/CHI.0b013e318179964f

Smith, T. J., Dillahunt-Aspillaga, C. J., & Kenney, R. M. (2017). Implementation of customized employment provisions of the workforce innovation and opportunity act within vocational rehabilitation systems. *Journal of Disability Policy Studies, 27*(4), 195–202. https://doi.org/10.1177/1044207316644412

Targett, P. S., Wehman, P. H., McKinley, W. O., & Young, C. L. (2004). Successful work supports for persons with SCI: Focus on job retention. *Journal of Vocational Rehabilitation, 21*(1), 19–26.

Tassé, M. J., & Grover, M. D. (2013). Normal curve. In F. R. Volkmar (Ed.), *Encyclopedia of autism spectrum disorders* (pp. 2059–2060). New York, NY: Springer.

Traustadóttir, R. (2006). Learning about self-advocacy from life history: A case study from the United States. *British Journal of Learning Disabilities, 34*(3), 175–180. https://doi.org/10.1111/j.1468-3156.2006.00414.x

Van Naarden Braun, K., Christensen, D., Doernberg, N., Schieve, L., Rice, C., Wiggins, L., … Yeargin-Allsopp, M. (2015). Trends in the prevalence of autism spectrum disorder, cerebral palsy, hearing loss, intellectual disability, and vision impairment, metropolitan atlanta, 1991-2010. *PLoS One, 10*(4), e0124120. https://doi.org/10.1371/journal.pone.0124120

Ward, M. J., & Meyer, R. N. (1999). Self-determination for people with developmental disabilities and autism: Two self-advocates' perspectives. *Focus on Autism and Other Developmental Disabilities, 14*(3), 133–139. https://doi.org/10.1177/108835769901400302

Yang, Q., Rasmussen, S. A., & Friedman, J. M. (2002). Mortality associated with Down's syndrome in the USA from 1983 to 1997: A population-based study. *Lancet, 359*(9311), 1019–1025.

Integration of Primary Care and Behavioral Health

Sara Haack, Jennifer M. Erickson, Matthew Iles-Shih, and Anna Ratzliff

General Overview and Rationale for Integrated Care

One of the great challenges facing health care over the last 50 years has been how to manage chronic medical problems. Medicine, as a system, has traditionally focused on swiftly addressing life-threatening illnesses, and, as a result, chronic, fluctuating, and slowly progressive disorders are often missed or inconsistently managed (Institute of Medicine, 2001). As medical technology has increased longevity, so too has it increased the number of people living with chronic medical conditions. This has led to a tipping point in the USA wherein many patients are receiving care for chronic medical conditions, but fewer than half of the patients seen for depression, hypertension, or diabetes are receiving appropriate treatment (Clark et al., 2000; Joint National Committee on Prevention, 1997; Young, Klap, Sherbourne, & Wells, 2001).

More concerning still is that this has now begun to negatively affect longevity, resulting, in the USA, in decreased life expectancy for the next generation (Olshansky et al., 2005). Specific to mental health, large population studies have found that major depressive disorder alone can decrease life expectancy by more than 10 years (Chang et al., 2011).

Since the 1980s, researchers have studied the impact of depression in primary care settings, with discouraging findings. It has been found that 5–12% of primary

S. Haack
University of Hawai'i John A. Burns School of Medicine, Department of Psychiatry, Honolulu, HI, USA
e-mail: SHaack@dop.hawaii.edu

J. M. Erickson (✉) · M. Iles-Shih · A. Ratzliff
University of Washington Medical Center, Department of Psychiatry and Behavioral Sciences, Seattle, WA, USA
e-mail: jericks@uw.edu

© Springer Nature Switzerland AG 2020
B. L. Levin, A. Hanson (eds.), *Foundations of Behavioral Health*,
https://doi.org/10.1007/978-3-030-18435-3_13

care patients at any point in time will meet criteria for major depressive disorder (Katon & Schulberg, 1992). Furthermore, early studies found depressed patients utilize health care twice as much as non-depressed patients, have greater functional impairment than that expected from their other medical conditions alone, and are more likely to have medically unexplained symptoms (Katon & Sullivan, 1990; Simon, Ormel, VonKorff, & Barlow, 1995; Simon & VonKorff, 1991; Wells et al., 1989). Since its initial investigation, depression remains the most common cause of disability worldwide and one of the most encountered diagnoses (Unützer & Park, 2012). Only half of patients with major depressive disorder are identified accurately in primary care, (Akincigil & Matthews, 2017; National Academies of Sciences, Engineering, & Medicine, 2015), and of those only half who are referred to specialty mental health care will make it to an appointment (Pace et al., 2018). In follow-up studies, this remains true and worsens in populations of ethnic minorities, older adults, medically complex patients, and men (Ettner et al., 2010; Gonzalez et al., 2010). When treated in primary care, patients may face client, provider, and health system barriers, including infrequent appointments, delays in medication adjustments, and discontinuation of antidepressants (Grembowski et al., 2002; Katon, Berg, Robins, & Risse, 1986; Ross et al., 2015; Simon, VonKorff, Wagner, & Barlow, 1993).

In addition to decreased life expectancy, mental disorders also lead to more frequent and severe chronic health conditions. Patients with psychiatric disorders have a threefold increase in the rate of diabetes, ten times the rate of heart disease, and 40 times the rate of cancer (Murray et al., 2012). The relationship between psychiatric and other medical conditions is likely complex. However, half of patients with a psychiatric concern struggle with adherence to medical recommendations (Murray et al., 2012).

Access to specialized mental health care is limited for primary care patients, and, inversely, access to primary care is limited for persons with severe mental illness. This can result in treatable medical problems affecting health, wellness, and life expectancy in mental health settings.

To improve outcomes in this population with frequent comorbid psychiatric and other medical needs, improvements are needed in care delivery methods. Systems pressures, including health care workforce shortages and the enactment of value-based care plans, greatly influence how any novel approach can function sustainably (Renders et al., 2001; Wagner et al., 2001). With a formidable workforce shortage in mental health care, 18% of US counties have an unmet need for non-prescribing mental health professionals (e.g., social workers, psychotherapists), while 96% of counties have a shortage of prescribers (e.g., psychiatrists, psychiatric nurse practitioners) (Thomas, Ellis, Konrad, Holzer, & Morrissey, 2009).

The concept of value-based care has developed to address the US high per capita health care costs that are coupled with lagging health metrics (Porter, 2009). Value-based care emphasizes the creation of tracking measurements to assess and improve outcomes in health care.

In response to these and other pressures, several models of integrated team-based care have developed, all of which aim to achieve improved clinical outcomes in a cost-effective manner. These models and common adaptations are discussed in the next section.

The Collaborative Care Model

Structure

The Collaborative Care Model (CoCM) is an evidence-based model of mental health service delivery in medical settings (Archer et al., 2012). The core CoCM team includes the patient, a primary care provider (PCP) or other treating medical providers, a behavioral health care manager (BHCM), and a psychiatric consultant. Depending on the resources of each clinic, teams may sometimes include other members, such as a psychologist or health navigator (see Fig. 1). Each team member has a clearly defined role (Centers for Medicare & Medicaid Services, 2018). The PCP is responsible for identifying patients in need of treatment, introducing the CoCM to the patient, and prescribing medications if needed. The BHCM provides care management by tracking behavioral health measures and response to treatment

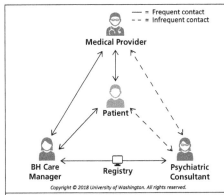

The solid arrows indicate regular direct communication between team members.

The dashed arrows indicate only as needed or indirect communication as part of care delivery.

Reprinted from "AIMS Center - Advancing Integrated Mental Health Solutions. *Collaborative Care - Team Structure* (2018). Available at: https://aims.uw.edu/collaborative-care/team-structure." Used with permission from the University of Washington AIMS Center.

Fig. 1 Typical team configuration of the CoCM team. The solid arrows indicate regular direct communication between team members. The dashed arrows indicate only as needed or indirect communication as part of care delivery. Collaborative Care Team Structure. Reprinted from "AIMS Center- Advancing Integrated Mental Health Solutions. (2018). Available at: https://aims.uw.edu/collaborative-care/team-structure." Used with permission from the University of Washington AIMS Center

in a registry and by delivering brief evidence-based behavioral interventions. The psychiatric consultant supports the other team members by providing expertise through weekly systematic case reviews with the BHCM to ensure appropriate diagnosis and development of care plans for common mental disorders.

A typical treatment course in the CoCM starts with identification of the patient needing treatment. This may be done through systematic screening, for example, for depression, or through the PCP's clinical assessment. Once the patient is identified, the BHCM is responsible for engaging the patient, completing an initial mental health assessment and adding the patient to a CoCM registry. The BHCM then meets with the patient at regular intervals, typically every 2 weeks in person or by phone to assess symptoms and provide evidence-based counseling/psychotherapy interventions like problem-solving therapy (PST), cognitive behavioral therapy (CBT), and behavioral activation (BA). The BHCM is also responsible for continuously engaging the patient in his care, repeating behavioral health assessment measures, such as the Patient Health Questionnaire-9 (PHQ-9), tracking response to treatment, and coordinating overall care for the patient.

The role of the BHCM is essential, with timely follow-up within the first 4 weeks strongly predicting clinically significant improvement in depression within 6 months and a shorter time to improvement (Bao, Druss, Jung, Chan, & Unützer, 2016). The psychiatric consultant may or may not be collocated with the primary care team and focuses the systematic weekly case review with the BHCM on intensifying the care plans for those patients who are not responding to initial treatment interventions.

Psychiatric case review in any given month is associated with twice the probability of receiving a new medication in the following month, indicating that systematic case review reduces clinical inertia in the treatment of depression (Sowa et al., 2018). A full-time BHCM within a typical CoCM team would have an active caseload of 50–80 patients and receive 1–2 h of support each week from the psychiatric consultant through case reviews of 5–8 patients.

Background and Evidence

There are over 80 randomized controlled trials demonstrating that the CoCM is more effective than care as usual for depression and anxiety disorders and a growing evidence base that CoCM is effective for other mental disorders, such as substance use disorders and bipolar disorder (Archer et al., 2012). The largest trial of CoCM, the IMPACT study, demonstrated that CoCM was twice as effective as usual care for treating depression in older adults in primary care settings (Unützer et al., 2002). Additional studies have demonstrated that CoCM can achieve the Quadruple Aim of health care system optimization: improved patient satisfaction, provider experience, patient outcomes, and cost-effectiveness of care (Archer et al., 2012).

The evidence base for CoCM continues to expand, and there is growing interest in understanding how the effectiveness of CoCM compares to that of other models of integration. For example, a recent small study demonstrated that more patients experienced a significant reduction in depression symptoms when treated in sites that used the CoCM compared with sites using the colocation model (Blackmore et al., 2018).

Target

CoCM has the strongest evidence base for its application in the treatment of depression and anxiety (Archer et al., 2012). However, a recent summary showed that other disorders can be effectively treated by CoCM including chronic pain, dementia, and depression with a variety of medical comorbidities including diabetes and cardiac risk factors (Huffman, Niazi, Rundell, Sharpe, & Katon, 2014).

More recently, studies have demonstrated that CoCM can effectively address substance use disorders in primary care settings (Watkins et al., 2017), ADHD in pediatric populations (Myers, Stoep, Thompson, Zhou, & Unützer, 2010), and adolescent depression (Richardson et al., 2014). CoCM has been shown to effectively treat mental health conditions in racially and ethnically diverse clinical populations (Angstman et al., 2015; Shao, Richie, & Bailey, 2016), including Blacks/African-Americans (Areán et al., 2005; Unützer et al., 2002), Hispanics/Latinos (Hay, Katon, Ell, Lee, & Guterman, 2012; Miranda et al., 2003; Unützer et al., 2002), and Asians/Asian-Americans (Ratzliff, Ni, Chan, Park, & Unützer, 2013).

Implementation and Resources Needed

The Collaborative Care Model is a complex intervention requiring significant resources for implementation. Successful collaborative care programs have all core team members in place and focus on five core principles: patient-centered team care, population-based care, measurement-based treatment to target, evidence-based treatment, and accountable care (AIMS Center, 2018b).

Patient-Centered Collaboration

Collaborative care starts with the patient, partnering with the PCP, BHCM, and psychiatric consultant to develop and follow a shared treatment plan. Clearly defined roles for each team member are essential to the provision of effective and efficient shared care.

Population-Based Care

The team must define the caseload of patients who are in active treatment for an identified mental health need. Using a registry to track this patient population allows the CoCM team to manage care proactively for these patients in a fundamental shift from treatment as usual, which often is provided reactively only to patients who consistently engage in treatment. A CoCM registry includes demographic information about the patient, behavioral health screening results (e.g., Patient Health Questionnaire (PHQ-9) for depression), and dates of clinical contacts.

Measurement-Based Treatment to Target

The CoCM team is structured to support the consistent use of measurement tools to guide active treatment until clinical target goals are achieved. The landmark STAR-D trial for depression showed that it can take up to four changes in treatment before 70% of the population will have a response to treatment (Rush, 2007). The routine implementation of measurement-based treatment to target, especially when measurements are appropriately timed to support clinical decision-making and prompt treatment changes, can improve clinical outcomes (Fortney et al., 2017).

Evidence-Based Care

Patients are offered evidence-based treatments in a biopsychosocial approach to mental health. The PCP initiates medication, the BHCM delivers behavioral or psychotherapeutic interventions, and the psychiatric consultant supports the PCP and BHCM to guide the evidence-based treatment most appropriate for the working diagnosis.

Accountable Care

CoCM is not only accountable to the individual patient but to the entire identified population. To achieve excellence in care, the whole team must commit to continuously improving the quality of care provided. This process starts with the team identifying goals and targets for collaborative care and then regularly reviewing program data to assess the effectiveness of treatments delivered. Quality measures might address processes (e.g., caseload size or number of actively engaged patients), outcomes (e.g., the percentage of patients achieving treatment response or remission of depression symptoms), and other important targets identified by the clinic (e.g., provider and patient satisfaction). The team monitors its progress and can use standard quality improvement strategies to address areas in need of improvement. High-quality CoCM delivery includes this continuous quality improvement process as standard practice.

There is now a growing literature on the factors that facilitate strong implementation of CoCM. One study examined the relationship between implementation factors, the likelihood that patients were engaged in CoCM care, and positive depression outcomes (Whitebird et al., 2014). It found that patient engagement was significantly correlated to the clinic having good leadership support, a strong PCP champion, a care manager whose role is both well-defined and implemented, and a care manager who is on-site and accessible. Depression remission was correlated with having an engaged psychiatrist, warm handoffs, and operating costs not being seen as a barrier.

Additionally, pay for performance metrics may improve outcomes in real-world implementation of CoCM (Unützer et al., 2012). In this analysis of safety-net clinics who implemented CoCM, it took 64 weeks to achieve clinically significant improvement in depression in 50% of patients. After the payer mandated that 25% of the payment to clinics for collaborative care be dependent on performance in five key quality metrics, time to depression improvement was reduced to 24 weeks. These types of strategies can help guide improvement efforts in clinical practices implementing the CoCM.

There are a number of national and federal resources that support implementation of CoCM. American Psychiatric Association (2018) offers resources on team training, implementation, and financing for CoCM. The UW AIMS Center (2018a) provides resources to support training and implementation. The American Medical Association provides a stepped approach to behavioral health integration (Drake & Valenstein, 2018) as do the Agency for Healthcare Research and Quality (Korsen et al., 2018) and the SAMHSA-HRSA Center for Integrated Health Solutions (2018). Interested readers should see additional books on CoCM team care delivery and its implementation (Raney, Bergman, Torous, & Hasselberg, 2017; Raney, Lasky, & Scott, 2017; Ratzliff, Unützer, Katon, & Stephens, 2016).

Challenges/Limitations

In addition to the steps required to successful implementation noted in the previous section, a common challenge for CoCM is obtaining adequate financial reimbursement of the costs of team-based approaches. Several of the team processes in CoCM, such as telephone outreach calls to patients, time spent on team communication, and the systematic case reviews, are not billable through traditional fee-for-service billing approaches. CoCM costs have been covered through a variety of strategies to date: grants, services delivered in fully capitated systems, partial capitated payment (i.e., the PCP continues fee-for-service billing, and the BHCM and psychiatric consultant are paid through adjusted case rate), bundled monthly payment rate, and billing fee-for-service for all billable services (Carlo, Unützer, Ratzliff, & Cerimele, 2018).

Encouragingly, a new payment opportunity was introduced in 2017 when CPT codes were introduced by Medicare to pay for the CoCM (Press et al., 2017). These codes are billed by and paid to the PCP for the work of the whole collaborative care team including the work of the BHCM and psychiatric consultant. The team must track minutes spent over the course of a calendar month and must deliver the core components of CoCM to be eligible to bill these codes (Centers for Medicare & Medicaid Services, 2018).

Real-World Program Example

The Depression Improvement Across Minnesota—Offering a New Direction (DIAMOND) is an example of a large real-world implementation of CoCM throughout Minnesota and western Wisconsin (Whitebird et al., 2014). The structure of the initiative was based largely on CoCM as it was tested in the IMPACT study. It focused on six components: (1) use of the PHQ-9 for assessment and ongoing monitoring; (2) use of a registry for systematic tracking of patients; (3) use of evidence-based guidelines to provide stepped care treatment modification/intensification; (4) relapse prevention education; (5) a care manager located in the clinic to provide education, care coordination, behavioral activation approaches, and support of medication management; and (6) a consulting psychiatrist to meet with the care manager for weekly case review and treatment change recommendations.

Training was provided by the Institute for Clinical Systems Improvement (ICSI), who systematically provided standardized training in implementing collaborative depression care and consultative support for primary care clinics over the course of 2 years. Payment for care delivery was provided through a partnership with nearly all commercial health plans in the state. Each clinic provided standardized monthly data reports through a common Internet portal about the number of patients seen by the care manager, the number enrolled in DIAMOND, and the PHQ-9 scores to monitor depression response and remission rates. On average, 23% of patients engaged in the program had remission from depression symptoms at 6 months.

Primary Care Behavioral Health Model

History/Background

The development of the Primary Care Behavioral Health (PCBH) model was a clinically based movement, with the goal of reducing the behavioral health services gap. Robinson and Strosahl (2009), two pioneers of the PCBH model, led integration efforts in the 1980s at Group Health Cooperative (GHC) of Puget Sound and then a consumer-owned and consumer-led Health Maintenance Organization (HMO) in Seattle, in response to an organizational leadership mandate to explore behavioral health integration.

This call for integration was itself a response to widespread GHC primary care provider dissatisfaction with the organization's existing mental health services. By shifting treatment away from diagnosis-based treatment toward a focus on the patient's functional outcomes and life satisfaction, creation of psychologist-led interventions for depression treatment that could be delivered in less than 3 h total, and the development of team-based behavioral health services in the primary care setting, the PCBH movement evolved.

Since its conception, the PCBH model of care has grown considerably over more than 30 years in a multitude of organizations. The US Air Force, US Navy, Kaiser Permanente, Veterans Health Administration, Cherokee Health System, and Southcentral Foundation are among the organizations that currently employ Behavioral Health Consultants (BHCs) in their primary care clinics. Perhaps largely due to the grassroots beginnings of the PCBH model, there are many variations in the models used in these and other facilities (Hunter et al., 2018).

As the model has grown, so have efforts to formally describe and measure the model. The first comprehensive text on the subject, *Behavioral Consultation and Primary Care*, written in 2007, is now in its second edition (Robinson & Reiter, 2016). Acknowledging the inconsistent use of terminology and varying model components, PCBH leaders have recently created a concise definition of the model, with the first part of this definition reproduced here (Reiter, Dobmeyer, & Hunter, 2018, p. 112):

> The PCBH model is a team-based primary care approach to managing behavioral health problems and biopsychosocially influenced health conditions. The model's main goal is to enhance the primary care team's ability to manage and treat such problems/conditions, with resulting improvements in primary care services for the entire clinic population. The model incorporates into the primary care team a behavioral health consultant (BHC), sometimes referred to as a behavioral health clinician, to extend and support the primary care provider (PCP) and team…

Evidence Base

Given the clinical grassroots inception of the PCBH model, its evidence base is still developing, but there is encouraging evidence of its impact on patient outcomes and implementation efficacy. Recently Hunter et al. (2018) summarized the available literature in a descriptive review of 20 articles that examined PCBH model outcomes, with most of the reviewed studies using a pre/post design.

The PCBH model has demonstrated improvements in clinical outcomes. Regarding specific disorders, PCBH patients have experienced improvements in depression, anxiety, and PTSD symptoms (Angantyr, Rimner, Norden, & Norlander, 2015; Cigrang et al., 2015; Hunter et al., 2018). There is also some initial evidence that the PCBH model addresses insomnia, tobacco use, and weight loss, with one study each indicating improvement in symptoms in small trials ($n = <30$) (Goodie, Isler, Hunter, & Peterson, 2009; Sadock, Auerbach, Rybarczyk, & Aggarwal, 2014).

However, within small samples, one of these same studies also failed to show improvement in sleep ($n= 4$) or pain ($n = 9$) (Sadock, et al., 2014). Suicidal ideation has also decreased in those receiving PCBH care (Bryan, Morrow, & Appolonio, 2009). These results demonstrate promising, albeit early, evidence of the PCBH model's efficacy.

Patients' overall functioning and care satisfaction has also improved with engagement in the PCBH model. One pediatric study indicated less global distress with PCBH care (Gomez et al., 2014). PCBH patients' satisfaction has been high in multiple studies, although one limitation of this conclusion is that most studies have used locally made self-questionnaires without psychometric data (Hunter et al., 2018).

Beyond patient-specific outcomes, the PCBH model also has been tested for its implementation properties. Fourteen studies have demonstrated a variety of implementation-related outcomes, including high provider satisfaction, positive shifts in PCP practice habits, and increased patient engagement in outside mental health referrals after involvement in the PCBH program (Hunter et al., 2018).

Lanoye et al. (2017) demonstrated decreases in preventable inpatient hospitalizations among those receiving PCBH care, which could be taken as encouraging evidence of cost-saving ability within the model. Gouge, Polaha, Rogers, and Harden (2016) also found the model demonstrated improved financial viability: a pediatrics practice was able to earn $1142 more on days with an on-site BHC, thought to be due to providers' increased efficiency in seeing more patients when BHCs were present and acting as "physician extenders."

Structure and Targets

Robinson and Reiter (2016) elucidate the PCBH components in the GATHER acronym (Table 1). BHCs aim to impact the health of a clinic's population through a *generalist* approach: they will effectively assist all patients with all problems, with a focus on concerns that are behaviorally or biopsychosocially influenced. Intervention examples include sleep hygiene habits for insomnia, behavioral

Table 1 GATHER acronym describing PCBH characteristics

Concept	Definition
Generalist	Assists all patients and health conditions
Accessible	Timely, ideally same-day, delivery of care to patient
Team-based	Shared clinic space, resources, and collaboration with team
High volume	Contributes to care for a large percentage of the clinic population
Educator	Improves the care team's biopsychosocial assessment and intervention skills and processes
Routine	Routine part of biopsychosocial care

Created by authors. Source: Robinson and Reiter (2016)

activation techniques for depression, mindfulness activities for anxiety disorders, and working on drinking diaries or action plans for alcohol misuse. Skills are delivered with a "here and now" approach, as the PCBH model prioritizes BHC *accessibility* to ensure the patient can have assistance in addressing his problem in real time, ideally the same day that he is referred.

Team-based refers to the integrated nature of the care delivery. While the BHC has a lead role in doing the behavioral intervention, they are still part of a care team that may include the primary care provider, nurse, and others. The team prioritizes regular communication about patients' care needs, has a consistent, integrated care plan for shared patients, and uses workflows that facilitate consistent and effective transitions between team members. With an integrated team approach and a population focus, *high volume* of care can be achieved. BHCs may see patients one or two times only for 15–30 min per interaction, averaging 10–14 patients per day with one visit being the modal number per patient served by a BHC (Reiter et al., 2018). In part due to this population-based approach, BHCs aim to provide active interventions and skills in each visit, including the first visit. Delivering effective interventions in only one visit enables the BHC to serve the entire clinical population more efficiently.

With the other GATHER pieces in place, the BHC role can also be that of an *educator*. By addressing a broad array of biopsychosocially influenced concerns with shared patients, the BHC can help the whole care team improve their behavioral health aptitude over time. When providers consistently and reliably involve BHCs in patients' care (*routine*) through standardized care pathways, this facilitates the educational component of the BHC's role, as providers will begin to see common interventional components for different behaviorally influenced concerns.

The BHC is often a psychologist or master's level therapist by training, growing from its beginnings as a psychologist-created model. Involvement from psychiatrists in this model is not classically discussed or consistent in practice, although many best practice sites do indeed involve psychiatric consultation in a collocated or integrated manner (Cohen, Davis, Hall, Gilchrist, & Miller, 2015).

Implementation and Resources Needed

Considerations for a successful PCBH program include organizational, interpersonal, and individual staff-level needs. Shifting the focus from providing resources to patients with only obvious or severe mental health concerns to care for all patients with behaviorally influenced conditions requires commitment from all stakeholders. On the organizational level, a truly integrated PCBH program must ensure the program's alignment with the organization's mission and values. This alignment enables quality improvement processes, financial backing, and appropriate staffing of the program to occur. An Agency for Healthcare Research and Quality report of exemplary programs noted that successful PCBH organizations supported their programs with structured clinical workflows, shared physical workspaces, and shared information infrastructures (e.g., electronic health records) (Cohen et al., 2015).

Examining interpersonal practices among programs, this same report found that effective PCBH models developed clinical workflows that included interdisciplinary communication and clear care pathways, as well as timely access to BHCs for both planned appointments and unplanned patient concerns. This last point requires a delicate balance of maintaining some scheduled visits, as well as allotting time for the BHC to contribute to unexpected care situations.

For the BHC specifically, initial and continued training needs is of utmost importance. Robinson and Reiter (2016) define the core competencies for BHCs as brief intervention skills, pathway service skills, documentation skills, consultation skills, team performance skills, practice management skills, and administrative knowledge and skills. These BHC core competencies have not traditionally been a focus of curricula for social work, psychology, or marriage or family therapy programs. This led to the development of a variety of training initiatives for both individuals still in training and those already licensed to practice who want to shift into a BHC role. Adding training to graduate programs, new certificate programs, curricula from the American Psychological Association, community-based trainings, and self-study options are some examples of these training approaches, with many of these resources outlined in a recent review (Serrano, Cordes, Cubic, & Daub, 2018). Once in practice as a BHC, ongoing supervision to ensure continued model fidelity and general support is also critical to the BHC's continued evolution of skills.

Real-World Program Example

The Southcentral Foundation (SCF), an Alaska Native-owned nonprofit health care organization based in Anchorage, Alaska, offers primary care and specialty services to nearly 65,000 Alaska Native and American Indian individuals (Southcentral Foundation, 2018). As a cornerstone of their integrated behavioral health services, the Southcentral Foundation trialed incorporation of BHCs into several primary care clinics over 10 years ago (Southcentral Foundation, 2017). With positive feedback from primary care providers and patients, the number and role of BHCs expanded, and they are now a presence throughout the organization's primary care clinics.

Starting in 2012, warm handoffs and same-day services were emphasized, which the organization has found reduced the wait time and need for traditional behavioral health service referrals. Southcentral Foundation customer owners (e.g., individuals referred to as patients in other health care organizations) may see a BHC one or more times, depending on the customer owner's specific needs. BHCs at SCF encounter patients with a variety of behaviorally influenced concerns, offering treatments ranging from biofeedback for enhancing mindfulness in an anxious individual to building a relationship with a customer owner with first-break psychosis to facilitate further behavioral health service engagement (author (SH) personal experience).

Time is balanced between scheduled appointments with customer owners and availability for immediate referrals from PCPs by employing a call schedule where the BHCs rotate who will be the "on call" providers for the day. BHC availability, along with other integrated strategies that include the presence of collocated psychiatrists within the primary care clinics, has led to improved wait times for customer owners who do need referrals to behavioral health services beyond what the BHCs can offer. Wait times have decreased from a 42 day average to a 7–28 day maximum post-BHC integration. BHCs also likely contribute to the high satisfaction rate of 96% among customer owners with the care they receive at (Southcentral Foundation, 2017).

Primary Care for Patients with Serious Mental Illnesses in Mental Health Care Settings

History and Background

Having a serious mental illness (SMI) elevates the risk for multiple medical issues and premature death (Alakeson, Frank, & Katz, 2010). SMI typically is defined as the subset of any mental illness that causes substantial functional impairment in one or more of life's domains. Psychotic disorders, such as schizophrenia, and mood disorders, such as major depressive or bipolar disorders, often fall within the SMI distinction. SMI's broad impact on health and risk for premature death may be partly due to limited access to preventative and primary care services (Cook et al., 2015). Patients with SMI are more often hospitalized for preventable medical illness and have chronic conditions that are poorly controlled (Druss & von Esenwein, 2006).

Multiple barriers can exist in obtaining primary care services for patients with SMI, including the impact of SMI on health behaviors and a patient's understanding of their health care needs, as well as perceived stigma in PCP settings toward patients with SMI (Alakeson et al., 2010; Cook et al., 2015; Druss & von Esenwein, 2006). Integrating primary care services into mental health clinics enables patients who may be engaged in care in their mental health center, but not in a primary care clinic, to receive integrated services simultaneously to address their mental health and other chronic health conditions in a more patient-centric manner.

To integrate services in this manner, a primary care provider (i.e., physician, nurse practitioner, or physician's assistant) typically is embedded in a mental health care clinic. Patients are often seen by a physically onsite PCP at the mental health care clinic, but they are also seen via telehealth in some programs. The

PCPs' provided services typically include annual physical exams and diagnosis and treatment of diabetes, hyperlipidemia, hypertension, and other chronic medical conditions.

There is a spectrum of integration within this care model. Some programs deliver primarily collocated care, with the primary care and behavioral health teams working independently or occasionally attending care team meetings together. When care is more integrated, patient panels may be formally co-managed, multidisciplinary team meetings regularly occur, and workflows are shared. To encourage shared management of patient needs, a registry may be used to track laboratory results and record return visit dates for patients.

Data and Evidence

The goals of integrating primary care services for patients with SMI are consistent with the Quadruple Aim's focus on improved clinical outcomes, cost-efficacy, patient satisfaction, and provider experience.

A study of 752 patients with SMI in 2 integrated behavioral health clinics, 1 established and 1 new, evaluated hospital utilization and costs (Breslau et al., 2018). In the established integrated care clinic, patients receiving integrated care services had reduced inpatient hospital admissions after enrollment in the integrated program, as compared to non-enrolled patients in the clinic. However, in the second clinic with a new integrated care program, this reduction in hospitalization did not materialize. A trend in decreased inpatient hospitalization costs for patients receiving integrated care services also occurred in the established clinic only. Neither clinic saw a reduction in emergency room visits or costs. These results indicate the benefit of an established integrated care program toward reducing hospital days and its costs.

Outcomes for several chronic medical conditions have also been evaluated within this model. A quasi-experimental difference of design study compared three primary care integrated behavioral health care sites to control clinics (Scharf et al., 2016). The patients in integrated care clinics possessed healthier cholesterol levels after 1 year, but no other significant impacts were demonstrated for other medical disorders. Another randomized controlled trial found that while the integrated model improved quality of care, it did not improve medical markers of health (Druss et al., 2017). Finally, a quasi-experimental study found that integrated primary care services resulted in a slight reduction in emergency department visits and psychiatric hospitalization, as well as an increase in diabetes monitoring (Rodgers et al., 2016). While this is a promising model, more data is needed to further assess its overall efficacy.

Implementation and Resources

Hiring, training, and logistical considerations all need be considered to develop a successful integration program. Related to hiring, this model requires hiring and/or training primary and preventative care staff to provide on-site assessments while also ensuring that the primary care and behavioral health providers have a basic understanding of each other's roles. When present, medical support staff, such as medical assistants or peer counselors, may also require training to provide services within the mental health care clinic.

Beyond hiring and training needs, infrastructure should also be thoughtfully developed. When a registry or panel is used for tracking patients' progress, this can require effort to create and implement. As part of seeing patients, the primary care provider will also need to have dedicated space with medical equipment that is usually not found in psychiatric clinics (e.g., an ophthalmoscope, a medical exam table, phlebotomy equipment).

For a more thorough discussion of the necessary pieces to launch integrated primary care in behavioral health settings, the reader is directed to the SAMHSA-HRSA Center for Integrated Health Solutions (2018).

Limitations

While integrating primary care into mental health settings demonstrates promise for lessening the health outcomes gaps between people with and without SMI, this model does have several challenges to address. Its evidence base is still developing, as it has limited controlled studies and outcomes data. One challenge to broadening the evidence base is that there is variability among the components and workflows of programs in practice. In terms of necessary resources, additional or repurposed space in a mental health care clinic is required, which can be challenging in some clinics. Finally, regular communication between the primary care and behavioral health team members can be difficult in busy clinics, which can lead to siloed care or unintegrated care plans (Rodgers et al., 2016).

Emerging Approaches to Integration

As was described in the chapter's introduction, integration can be understood as a spectrum of strategies for overcoming systemic care fragmentation. While CoCM and PCBH represent two of the more widespread and recognized models of integrated behavioral health care, the wider universe of potential approaches is always expanding. This section seeks to highlight several constellations of approaches and practices that hint at the range of possible forms of integration.

Elaborating on Existing Models

Some integration approaches share significant overlap with the models described above. For example, it is possible to create programs that effectively "blend" key elements of CoCM and PCBH models, providing access to both (1) rapid assessment and management of acute, time-limited stressors, or crises and (2) the capacity for assessment and treatment of identified psychiatric conditions within a more comprehensive, population-based behavioral health program. While such "blended" approaches have not yet been rigorously studied, pragmatic experimentation in this area is ongoing and encouraged by leaders in the field (Unützer, 2016).

Other approaches have already received more rigorous study, such as TEAMcare, which like CoCM, was built upon Wagner's chronic care model. In Katon et al.'s (2010) seminal single-blind randomized controlled trial, a TEAMcare intervention versus usual care was studied in 14 primary care clinics and included 214 adult patients with comorbid depression and coronary heart disease and/or poorly controlled diabetes. The intervention sought to provide patients and their primary care teams with a combination of enhanced behavioral health and general medical treatment support using an on-site nurse who was supported by primary care physicians and psychiatrists through population-based consultation. As with CoCM, the TEAMcare approach was shown to facilitate active treatment changes and lead to improved metabolic (A1c, cholesterol), cardiovascular (systolic blood pressure), and depression (SCL-20) measures while also increasing patients' satisfaction with care and improving their overall quality of life (Katon et al., 2010; Ratzliff et al., 2016).

There is also the potential to develop fully integrated health homes and even larger-scale community-level integrated health programs, wherein a nearly complete range of integrated general medical and behavioral health services are provided directly in the same clinical and community settings. Particularly in environments, such as US health care systems, where behavioral health and general medical care have historically occupied rather distinct institutional and cultural spaces, developing such fully integrated programs requires extensive coordination, planning, institutional support, financial realignment, and cultural shifts. Successful ongoing efforts to create and develop such systems in the US context include Cherokee Health Systems (2018) and the state of Vermont (2018).

Alternatively, there may be other situations in which an upskilled primary care workforce is called upon to provide integrated general medical and behavioral health care without ready access to other professionals. Such circumstances include situations in which (1) symptom severity and complexity are sufficiently low, (2) access to local specialists or other integrated care resources are limited, and/or (3) a patient's care preferences limit access to other forms of integration. In such instances, additional support in terms of training and clinical resources can be invaluable (American Academy of Family Physicians, 2018).

Innovating for Specific Populations and Conditions

It is possible, as well, to develop integrated approaches that respond to the unique needs and circumstances of specific populations, with the population defined by some combination of behavioral health conditions and sociocultural factors. This was noted, above, in discussing the implementation of primary care services within mental health settings for individuals with SMI wherein specialty mental health clinics were identified by patients as their primary health home.

The integrated treatment of substance use disorders (SUDs) represents another such example. Due to factors such as elevated social stigma and institutional-structural features of health care systems, the treatment of SUDs is often separated from other general outpatient medical care (Office of the Surgeon General, 2016). However, experience in primary care and with partial integration efforts, such as Screening Brief Intervention and Referral to Treatment (SBIRT) programs, have demonstrated that referral to treatment in separate specialty addictions treatment centers constitutes a significant barrier to initiating and maintaining patients in treatment for SUDs (Kim et al., 2017; Saitz et al., 2014).

In response, there have been efforts to incorporate treatment directly into primary care that have demonstrated improved health outcomes. For example, in one study of US military veterans diagnosed with alcohol use disorder (AUD) in US Veterans Administration Medical Centers (VAMC), primary care clinics were randomized to two groups. One group was comprised of intervention clinics who offered patients with AUD primary care-based treatment (i.e., counseling and access to oral naltrexone to alcohol curb cravings); the second group was usual care clinics who offered referrals to a VAMC outpatient specialty addictions clinic's intensive outpatient treatment program. Patients treated in primary care demonstrated improved treatment engagement and reduction in heavy drinking days relative to those referred to traditional specialty care (Oslin et al., 2014). This finding appears to be driven largely by the low rate of successful initial engagement after referral to non-primary care-based treatment, as opposed to a deficiency in the treatment provided for those who were able to engage in specialty care.

Others have sought to adapt CoCM principles and techniques to SUD treatment. The SUMMIT trial showed increased receipt of evidence-based treatments and self-reported 30-day abstinence among patients with AUD and/or opioid use disorder (OUD) who were randomized to CoCM versus usual care. These benefits were observed despite surprisingly low use of medication-assisted treatment in both groups (Watkins et al., 2017).

The successful and more widely disseminated Massachusetts Model of Collaborative Care for OUD relies heavily on primary care-based nurse care managers, working in coordination with their clinic's primary care providers and a program-level coordinator, to support, monitor, and manage of patients with OUD who are being treated with buprenorphine-naloxone in primary care. This scalable and efficient approach shows evidence of greater than 50% retention in treatment at

1 year with 95% reduction in illicit opioid use for those remaining in treatment (Alford et al., 2011; LaBelle, Han, Bergeron, & Samet, 2016).

Finally, the Vermont Hub-and-Spoke model for OUD treatment relies on larger health care system redesign that enables integration of specialty addictions treatment and primary care and facilitates a more seamless flow of patients and resources across a continuum of treatment contexts, according to an individual patient's clinical needs. In this model, regional specialty addictions centers serve as hubs that provide assessment, assistance with treatment initiation, ongoing education, and coordination-of-care transfers to support networks, or "spokes," of primary care clinics (Vermont Agency of Human Services & Vermont Blueprint for Health, 2012).

Spokes are eligible for in-clinic nurse and case manager staff assistance, as well as access to hub-based addiction treatment expertise and the opportunity to participate in a statewide virtual "learning collaborative." This program has facilitated primary care workforce expansion, allowed for same-day access to treatment in many regions, increased access to and appropriate use of OUD medication-assisted treatment, facilitated retention in treatment, and enabled timely care transitions between specialty and primary care settings (Cimaglio, 2015; State of Vermont, 2018; Vermont Agency of Human Services & Vermont Blueprint for Health, 2012).

Leveraging Technology

Finally, the increasing role of information and communication technologies (ICTs) in facilitating multiple different approaches to care integration should be acknowledged. Even beyond the use of electronic health records and clinical registries that support CoCM and other established integrated care approaches, ICTs, in the form of a rapidly expanding array of "telehealth" modalities, are being leveraged to bring behavioral health into non-behavioral clinical and community settings.

The oldest of these is synchronous two-way interactive video-based virtual encounters between patients and behavioral health specialists, often referred to as telepsychiatry (Shore, 2015). Early experimentation in the late 1950s and 1960s with closed circuit analog videoconferencing was followed by decades of limited use, before telepsychiatry and telemental health, more generally, saw a resurgence in the 1990s and 2000s. In recent years, this has been accelerated though access to digital web-based platforms (Chan, Parish, & Yellowlees, 2015).

Today, direct patient-to-clinician synchronous videoconferencing is incorporated into multiple integrated care approaches, including CoCM (Fortney et al., 2015; Turvey & Fortney, 2017). In addition, there is a growing use of digital electronic consultation platforms used for both (1) synchronous and asynchronous consultation between a remote behavioral health specialist and a primary care clinician regarding the clinical care of individual patients in primary care and (2) population-based consultation through "remote telehubs" (Raney, Lasky, et al., 2017). While the former has not yet been rigorously studied, there are high-quality studies indicating the effectiveness of the latter in CoCM (Fortney et al., 2013). There is also increasing experience with and emerging evidence for the use of learning collaboratives, such as Project ECHO, to facilitate telementoring and shared learning among behavioral health experts and primary care clinicians with the goal of supporting local practice change and improved patient outcomes (Fisher et al., 2017; Hager et al., 2018).

Finally, there are emerging opportunities to leverage access to patients outside of traditional clinical settings. In recent years, this has been an area of significant research and commercial interest, expanding in large part through the proliferation of sophisticated mobile devices and other web-based technologies. These devices and technologies enable new patterns of communication and can generate complex mixed datasets using patient-generated and passively collected data. These, in combination with powerful new data management and analysis techniques, are beginning to generate new opportunities for diagnostic clarification, decision support, treatment delivery, and monitoring treatment progress (Hallgren, Bauer, & Atkins, 2017; Raney, Bergman, et al., 2017).

Implications for Behavioral Health

The established models and emerging approaches described in this chapter attest to the range of possibilities for integrating of primary care and behavioral health services (Table 2). Many of the challenges that led to the need for integration initially remain true to this day. These include behavioral health workforce shortages, stigma related to mental health conditions, lack of coordination among treatment teams, high rates of undetected and untreated psychiatric conditions, and rising health care costs, among other ongoing issues. Different integrated care models offer a variety of innovative responses to these challenges, with strengths and limitations specific to each model. Although CoCM has achieved a strong evidence base, it still requires significant resources to appropriately implement and maintain a high-fidelity program.

While there is a less-established evidence base for the PCBH model, there is nonetheless some compelling evidence, as well as an implicit endorsement of the PCBH model's utility, as evidenced by its use in many large US health care systems. For individuals with SMI, integrating primary care services into the behavioral health settings that patients are comfortable in can enable the delivery of fundamental primary and preventative services for this vulnerable population. Blended approaches to integration also exist beyond these models, with variations on the strategies and practices used to deliver comprehensive care to patients.

Innovations in integrated care will continue. Ideally, this movement will be guided by a balance in employing evidence-based approaches while also acknowledging that each organization's culture, resources, and other unique features will

Table 2 Overview of integrated care models

Model	Target population	Primary goal	Involved personnel	Unique integration components	Strengths	Limitations
Collaborative care	– Primary care patients with diagnosable mental health conditions – Strongest evidence for depression, anxiety	To treat to target common mental health disorders such as depression and anxiety; additional target conditions include substance use disorders, dementia, chronic pain, ADHD, and bipolar disorder	– Primary care provider (primary relationship; prescribing function) – Behavioral health care manager (care management; delivery of evidence-based brief behavioral interventions) – Psychiatric consultant (provides indirect care through systematic case review)	– Regular use of behavioral health measures – Use of registry to identify patient in need of intervention and drive treatment to target	– Strong evidence base – Leverages scarce psychiatric resources	– Complex intervention which makes implementation more challenging – Financial sustainability for team-based care is limited

Primary behavioral health consultant	Primary care patients with any biopsychosocially influenced health condition	"To enhance the primary care team's ability to managed and treat behavioral health problems and influenced conditions, with resulting improvements in primary care services for the entire clinic population" (Serrano et al., 2018)	– Behavioral health consultant (provides brief behavioral interventions) – Primary care provider (referring physician, collaborates on care with the BHC)	– Model focuses on extending beyond diagnoses – Identifies and treats patients with any type of biopsychosocially-influenced concern – Uses warm handoffs	– Available to all patients – Not focusing on a diagnosis can be helpful to patients who do not identify as having a psychiatric issue – Focused on immediate care delivery	– Workforce shortage of trained BHCs – Traditionally, there are no psychiatrists involved in the model to provide expertise on medication management
Primary care in behavioral health settings	Patients with psychiatric conditions who have other untreated medical needs	To decrease the amount of untreated medical comorbidity in psychiatric clinics	– Primary care provider (provides medical care for chronic and acute medical conditions) – Behavioral health provider/s (collaborates on patient's health care needs with primary care personnel)	– The clinic location is within a mental health center – Integration of primary care services into a non-primary care setting	– Provides primary care services to patients who often do not regularly engage in primary care services	– Requires additional clinic space – Requires team members with experience in medical presentations in patients with psychiatric conditions

inevitably lead to continued development of integrated care models. This evolution will be carried out with the ambitious, but achievable, goal of providing cost- and clinically- effective patient care in a system that gets the approval of patient and clinical stakeholders alike.

References

AIMS Center. (2018a). *Advancing integrated mental health solutions in integrated care* [Web page]. Seattle, Washington: University of Washington, Department of Psychiatry and Behavioral Sciences, Division of Population Health. https://aims.uw.edu/

AIMS Center. (2018b). *Principles of collaborative care* [Web page]. Seattle, Washington: University of Washington, Department of Psychiatry and Behavioral Sciences, Division of Population Health. https://aims.uw.edu/collaborative-care/principles-collaborative-care

Akincigil, A., & Matthews, E. B. (2017). National rates and patterns of depression screening in primary care: Results from 2012 and 2013. *Psychiatric Services, 68*(7), 660–666. https://doi.org/10.1176/appi.ps.201600096

Alakeson, V., Frank, R. G., & Katz, R. E. (2010). Specialty care medical homes for people with severe, persistent mental disorders. *Health Affairs, 29*(5), 867–873. https://doi.org/10.1377/hlthaff.2010.0080

Alford, D. P., LaBelle, C. T., Kretsch, N., Bergeron, A., Winter, M., Botticelli, M., & Samet, J. H. (2011). Collaborative care of opioid-addicted patients in primary care using buprenorphine: Five-year experience. *Archives of Internal Medicine, 171*(5), 425–431. https://doi.org/10.1001/archinternmed.2010.541

American Academy of Family Physicians. (2018). *Mental health care services by family physicians (Position paper)*. Leawood, KS: Author. https://www.aafp.org/about/policies/all/mental-services.html

American Psychiatric Association. (2018). *Integrated care* [Web page]. Chicago, IL: American Psychiatric Association. https://www.psychiatry.org/psychiatrists/practice/professional-interests/integrated-care

Angantyr, K., Rimner, A., Norden, T., & Norlander, T. (2015). Primary care behavioral health model: Perspectives of outcome, client satisfaction, and gender. *Social Behavior and Personality: An International Journal, 43*(2), 287. https://doi.org/10.2224/sbp.2015.43.2.287

Angstman, K. B., Phelan, S., Myszkowski, M. R., Schak, K. M., DeJesus, R. S., Lineberry, T. W., & van Ryn, M. (2015). Minority primary care patients with depression: Outcome disparities improve with collaborative care management. *Medical Care, 53*(1), 32–37. https://doi.org/10.1097/mlr.0000000000000280

Archer, J., Bower, P., Gilbody, S., Lovell, K., Richards, D., Gask, L., … Coventry, P. (2012). Collaborative care for depression and anxiety problems. *Cochrane Database of Systematic Reviews, 10*, Cd006525. https://doi.org/10.1002/14651858.CD006525.pub2

Areán, P. A., Ayalon, L., Hunkeler, E., Lin, E. H., Tang, L., Harpole, L., … Unutzer, J. (2005). Improving depression care for older, minority patients in primary care. *Medical Care, 43*(4), 381–390.

Bao, Y., Druss, B. G., Jung, H. Y., Chan, Y. F., & Unützer, J. (2016). Unpacking collaborative care for depression: Examining two essential tasks for implementation. *Psychiatric Services, 67*(4), 418–424. https://doi.org/10.1176/appi.ps.201400577

Blackmore, M. A., Carleton, K. E., Ricketts, S. M., Patel, U. B., Stein, D., Mallow, A., … Chung, H. (2018). Comparison of collaborative care and colocation treatment for patients with clinically significant depression symptoms in primary care. *Psychiatric Services, 69*(11), 1184–1187. https://doi.org/10.1176/appi.ps.201700569

Breslau, J., Leckman-Westin, E., Han, B., Pritam, R., Guarasi, D., Horvitz-Lennon, M., … Yu, H. (2018). Impact of a mental health based primary care program on emergency department visits and inpatient stays. *General Hospital Psychiatry, 52*, 8–13. https://doi.org/10.1016/j.genhosppsych.2018.02.008

Bryan, C. J., Morrow, C., & Appolonio, K. K. (2009). Impact of behavioral health consultant interventions on patient symptoms and functioning in an integrated family medicine clinic. *Journal of Clinical Psychology, 65*(3), 281–293. https://doi.org/10.1002/jclp.20539

Carlo, A. D., Unützer, J., Ratzliff, A. D. H., & Cerimele, J. M. (2018). Financing for collaborative care: A narrative review. *Current Treatment Options in Psychiatry, 5*(3), 334–344. https://doi.org/10.1007/s40501-018-0150-4

Centers for Medicare & Medicaid Services. (2018). *Behavioral health integration services* (Medicare Learning Network Factsheet). Washington, DC: Centers for Medicare & Medicaid Services. https://www.cms.gov/Outreach-and-Education/Medicare-Learning-Network-MLN/MLNProducts/Downloads/BehavioralHealthIntegration.pdf

Chan, S., Parish, M., & Yellowlees, P. (2015). Telepsychiatry today. *Current Psychiatry Reports, 17*(11), 89. https://doi.org/10.1007/s11920-015-0630-9

Chang, C. K., Hayes, R. D., Perera, G., Broadbent, M. T., Fernandes, A. C., Lee, W. E., … Stewart, R. (2011). Life expectancy at birth for people with serious mental illness and other major disorders from a secondary mental health care case register in London. *PLoS One, 6*(5), e19590. https://doi.org/10.1371/journal.pone.0019590

Cherokee Health Systems. (2018). *Together enhancing life*. Knoxville, TN: Author. https://www.cherokeehealth.com/

Cigrang, J. A., Rauch, S. A., Mintz, J., Brundige, A., Avila, L. L., Bryan, C. J., … Peterson, A. L. (2015). Treatment of active duty military with PTSD in primary care: A follow-up report. *Journal of Anxiety Disorders, 36*, 110–114. https://doi.org/10.1016/j.janxdis.2015.10.003

Cimaglio, B. (2015, October). *Vermont's approach: Treating the opiate epidemic*. Paper presented at the meeting of the National Governor's Association, Salt Lake City, UT. Retrieved from https://docplayer.net/19951621-Vermont-s-approach-treating-the-opiate-epidemic-barbara-cimaglio-deputy-commissioner-vermont-department-of-health.html

Clark, C. M., Fradkin, J. E., Hiss, R. G., Lorenz, R. A., Vinicor, F., & Warren-Boulton, E. (2000). Promoting early diagnosis and treatment of type 2 diabetes: The National Diabetes Education Program. *JAMA, 284*(3), 363–365. https://doi.org/10.1001/jama.284.3.363

Cohen, D. J., Davis, M. M., Hall, J. D., Gilchrist, E. C., & Miller, B. F. (2015, March). *A guidebook of professional practices for behavioral health and primary care integration: Observations from exemplary sites*. Rockville, MD: Agency for Healthcare Research and Quality. https://integrationacademy.ahrq.gov/sites/default/files/AHRQ_AcademyGuidebook.pdf

Cook, J. A., Razzano, L. A., Swarbrick, M. A., Jonikas, J. A., Yost, C., Burke, L., … Santos, A. (2015). Health risks and changes in self-efficacy following community health screening of adults with serious mental illnesses. *PLoS One, 10*(4), e0123552. https://doi.org/10.1371/journal.pone.0123552

Drake, E., & Valenstein, M. (2018). *Behavioral health integration into ambulatory practice* [Web page]. Chicago, IL: American Medical Association. https://www.stepsforward.org/modules/integrated-behavioral-health

Druss, B. G. (2004). A review of HEDIS measures and performance for mental disorders. *Managed Care, 13*(6 Suppl Depression), 48–51. https://www.managedcaremag.com/linkout/2004/6%20Suppl%20Depression/48

Druss, B. G., & von Esenwein, S. A. (2006). Improving general medical care for persons with mental and addictive disorders: systematic review. *General Hospital Psychiatry, 28*(2), 145–153. https://doi.org/10.1016/j.genhosppsych.2005.10.006

Druss, B. G., von Esenwein, S. A., Glick, G. E., Deubler, E., Lally, C., Ward, M. C., & Rask, K. J. (2017). Randomized trial of an integrated behavioral health home: The Health Outcomes Management and Evaluation (HOME) Study. *American Journal of Psychiatry, 174*(3), 246–255. https://doi.org/10.1176/appi.ajp.2016.16050507

Ettner, S. L., Azocar, F., Branstrom, R. B., Meredith, L. S., Zhang, L., & Ong, M. K. (2010). Association of general medical and psychiatric comorbidities with receipt of guideline-concordant care for depression. *Psychiatric Services, 61*(12), 1255–1259. https://doi.org/10.1176/ps.2010.61.12.1255

Fisher, E., Hasselberg, M., Conwell, Y., Weiss, L., Padron, N. A., Tiernan, E., ... Pagan, J. A. (2017). Telementoring primary care clinicians to improve geriatric mental health care. *Population Health Management, 20*(5), 342–347. https://doi.org/10.1089/pop.2016.0087

Fortney, J. C., Enderle, M. A., Clothier, J. L., Otero, J. M., Williams, J. S., & Pyne, J. M. (2013). Population level effectiveness of implementing collaborative care management for depression. *General Hospital Psychiatry, 35*(5), 455–460. https://doi.org/10.1016/j.genhosppsych.2013.04.010

Fortney, J. C., Pyne, J. M., Kimbrell, T. A., Hudson, T. J., Robinson, D. E., Schneider, R., ... Schnurr, P. P. (2015). Telemedicine-based collaborative care for posttraumatic stress disorder: a randomized clinical trial. *JAMA Psychiatry, 72*(1), 58–67. https://doi.org/10.1001/jamapsychiatry.2014.1575

Fortney, J. C., Unützer, J., Wrenn, G., Pyne, J. M., Smith, G. R., Schoenbaum, M., & Harbin, H. T. (2017). A tipping point for measurement-based care. *Psychiatric Services, 68*(2), 179–188. https://doi.org/10.1176/appi.ps.201500439

Gomez, D., Bridges, A. J., Andrews Iii, A. R., Cavell, T. A., Pastrana, F. A., Gregus, S. J., & Ojeda, C. A. (2014). Delivering parent management training in an integrated primary care setting: Description and preliminary outcome data. *Cognitive and Behavioral Practice, 21*(3), 296–309. https://doi.org/10.1016/j.cbpra.2014.04.003

Gonzalez, H. M., Vega, W. A., Williams, D. R., Tarraf, W., West, B. T., & Neighbors, H. W. (2010). Depression care in the United States: Too little for too few. *Archives of General Psychiatry, 67*(1), 37–46. https://doi.org/10.1001/archgenpsychiatry.2009.168

Goodie, J. L., Isler, W. C., Hunter, C., & Peterson, A. L. (2009). Using behavioral health consultants to treat insomnia in primary care: A clinical case series. *Journal of Clinical Psychology, 65*(3), 294–304. https://doi.org/10.1002/jclp.20548

Gouge, N., Polaha, J., Rogers, R., & Harden, A. (2016). Integrating behavioral health into pediatric primary care: Implications for provider time and cost. *Southern Medical Journal, 109*(12), 774–778. https://doi.org/10.14423/smj.0000000000000564

Grembowski, D. E., Martin, D., Patrick, D. L., Diehr, P., Katon, W., Williams, B., ... Goldberg, H. I. (2002). Managed care, access to mental health specialists, and outcomes among primary care patients with depressive symptoms. *Journal of General Internal Medicine, 17*(4), 258–269. https://www.ncbi.nlm.nih.gov/pmc/articles/PMC1495032/

Hager, B., Hasselberg, M., Arzubi, E., Betlinski, J., Duncan, M., Richman, J., & Raney, L. E. (2018). Leveraging behavioral health expertise: Practices and potential of the Project ECHO approach to virtually integrating care in underserved areas. *Psychiatric Services, 69*(4), 366–369. https://doi.org/10.1176/appi.ps.201700211

Hallgren, K. A., Bauer, A. M., & Atkins, D. C. (2017). Digital technology and clinical decision making in depression treatment: Current findings and future opportunities. *Depression and Anxiety, 34*(6), 494–501. https://doi.org/10.1002/da.22640

Hay, J. W., Katon, W. J., Ell, K., Lee, P. J., & Guterman, J. J. (2012). Cost-effectiveness analysis of collaborative care management of major depression among low-income, predominantly Hispanics with diabetes. *Value in Health, 15*(2), 249–254. https://doi.org/10.1016/j.jval.2011.09.008

Huffman, J. C., Niazi, S. K., Rundell, J. R., Sharpe, M., & Katon, W. J. (2014). Essential articles on collaborative care models for the treatment of psychiatric disorders in medical settings: A publication by the Academy of Psychosomatic Medicine Research and Evidence-Based Practice Committee. *Psychosomatics, 55*(2), 109–122. https://doi.org/10.1016/j.psym.2013.09.002

Hunter, C. L., Funderburk, J. S., Polaha, J., Bauman, D., Goodie, J. L., & Hunter, C. M. (2018). Primary Care Behavioral Health (PCBH) model research: Current state of the science and a call to action. *Journal of Clinical Psychology in Medical Settings, 25*(2), 127–156. https://doi.org/10.1007/s10880-017-9512-0

Institute of Medicine. (2001). *Crossing the quality chasm: A new health system for the twenty-first century*. Washington, DC: National Academy Press.

Joint National Committee on Prevention. (1997). The sixth report of the Joint National Committee on prevention, detection, evaluation, and treatment of high blood pressure. *Archives of Internal Medicine, 157*(21), 2413–2446. https://doi.org/10.1001/archinte.1997.00440420033005

Katon, W., Berg, A. O., Robins, A. J., & Risse, S. (1986). Depression: Medical utilization and somatization. *Western Journal of Medicine, 144*(5), 564–568. https://www.ncbi.nlm.nih.gov/pmc/articles/PMC1306704/

Katon, W., & Schulberg, H. (1992). Epidemiology of depression in primary care. *General Hospital Psychiatry, 14*(4), 237–247. https://doi.org/10.1016/0163-8343(92)90094-Q

Katon, W., & Sullivan, M. D. (1990). Depression and chronic medical illness. *Journal of Clinical Psychiatry, 51*(*Suppl*), 3–11; discussion 12–14.

Katon, W. J., Lin, E. H., Von Korff, M., Ciechanowski, P., Ludman, E. J., Young, B., … McCulloch, D. (2010). Collaborative care for patients with depression and chronic illnesses. *New England Journal of Medicine, 363*(27), 2611–2620. https://doi.org/10.1056/NEJMoa1003955

Kim, T. W., Bernstein, J., Cheng, D. M., Lloyd-Travaglini, C., Samet, J. H., Palfai, T. P., & Saitz, R. (2017). Receipt of addiction treatment as a consequence of a brief intervention for drug use in primary care: A randomized trial. *Addiction, 112*(5), 818–827. https://doi.org/10.1111/add.13701

Korsen, N., Blount, A., Peek, C. J., Kathol, R., Narayanan, V., Teixeira, N., … Miller, B. F. (2018). *AHRQ academy playbook* [Web page]. Rockville, MD: Agency for Healthcare Research & Quality. https://integrationacademy.ahrq.gov/products/playbook/about-playbook

LaBelle, C. T., Han, S. C., Bergeron, A., & Samet, J. H. (2016). Office-Based Opioid Treatment with Buprenorphine (OBOT-B): Statewide implementation of the Massachusetts Collaborative Care Model in community health centers. *Journal of Substance Abuse Treatment, 60*, 6–13. https://doi.org/10.1016/j.jsat.2015.06.010

Lanoye, A., Stewart, K. E., Rybarczyk, B. D., Auerbach, S. M., Sadock, E., Aggarwal, A., … Austin, K. (2017). The impact of integrated psychological services in a safety net primary care clinic on medical utilization. *Journal of Clinical Psychology, 73*(6), 681–692. https://doi.org/10.1002/jclp.22367

Miranda, J., Duan, N., Sherbourne, C., Schoenbaum, M., Lagomasino, I., Jackson-Triche, M., & Wells, K. B. (2003). Improving care for minorities: Can quality improvement interventions improve care and outcomes for depressed minorities? Results of a randomized, controlled trial. *Health Services Research, 38*(2), 613–630. https://doi.org/10.1111/1475-6773.00136

Murray, C. J., Vos, T., Lozano, R., Naghavi, M., Flaxman, A. D., Michaud, C., … Memish, Z. A. (2012). Disability-adjusted life years (DALYs) for 291 diseases and injuries in 21 regions, 1990–2010: A systematic analysis for the Global Burden of Disease Study 2010. *Lancet, 380*(9859), 2197–2223. https://doi.org/10.1016/s0140-6736(12)61689-4

Myers, K., Stoep, A. V., Thompson, K., Zhou, C., & Unützer, J. (2010). Collaborative care for the treatment of Hispanic children diagnosed with attention-deficit hyperactivity disorder. *General Hospital Psychiatry, 32*(6), 612–614. https://doi.org/10.1016/j.genhosppsych.2010.08.004

National Academies of Sciences, Engineering, & Medicine. (2015). *Improving diagnosis in health care*. Washington, DC: The National Academies Press.

Office of the Surgeon General. (2016). *Facing addiction in America: The Surgeon General's report on alcohol, drugs, and health* (Reports of the Surgeon General). Washington, DC: US Department of Health and Human Services. https://addiction.surgeongeneral.gov/surgeon-generals-report.pdf

Olshansky, S. J., Passaro, D. J., Hershow, R. C., Layden, J., Carnes, B. A., Brody, J., … Ludwig, D. S. (2005). A potential decline in life expectancy in the United States in the 21st century. *New England Journal of Medicine, 352*(11), 1138–1145. https://doi.org/10.1056/NEJMsr043743

Oslin, D. W., Lynch, K. G., Maisto, S. A., Lantinga, L. J., McKay, J. R., Possemato, K., … Wierzbicki, M. (2014). A randomized clinical trial of alcohol care management delivered in Department of Veterans Affairs primary care clinics versus specialty addiction treatment. *Journal of General Internal Medicine, 29*(1), 162–168. https://doi.org/10.1007/s11606-013-2625-8

Pace, C. A., Gergen-Barnett, K., Veidis, A., D'Afflitti, J., Worcester, J., Fernandez, P., & Lasser, K. E. (2018). Warm handoffs and attendance at initial integrated behavioral health appointments. *Annals of Family Medicine, 16*(4), 346–348. https://doi.org/10.1370/afm.2263

Porter, M. E. (2009). A strategy for health care reform: Toward a value-based system. *New England Journal of Medicine, 361*(2), 109–112. https://doi.org/10.1056/NEJMp0904131

Press, M. J., Howe, R., Schoenbaum, M., Cavanaugh, S., Marshall, A., Baldwin, L., & Conway, P. H. (2017). Medicare payment for behavioral health integration. *New England Journal of Medicine, 376*(5), 405–407. https://doi.org/10.1056/NEJMp1614134

Raney, L., Bergman, D., Torous, J., & Hasselberg, M. (2017). Digitally driven integrated primary care and behavioral health: How technology can expand access to effective treatment. *Current Psychiatry Reports, 19*(11), 86. https://doi.org/10.1007/s11920-017-0838-y

Raney, L. E., Lasky, G. B., & Scott, C. (2017). *Integrated care: A guide for effective implementation*. Chicago, IL: American Psychiatric Association Press.

Ratzliff, A., Unützer, J., Katon, W., & Stephens, K. A. (2016). *Integrated care: Creating effective mental and primary health care teams*. Hoboken, NJ: John Wiley & Sons, Inc.

Ratzliff, A. D. H., Ni, K., Chan, Y. F., Park, M., & Unützer, J. (2013). A collaborative care approach to depression treatment for Asian Americans. *Psychiatric Services, 64*(5), 487–490. https://doi.org/10.1176/appi.ps.001742012

Reiter, J. T., Dobmeyer, A. C., & Hunter, C. L. (2018). The Primary Care Behavioral Health (PCBH) model: An overview and operational definition. *Journal of Clinical Psychology in Medical Settings, 25*(2), 109–126. https://doi.org/10.1007/s10880-017-9531-x

Renders, C. M., Valk, G. D., Griffin, S., Wagner, E. H., Eijk, J. T., & Assendelft, W. J. (2001). Interventions to improve the management of diabetes mellitus in primary care, outpatient and community settings. *Cochrane Database of Systematic Reviews, 1*, Cd001481. https://doi.org/10.1002/14651858.cd001481

Richardson, L. P., Ludman, E., McCauley, E., Lindenbaum, J., Larison, C., Zhou, C., … Katon, W. (2014). Collaborative care for adolescents with depression in primary care: A randomized clinical trial. *JAMA, 312*(8), 809–816. https://doi.org/10.1001/jama.2014.9259

Robinson, P., & Reiter, J. T. (2016). *Behavioral consultation and primary care: A guide to integrating services*. Seattle, WA: Springer.

Robinson, P. J., & Strosahl, K. D. (2009). Behavioral health consultation and primary care: Lessons learned. *Journal of Clinical Psychology in Medical Settings, 16*(1), 58–71. https://doi.org/10.1007/s10880-009-9145-z

Rodgers, M., Dalton, J., Harden, M., Street, A., Parker, G., & Eastwood, A. (2016). *Integrated care to address the physical health needs of people with severe mental illness: A rapid review* (Health Services and Delivery Research, no. 4.13). Southampton, UK: HS&DR Evidence Synthesis Centre. https://www.ncbi.nlm.nih.gov/books/NBK355962/

Ross, L. E., Vigod, S., Wishart, J., Waese, M., Spence, J. D., Oliver, J., … Shields, R. (2015). Barriers and facilitators to primary care for people with mental health and/or substance use issues: A qualitative study. *BMC Family Practice, 16*, 135. https://doi.org/10.1186/s12875-015-0353-3

Rush, A. J. (2007). STAR*D: What have we learned? *American Journal of Psychiatry, 164*, 201–204.

Sadock, E., Auerbach, S. M., Rybarczyk, B., & Aggarwal, A. (2014). Evaluation of integrated psychological services in a university-based primary care clinic. *Journal of Clinical Psychology in Medical Settings, 21*(1), 19–32. https://doi.org/10.1007/s10880-013-9378-8

Saitz, R., Palfai, T. P., Cheng, D. M., Alford, D. P., Bernstein, J. A., Lloyd-Travaglini, C. A., … Samet, J. H. (2014). Screening and brief intervention for drug use in primary care: The ASPIRE randomized clinical trial. *JAMA, 312*(5), 502–513. https://doi.org/10.1001/jama.2014.7862

SAMHSA-HRSA Center for Integrated Health Solutions. (2018). *About CIHS* [Web page]. Rockville, MD: Author. https://www.integration.samhsa.gov/

Scharf, D. M., Schmidt Hackbarth, N., Eberhart, N. K., Horvitz-Lennon, M., Beckman, R., Han, B., … Burnam, M. A. (2016). General medical outcomes from the Primary and Behavioral Health Care Integration grant program. *Psychiatric Services, 67*(11), 1226–1232. https://doi.org/10.1176/appi.ps.201500352

Serrano, N., Cordes, C., Cubic, B., & Daub, S. (2018). The state and future of the Primary Care Behavioral Health model of service delivery workforce. *Journal of Clinical Psychology in Medical Settings, 25*(2), 157–168. https://doi.org/10.1007/s10880-017-9491-1

Shao, Z., Richie, W. D., & Bailey, R. K. (2016). Racial and ethnic disparity in major depressive disorder. *Journal of Racial and Ethnic Health Disparities, 3*(4), 692–705. https://doi.org/10.1007/s40615-015-0188-6

Shore, J. (2015). The evolution and history of telepsychiatry and its impact on psychiatric care: Current implications for psychiatrists and psychiatric organizations. *International Review of Psychiatry, 27*(6), 469–475. https://doi.org/10.3109/09540261.2015.1072086

Simon, G., Ormel, J., VonKorff, M., & Barlow, W. (1995). Health care costs associated with depressive and anxiety disorders in primary care. *American Journal of Psychiatry, 152*(3), 352–357. https://doi.org/10.1176/ajp.152.3.352

Simon, G. E., & VonKorff, M. (1991). Somatization and psychiatric disorder in the NIMH Epidemiologic Catchment Area study. *American Journal of Psychiatry, 148*(11), 1494–1500. https://doi.org/10.1176/ajp.148.11.1494

Simon, G. E., VonKorff, M., Wagner, E. H., & Barlow, W. (1993). Patterns of antidepressant use in community practice. *General Hospital Psychiatry, 15*(6), 399–408. https://doi.org/10.1016/0163-8343(93)90009-D

Southcentral Foundation. (2017). *Behavioral health integration at Southcentral Foundation* [Web page]. Anchorage, AK: SCFNuka. https://scfnuka.com/behavioral-health-integration-southcentral-foundation/

Southcentral Foundation. (2018). *Our story: Southcentral Foundation Nuka system of care* [Web page]. Anchorage, AK: SCFNuka. https://scfnuka.com/our-story/

Sowa, N. A., Jeng, P., Bauer, A. M., Cerimele, J. M., Unützer, J., Bao, Y., & Chwastiak, L. (2018). Psychiatric case review and treatment intensification in collaborative care management for depression in primary care. *Psychiatric Services, 69*(5), 549–554. https://doi.org/10.1176/appi.ps.201700243

State of Vermont. (2018). *Blueprint for health* [Web page]. Waterbury, VT: Author. http://blueprintforhealth.vermont.gov/

Thomas, K. C., Ellis, A. R., Konrad, T. R., Holzer, C. E., & Morrissey, J. P. (2009). County-level estimates of mental health professional shortage in the United States. *Psychiatric Services, 60*(10), 1323–1328. https://doi.org/10.1176/ps.2009.60.10.1323

Turvey, C., & Fortney, J. (2017). The use of telemedicine and mobile technology to promote population health and population management for psychiatric disorders. *Current Psychiatry Reports, 19*(11), 88. https://doi.org/10.1007/s11920-017-0844-0

Unützer, J. (2016). All hands on deck. *Psychiatric News, 51*(5), 1. https://doi.org/10.1176/appi.pn.2016.3a28

Unützer, J., Chan, Y. F., Hafer, E., Knaster, J., Shields, A., Powers, D., & Veith, R. C. (2012). Quality improvement with pay-for-performance incentives in integrated behavioral health care. *American Journal of Public Health, 102*(6), e41–e45. https://doi.org/10.2105/ajph.2011.300555

Unützer, J., Katon, W., Callahan, C. M., Williams, J. W., Jr., Hunkeler, E., Harpole, L., … Langston, C. (2002). Collaborative care management of late-life depression in the primary care setting: a randomized controlled trial. *JAMA, 288*(22), 2836–2845. https://doi.org/10.1001/jama.288.22.2836

Unützer, J., & Park, M. (2012). Strategies to improve the management of depression in primary care. *Primary Care, 39*(2), 415–431. https://doi.org/10.1016/j.pop.2012.03.010

Vermont Agency of Human Services, & Vermont Blueprint for Health. (2012). *Planning guidance to expand Blueprint community health teams with "spoke staffing" for treatment of opioid dependence.* Waterbury, VT: Authors. https://blueprintforhealth.vermont.gov/sites/bfh/files/Vermont%20Blueprint%20for%20Health%202012%20Annual%20Report%20Supporting%20Document%20-%20Planning%20Guidance%20to%20Expand%20Blueprint%20CHTs%20with%20Spoke%20Staffing%20for%20Treatment%20of%20Opioid%20Dependence.pdf

Wagner, E. H., Austin, B. T., Davis, C., Hindmarsh, M., Schaefer, J., & Bonomi, A. (2001). Improving chronic illness care: translating evidence into action. *Health Affairs, 20*(6), 64–78. https://doi.org/10.1377/hlthaff.20.6.64

Watkins, K. E., Ober, A. J., Lamp, K., Lind, M., Setodji, C., Osilla, K. C., ... Pincus, H. A. (2017). Collaborative care for opioid and alcohol use disorders in primary care: The SUMMIT randomized clinical trial. *JAMA Internal Medicine, 177*(10), 1480–1488. https://doi.org/10.1001/jamainternmed.2017.3947

Wells, K. B., Stewart, A., Hays, R. D., Burnam, M. A., Rogers, W., Daniels, M., ... Ware, J. (1989). The functioning and well-being of depressed patients. Results from the Medical Outcomes Study. *JAMA, 262*(7), 914–919. https://doi.org/10.1001/jama.1989.03430070062031

Whitebird, R. R., Solberg, L. I., Jaeckels, N. A., Pietruszewski, P. B., Hadzic, S., Unützer, J., ... Rubenstein, L. V. (2014). Effective implementation of collaborative care for depression: What is needed? *American Journal of Managed Care, 20*(9), 699–707. https://www.ajmc.com/journals/issue/2014/2014-vol20-n9/effective-implementation-of-collaborative-care-for-depression-what-is-needed

Young, A. S., Klap, R., Sherbourne, C. D., & Wells, K. B. (2001). The quality of care for depressive and anxiety disorders in the United States. *Archives of General Psychiatry, 58*(1), 55–61. https://doi.org/10.1001/archpsyc.58.1.55

Rural Behavioral Health Services

Bruce Lubotsky Levin and Ardis Hanson

Introduction

Health and behavioral health care in America have come under increasing scrutiny during the last half of the twentieth century and beginning of the twenty-first century from a vast array of stakeholders, including consumers, providers, employers, community leaders, policymakers, administrators, educators, as well as lawmakers at the state and federal levels of government. Proposals for national and state health care reform have been encouraged, in part, by the need to control the rising costs of health and behavioral health care and to address the obstacles and inequities in accessing health and behavioral health services. Although the United States Congress passed major comprehensive health care reform legislation in 2010 with the Patient Protection and Affordable Care Act (ACA, PL 111–148), significant health care initiatives (particularly in association with entitlement programs) have been proposed and implemented by various individual states.

Historically, individuals who live in rural and frontier areas in America have significant and often times distinct health and behavioral health care needs, but have experienced numerous obstacles in obtaining these services. These numerous challenges include the lack of accessible services (e.g., social isolation, significant geographical distances, and inhospitable climates), a general scarcity of resources and

B. L. Levin (✉)
Department of Child and Family Studies, College of Behavioral and Community Sciences, University of South Florida, Tampa, FL, USA

Behavioral Health Concentration, College of Public Health, University of South Florida, Tampa, FL, USA
e-mail: levin@usf.edu; levin@health.usf.edu

A. Hanson
Research and Education Unit, Shimberg Health Sciences Library, University of South Florida, Tampa, FL, USA
e-mail: hanson@health.usf.edu

© Springer Nature Switzerland AG 2020
B. L. Levin, A. Hanson (eds.), *Foundations of Behavioral Health*,
https://doi.org/10.1007/978-3-030-18435-3_14

the absence of a human services infrastructure, severe shortages of service providers, the absence of service specialization (availability of services), the inappropriate organization of services based upon urban (metropolitan) delivery system models, and inefficient communication (including diversity of languages and sub-cultures) to disseminate information and coordinate care.

These rural health care delivery barriers become even more complex with the provision of rural (and particularly frontier) behavioral health services, since behavioral health services delivery has historically faced problems of stigma (among health providers, consumers, and employers), poor integration with physical (or somatic) health services, unique language and cultural challenges to treatment, as well as substantial reliance on public sector funding.

This chapter presents an overview of the major challenges in the provision of rural behavioral health services in the United States. It also identifies what we see as the most important issues facing rural behavioral health services delivery in the foreseeable future.

Defining Rural and Frontier Areas

Rural America encompasses 97% of the land area of the United States and contains 60 million residents (19% of the U.S. population) (Ratcliffe, Burd, Holder, & Fields, 2016). Furthermore, 10 states in the United States have 40% or more of their population who live in rural or frontier areas.[1] The most rural populations of America are spread across almost 2500 counties heavily concentrated in the South and the Midwest.

Factors contributing to the decrease in rural America include migration of young adults to more urban areas, fewer births, increased mortality among working adults, an aging population, and re-classification of previously rural areas to urbanized and urban areas (Cromartie, 2017).

Basing its definition upon residential population density and land-use characteristics, the U.S. Census Bureau defines rural as "all population, housing, and territory not included within an urbanized area or urban cluster" (Ratcliffe et al., 2016, p. 3). The Census Bureau defines territory within tracts, which may contain both rural and urban areas, and its Rural-Urban Commuting Area Codes characterize the nation's Census tracts. Since the U. S. rural population abides in housing subdivisions on the edge of urban centers, in densely settled small towns, and in sparsely populated or remote areas, rural categories can be classed as mostly urban, mostly rural, or completely rural.

The Census Bureau also uses other measures to assist others in understanding the socioeconomic diversity of rural America. These include the Rural-Urban Continuum Codes, Urban-Influence Codes, Natural Amenities Scale, and the ERS

---

[1](Maine (61%), Vermont (61%), West Virginia (51%), Mississippi (50%), Montana (44%), Arkansas (43%), South Dakota (43%), Kentucky (41%), Alabama (40%), and North Dakota (40%).

Typology Codes. Of especial interest to behavioral health are the ERS Typologies Codes, which examine six policy-relevant class areas (education, employment, persistent poverty and persistent child poverty, population loss, and retirement destination) in addition to six economic dependence categories (Cromartie, 2017). This can make understanding rural issues challenging.

To further complicate matters, there is no standard, universally used definition for frontier and remote (FAR) areas. While a FAR is commonly defined as six or fewer people per square mile, there are other factors that also may define an area as a FAR. In addition to population density, other factors include distance from a specific service point or a population center, travel time, availability of paved roads, and seasonal changes that may affect access to services. In 2007, the National Center for Frontier Communities (2007) created a consensus definition using a weighted matrix that utilized density (persons per square mile), distance (miles to supermarket), and travel time (minutes to supermarket). Building upon this model, the Office of Rural Health Policy (ORHP) and the U.S. Department of Agriculture (USDA) developed the Frontier and Remote Areas (FAR) methodology, which uses ZIP-code-level frontier and remote area (FAR) codes to assist with policy and research (Economic Research Service, 2017). The FAR methodology utilizes travel time to nearby urban areas (population centers) to create a four-level categorical schema. The levels are based on access to high order services (level one), low order services (level four), and intermediate order services (levels two and three). Section 10324(B1-II) of the ACA defines a "Frontier State" where "at least 50 percent of the counties in the State are frontier counties…counties in which the population per square mile is less than 6" (p. 841).

Rural Behavioral Health Services

Historically, health and behavioral health services have been largely concentrated in large, urban areas of America. Hence, the basic organizational models for health and behavioral health services delivery have been based upon urban at-risk populations. The same can be said of professional and graduate education and training programs for health and behavioral health practitioners, many of which evolved in major metropolitan universities and hospitals. Few graduate training programs have concentrations in rural behavioral health, separate certification, or other credentialing programs.

There is significant variability and heterogeneity in rural environments throughout the United States. Every rural community is unique, with its own at-risk populations as well as its underlying economic, historical, political, cultural, and social structures, collectively contributing to diverse patterns of health and behavioral health problems. Population characteristics and the economic base in the rural Southwest will differ significantly when compared to population characteristics in rural Appalachia, Northern New England, the South, the Great Plains, or in the Frontier West. Moreover, no single systems delivery model of rural health and behavioral health services could be expected to serve all rural and frontier areas in the United States, just as there is no single systems delivery model for urban health and behavioral health services.

Collectively, rural populations in America have unique characteristics that impact issues of accessibility, availability, and acceptability of health and behavioral health services. Issues include sociodemographic differences (e.g., income, poverty, and education), geographic differences (distance to care), cultural differences (rural vs. urban), and perceptual differences (e.g., stigma surrounding mental illnesses).

Hospitals in rural areas tend to be smaller, older facilities that serve a higher proportion of unemployed, lower income, uninsured, or publicly insured individuals compared to urban hospitals (Phillips & Moylan, 2017). Hence, rural areas often have disproportionate populations dependent upon Medicare and Medicaid programs (Foutz, Artiga, & Garfield, 2017). Nearly two-thirds of uninsured people in rural areas live in a state that did not implement the ACA Medicaid expansion. Since uninsured or underinsured rural individuals are disproportionally affected by state decisions to not implement the expansion option, they may have fewer affordable coverage options to obtain care early (prevention) or until they are in a crisis mode (Newkirk & Damico, 2014).

More basic problems, such as insufficient transportation, electricity, water, and communication systems, have only complicated the process of providing and using rural health and behavioral health services.

Investment in health infrastructure is critical to improving quality of care and reducing disparities in the delivery of care to rural Americans (Seigel, 2018). This investment is critical to care for the number of rural residents who suffer from mental illnesses, alcohol abuse, and substance use disorders.

Epidemiology

Rural populations have historically experienced increased rates of alcohol abuse, substance use, child and spousal abuse, and depression. However, one of the basic problems facing the rural behavioral health services research field involves the estimation of the prevalence of behavioral disorders in individuals who live in rural and frontier areas as well as subsequent rural versus urban prevalence comparisons. The lack of definitive conclusions and study findings have been attributed, in part, to the variability in definitions (of both rural/urban areas and of behavioral disorders), sampling design (including potential differences in the age, ethnicity, and/or racial characteristics of the population), measurement (e.g., treated prevalence versus true prevalence), source of data, and the type of instrument utilized in rural behavioral health studies. Studies on mental illnesses may or may not include substance use disorders or co-occurring disorders. Studies may fail to address what level of severity is being examined (mild, moderate, or serious) and whether the population is being examined over a 12-month period or a lifetime.

Of the total percent of adults identified with a mental disorder in the United States, for example, it is estimated that 40.4% experienced mild disorders, 37.3% experienced moderate disorders, and 22.3% experienced serious mental disorders (Bagalman & Napili, 2018). Estimates of 12-month prevalence of mental illnesses are 24.8% among adults and estimates of 12-month prevalence of mental illnesses including substance use disorders among adults are 32.4% (Druss et al., 2009). However, these estimates may not always differentiate among rural, urban, or suburban populations or areas.

SAMHSA reports almost 20% (over 6.5 million) of residents living in non-metropolitan counties suffered from one or more behavioral health problems during 2016 (Center for Behavioral Health Statistics and Quality, 2017). Symptoms related to anxiety disorders, trauma, cognitive disorders, behavioral disorders, and psychotic disorders are often comparable to urban residents (CBHSQ, 2017), however, suicide rates in rural areas have surpassed urban suicide rates (Ivey-Stephenson, Crosby, Jack, Haileyesus, & Kresnow-Sedacca, 2017).

In addition, the highest per capita rates of complex co-occurring disorders (COD) were found in rural areas (Somers, Moniruzzaman, Rezansoff, Brink, & Russolillo, 2016). Further, rural residents who are female, poor, elderly, belong to a cultural, racial, or ethnic minority, or who are unemployed have an increased likelihood of experiencing behavioral health problems (Bardach, Tarasenko, & Schoenberg, 2011; Burholt & Scharf, 2014; Cummings, Wen, Ko, & Druss, 2013, 2014; Tjaden, 2015; Wielen et al., 2015).

The stress of ranching and farming has been a major problem in selected rural areas of America. The threat of losing family land, a home, a family, experiencing severe weather problems, and the constant preoccupation with uncertain crop production creates major stressors on many ranch and farm families. Accidents, equipment problems, social isolation, and irregular cash flow can produce unhealthy emotional reactions, often in association with behavioral and/or somatic disorders. Added stress and depression, suicidal tendencies, and substance abuse all increase the probability of already above average work-related accidents and contribute to the exacerbation of physical health conditions.

Obstacles to Services Delivery

The number of obstacles rural residents face in obtaining behavioral health services results in increased disparities compared to urban residents. It is well-established the need to implement adequate services in non-metropolitan areas was and remains a critical national behavioral health imperative (Roberts, Battaglia, & Epstein, 1999; Seigel, 2018; Wilson, Bangs, & Hatting, 2015). The availability of behavioral health services and service providers, the accessibility to services, the acceptability of these services to rural residents, and the utilization and costs of specialty services remain critical factors in rural behavioral health services delivery.

Rural American families have difficulty managing multiple health care needs due to a number of structural reasons. These challenges include: higher numbers of individuals without health care insurance or who are underinsured; fewer primary and specialty providers; time, geography, and transportation challenges; and community and employment disenfranchisement (Barker, Londeree, McBride, Kemper, & Mueller, 2013; Chavez, Kelleher, Matson, Wickizer, & Chisolm, 2018; Monnat & Beeler Pickett, 2011; Weinhold & Gurtner, 2014).

Rural poverty and persistent rural poverty are problematic. Across all four regions of the United States (Northeast, Midwest, South, and West), poverty rates were consistently higher for those living in rural areas (Semega, Fontenot, & Kollar, 2017). Further, persistent poverty, defined as a poverty rate of 20% or greater for at least four consecutive decades, is primarily a rural phenomenon, and 301 (85.3%) counties experiencing persistent poverty in the USA are rural (Economic Research Service, 2018). These structural barriers exacerbate the social determinants of health for rural populations (National Advisory Committee on Rural Health and Human Services, 2017).

It is not surprising the overall availability and volume of behavioral health services, programs, and providers increases with the population density of a community or area. Thus, the growth of behavioral health services in rural areas remains limited. Residents of rural jurisdictions face significant health challenges, including some of the highest rates of risky health behaviors and worst health outcomes of any at-risk population in the country.

In the next four sections, we borrow the framework of availability, accessibility, affordability, and acceptability, first developed by Bushy and still relevant today, at the level of national rural policy (Bushy, 1997; Wilson et al., 2015). *Availability* examines staffing or service shortages which often limit the receipts of services. *Accessibility* looks at coordination of services across the many sectors of the health, behavioral health, and social service systems and transportation to those service providers and/or facilities. *Affordability* involves the costs of care, such as direct and indirect costs, and affording insurance that covers one's needs. *Acceptability* addresses the persistent discrimination, perception, and stigma attached to the receipt of or need for behavioral health services.

Availability (Facilities and Staffing)

Rural America has suffered from continual shortages of available behavioral health and supportive services that, in turn, have restricted the array of behavioral health services in rural areas. The availability of specialty behavioral health services has been partially dependent upon the existence and availability of professionally trained behavioral health providers. The Health Resources and Services Administration uses Health Professional Shortage Areas (HPSAs) to define areas with shortages of primary medical care, dental, or mental health providers and may be geographic in nature (e.g., county or service area), population (e.g., low income,

Medicaid eligible), or facilities (e.g., federally qualified health center). The Federal definition for mental health HPSA requires the population-to-provider ratio must be at least 30,000–1 (20,000 to 1 if there are unusually high needs in the community). Mental health designations may qualify for designation based upon three criteria: (1) the population to psychiatrist ratio, (2) the population to core mental health provider (psychiatrists, clinical psychologists, clinical social workers, psychiatric nurse specialists, and marriage and family therapists) ratio, or (3) the population to both psychiatrist and core mental health provider ratios (Bureau of Health Workforce, 2018).

Over 60% of rural areas in the United States have been designated as federal mental health professional shortage areas (MH HPSAs). Of the 5119 MH HPSAs in the United States as of December 2017, there were 2718 rural MH HPSAs and 467 Partially Rural MH HPSAs across the ten HRSA regions. The total number of MH practitioners needed to remove the HPSA designation are 5985 and 2257, respectively. To achieve target ratios of 10,000:1, an additional 5985 practitioners would be required.

Unfortunately, the sparseness of rural populations as well as geography limit both the number of behavioral health providers as well as the diversity of behavioral health specialists in rural areas. In turn, these shortages in behavioral health providers as well as services significantly impact the organization and delivery of rural behavioral health services. There are proportionately fewer behavioral health

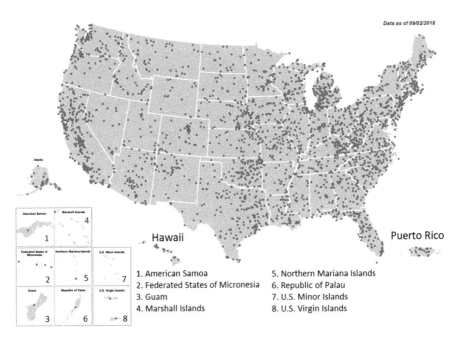

Fig. 1 HRSA Health Professional Shortage Area (HPSAs) facilities – mental health. Used with permission. Retrieved from the HRSA Map Gallery https://data.hrsa.gov/maps/map-gallery [ExportedMaps/HPSAs/HGDWMapGallery_HPSAs_MH_Facilities.pdf]

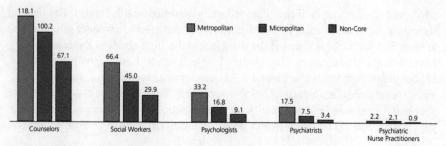

Data Sources: National Plan and Provider Enumeration System (NPPES) National Provider Identifier (NPI) data, October 2015, the U.S. Department of Agriculture Economic Research Service (ERS) Urban Influence Codes, 2013, and the 2014 Claritas U.S. population data.

Fig. 2 Behavioral health providers per 100,000 population in U.S. Counties by Urban Influence Category. Used with permission of the WWAMI Rural Health Center, University of Washington (Larson, Patterson, Garberson, & Andrilla, 2016). Note: Micropolitan and Non-Core are rural designations

providers (psychologists, social workers, and counselors) living in rural areas, regardless of education and training levels (Figs. 1 and 2).

With the rise of integrated health and behavioral health care, 40% of primary care physicians were geographically co-located with behavioral health providers in urban areas compared with co-located primary and behavioral health providers in isolated rural areas (22.8%) and in frontier areas (26.5%) (Miller et al., 2014). Although physicians often provide behavioral health care in the absence of behavioral health specialty providers, there are concerns by physicians they may not be trained sufficiently to diagnosis or treat mental or substance use disorders. A survey of family medicine physicians in rural Montana reported a number of self-limitations in behavioral health services delivery, including lack of confidence or competence and inadequate knowledge or training (Robohm, 2017).

Even rural health clinics struggle to provide mental health services (Harris et al., 2016; Kosteniuk et al., 2014; Wright, Damiano, & Bentler, 2015). A survey of Iowa rural health centers reported difficulty hiring and retaining physicians (80%), physician assistants, and nurse practitioners (both 50%), with referrals to specialists being common. With the implementation of the ACA, almost 60% of respondents also anticipated an increase in the size of their patient load; however, only 19% believed they had the human, financial, and material resources necessary to respond to those challenges (Wright et al., 2015).

Despite continuing efforts to recruit, staff, and retain rural behavioral health professionals from social work, psychology, psychiatry, and psychiatric nursing, efforts at meeting the special needs of these behavioral health professionals have been isolated and have focused on relatively few geographic areas in rural and frontier areas of the United States.

Accessibility (Coordination of Care and Community and Social Supports)

Rural residents often live farther away from health care resources and providers and therefore must travel farther to obtain needed services (Meit et al., 2014). With only a quarter of rural and frontier primary and behavioral health care providers co-located, there is an increased need for coordination of hospital, provider, and community-based services for persons with mental and substance use disorders. Since patients receiving care in the specialty mental health sector are much more likely to receive adequate care than patients receiving care in the general medical sector only, rural individuals often receive poorer quality care (Agency for Healthcare Research and Quality (AHRQ), 2017).

Emergency Room as Primary Care

It is not uncommon for individuals living in rural areas to travel hundreds of miles to seek inpatient behavioral health care because of the absence of emergency/24 h behavioral health services in their rural communities as well as the stigma still attached to the treatment of mental illnesses. While approximately 30% of rural individuals identified a hospital, emergency room, or clinic as a source of ongoing care (AHRQ, 2017), 12% of rural residents use the emergency room (ER) for behavioral health treatment (Schroeder & Leigh-Peterson, 2017). Approximately 75% of rural residents present at the ER with a primary diagnosis of a mental disorder and approximately 60% present with a primary diagnosis of a mental or substance use disorder were more likely to be on public insurance. In addition, approximately 25% of rural elderly present to the ER with a mental health problem (Schroeder & Leigh-Peterson, 2017).

The requirement to drive so far away to receive care and not be able to receive referrals for continuity of care in one's local communities reduces rural residents' ability to have consistency in care, follow-up, and provider. Further, rural behavioral health providers and agencies, often over-extended with large client caseloads, may not have the time or expertise to seek additional or supplemental support for needed programs, especially outside of their standard service area(s) or case management partnerships, or for complex, co-occurring disorders (Mowbray, McBeath, Bank, & Newell, 2016; Nover, 2014). Mowbray et al. (2016) describe the challenges of coordinating behavioral health and social services to rural corrections-involved populations.

Integrated Care Coordination

There remains heterogeneity in the organizational models of behavioral health services delivery. For example, while some states and communities organize behavioral health services together with substance abuse services in a single agency, other states have separate agencies for behavioral health and substance abuse services. In addition, selected states house behavioral health and substance abuse services in an umbrella human services agency.

Nevertheless, the scarcity of rural behavioral health services and rural behavioral health providers together with continual changes in the organization, financing, and delivery of health and behavioral health services (through provider networks and managed care) provides strong incentives for linking or integrating behavioral health services with primary health care. Models include integrated provider teams and collaboration and partnerships between behavioral health services and other human services organizations through co-locations, site visits, shared facilities, and joint staff activities. One benefit of integrated care is the "medical cost offset effect", or the decrease in medical care utilization and costs after the introduction of an integrated behavioral health component within a comprehensive health care program, which can assist with the coordination of care for complex co-morbid conditions (Cummings, O'Donohue, & Cummings, 2009).

Individuals with serious mental illness are at an increased risk for developing co-morbid chronic physical illnesses. The CalMEND Pilot Collaborative to Integrate Primary Care and Mental Health Services was an attempt to address the needs of this population (Nover, 2014). Focused on quality assurance, intra- and inter-agency teamwork, and access to adequate primary care for this population, the CalMEND Pilot showed it was able to improve collaboration among the six CPCI pilot partnerships by unifying primary care and behavioral health providers. It focused on team-driven care with the design, development, and running of effective care teams, implementing clinical workflows supportive of integrated care, and improved care management among persons with complex, co-occurring disorders (Nover, 2014). For additional reading on the integration of physical and behavioral health care, see Chapter "Integration of Primary Care and Behavioral Health" in this volume.

Safety Net Clinics

There are numerous challenges common to safety net clinics. These include limited access to specialists for Medicaid and uninsured patients, difficulty communicating with external providers, and payment models with limited support for care integration activities (Derrett et al., 2014). A study of clinicians in 150 safety net primary care clinics in Washington State, primarily Federally Qualified Health Centers or Rural Health Clinics, found that most respondents believed the integrated health/ behavioral health program was beneficial (Williams, Eckstrom, Avery, & Unützer, 2015). Rural respondents approved of the flexibility of the program when planning care. However, social service limitations (e.g., housing or transportation services) were identified more often as program limitations and a lack of awareness of program resources by other team members (Williams et al., 2015).

Telehealth, e-Health, and m-Health

Considering many of the challenges in accessibility for residents of rural and frontier areas, telehealth and emerging e-/m-health technologies may be able to surmount these barriers. In their retrospective review of Medicare data, Mehrotra et al. (2017) found the number of telemental health visits not only grew on average 45.1% annually but by 2014, there were 5.3 and 11.8 telemental health visits per 100 rural residents with mental illnesses. Residents who received telemental health services tended to be younger, have disabilities, and live in poorer communities.

Also, states with telemedicine parity laws and regulatory environments had significantly higher utilization than other states. In their review of Medicaid data in the 22 states with telehealth reimbursement, Douglas et al. (2017) found the highest utilization of telemedicine (95%) was predominantly used to treat persons with behavioral health diagnoses. Patients were more likely to live in a rural area with a managed care plan, have an aged, blind, and disabled criteria, and be males 45–64 years of age. Douglas and colleagues also determined that reimbursement alone was not enough to drive the use of telemedicine; it is critical to more closely examine state-specific reimbursement and licensure policies on telemedicine.

These studies, with others, illustrate the challenges and issues involved in licensing, liability, and accreditation when it comes to the provision of mental health and substance use services. For example, when six states in the nation allowed telemental health counseling across state lines with full and reciprocal privileges, but due to the states' interpretation of Medicare/Medicaid rulings on telehealth reimbursement, providers receive unequal reimbursement for services rendered.

Health care professionals have to address limitations in scope of practice, difficulties with in-state and interstate credentialing, lack of portability of practitioner licenses, remote prescribing, not to mention immunity and liability issues that may occur when dealing with emergency or crisis events. However, there is progress being made. Since 2016, more states have addressed these key regulatory questions. For example, Arkansas, Hawaii, Indiana, Louisiana, and Maine established regulations that allow patient relationships and evaluations to be established via real-time audio and visual telehealth technologies (Epstein Becker Green, 2017).

Affordability (Individual and System)

Affordability involves the costs of care, and for many that centers on the affordability of health insurance. For others, affordability also examines system issues that affect affordability of care, such as provider reimbursement, which affect availability of services and resources.

Historically, individuals living in rural areas were more likely to have their mental health services paid for by public insurance and less likely paid by private insurance than individuals living in more urban areas. Today, rural individuals with serious or persistent mental illnesses (SMI/SPMI) still remain more likely to have their mental health services paid by public insurance. They were also more likely to pay out-of-pocket costs compared to individuals with SMI living in urban areas (Harman, Fortney, Dong, & Xu, 2010).

With the implementation of the Patient Protection and Affordable Care Act in 2010 and Medicaid expansion, there have been more opportunities for rural individuals to obtain health coverage for behavioral disorders. However, states that did not accept Medicaid expansion created significant gaps in coverage as households, with incomes between 18% and 99% of the federal poverty level (FPL) were ineligible for Medicaid or to enroll in the health insurance exchange (HIE) marketplace. Rural residents were less likely than urban residents to use the Marketplace.

In states, such as Texas, there were 1,101,000 adults in the insurance gap, accounting for almost a quarter of all uninsured persons in Texas (Gong, Huey, Johnson, Curti, & Philips, 2016, 2017). The gap was significantly higher in rural East and South Texas and in Texas as a whole. One-third of the enrollees previously had private or employer-based insurance before enrollment into the Marketplace. By 2014, the number of uninsured adults was reduced by 710,000, with two-thirds of the enrollees in the Marketplace (Gong et al., 2016, 2017). In rural Wisconsin, enrollments in public insurance led to substantial increases in outpatient visits but not mental health visits (Burns et al., 2014).

How individuals chose health insurance plans may be related to a number of factors, including comprehension of insurance terminology and language, numeracy, consistency of options across choices, and the number of available plans. Hence, the ability of an individual to choose an affordable option may depend upon improving the consumer's ability to comprehend the intricacies of health insurance (Barnes, Hanoch, & Rice, 2015, 2016).

Interventions designed to improve rates of mental health treatment, such as the collaborative care models, are usually based on private payers, such as managed care organizations which are less likely to operate in rural areas. However, in addition to shortages of providers, third party payers have placed restrictions on both the delivery and reimbursement of behavioral health services. For rural behavioral health settings, this has primarily affected Medicare and Medicaid entitlement programs. Although licensed behavioral health practitioners from various disciplines may be reimbursed for behavioral health services, physicians continue to receive supervisory and medication authority, legal responsibility, and accountability for behavioral health treatment, despite the severe shortage of physicians trained and/or interested in behavioral health treatment in rural areas. Furthermore, the particular behavioral health providers who are "approved" to deliver behavioral health services vary in terms of the health and behavioral health service settings, states, and funding sources. This has been particularly important with the introduction of new health care strategies and developing provider networks in rural areas in America.

Acceptability (Values, Traditions, Culture)

Acceptability refers to the provision of behavioral health services in a way that is compatible with the values of the populations at-risk. Rural values, attitudes, and traditions may limit the utilization of behavioral health services. Given the racial, ethnic, and cultural diversity among rural populations, acceptability of behavioral health services may be difficult to achieve for a number of reasons, including: established self-care practices; specific behavioral health etiologic beliefs; the lack of knowledge about behavioral health services, gatekeeping, and treatment for these services; and the location of behavioral health treatment settings.

Acceptability of rural behavioral health services may also be influenced by the urban education and training orientation of behavioral health providers. How practitioners learn to work with rural populations potentially affects the establishment of trust during the construction of the behavioral health provider-consumer relationship. This relationship directly impacts the success of rural behavioral health outreach and aftercare programs. If the rural behavioral health outreach providers are viewed as community outsiders, then the helping relationship will not be established. Thus, careful recruiting and retaining of behavioral health professionals for work in rural areas is critical in planning and implementing rural behavioral health programs.

Community acceptability is also critical for the survival and effectiveness of rural behavioral health programs (Bushy, 1997). To help ensure that a program is acceptable by a population at-risk for behavioral disorders, a community needs assessment should be conducted prior to the planning and implementation of a new rural behavioral health program. The collection and thorough understanding of cultural data is critical so that the provision of rural behavioral health services will be made available in a manner consistent with the cultures of at-risk populations.

Behavioral health providers should consider a number of factors for a rural behavioral health needs assessment initiative, including: population density; travel; time and work-related issues; customs, values, and traditions related to behavioral health services; and patterns of natural events. Thus, behavioral health programs will not thrive unless personal, employment, cultural, and enviro-behavioral factors are taken into consideration.

Implications for Behavioral Health

The shortage of rural behavioral health professionals, the limited availability of behavioral health services, and the relative dependence upon government entitlement programs for the financing of rural and frontier behavioral health services has contributed to significant problems for rural communities. These problems include: rural residents not receiving needed behavioral health services; rural individuals not receiving timely behavioral health services, potentially increasing the cost, duration, and level of behavioral health care; and the provision of treatment for behavioral disorders in service settings far from the home community.

The Rural Healthy People 2020 survey found that mental health and mental disorders remain the fourth most often identified rural health priority (Bolin et al., 2015). Many of the basic service delivery issues and challenges in the organization and delivery of rural behavioral health services have not been addressed effectively or consistently by policymakers and legislators.

Two decades ago, Roberts et al. (1999) concluded the "implementation of adequate services in non-metropolitan areas is a critical national health imperative." The California Rural Health Policy Council (1998) defined the ideal rural health care delivery system as addressing three components. First, the system would integrate fully locally defined health- and prevention-related services. Second, it would incorporate broad community engagement and collaboration. Finally, strategic planning would be locally driven with measurable outcomes for the community.

More recent recommendations, such as the emphasis on (re)building rural infrastructure from the National Rural Health Association (Seigel, 2018), again reinforce what behavioral health providers, consumers, advocates, and researchers have known for some time: although health care in the United States is generally viewed by most in society as a right (of citizenship), behavioral health care is not a part of that right.

Nevertheless, the era of tremendous change in health and behavioral health care will continue in the foreseeable future. While challenges remain in addressing severe shortages in rural behavioral health providers as well as building successful models of rural managed behavioral health services delivery, we see a strategic rural focus on the following key elements in behavioral health services delivery:

1. continued consumer and family involvement in program, policy, and clinical decision making and outcomes (MacDonald-Wilson, Schuster, & Wasilchak, 2015; Nelson, Barr, & Castaldo, 2015);
2. integration models that address patient centeredness and normative aspects of care across functional, organizational, professional and service components within integrated primary care/mental health programs (Bachrach, Boozang, & Davis, 2017; Bird, Lambert, Hartley, Beeson, & Coburn, 1998; van der Klauw, Molema, Grooten, & Vrijhoef, 2014), and,
3. clinical, service provision, cultural, and management competence (or rural practice expertise) of rural behavioral health providers, especially in the adoption and implementation of evidence-based practices (Dotson et al., 2014; Weaver, Capobianco, & Ruffolo, 2015).

Through public and private services delivery partnerships, coalitions of consumers and providers, integration of health and behavioral health providers and services, telecommunication technologies, and targeted as well as experiential education and training programs for practitioners, rural and frontier communities have the potential of building stronger, more vital behavioral health services.

References

Agency for Healthcare Research and Quality (AHRQ). (2017, October). *National healthcare quality and disparities report: Chartbook on rural health care*. Rockville, MD: Author. Retrieved from https://www.ahrq.gov/sites/default/files/wysiwyg/research/findings/nhqrdr/chartbooks/qdr-ruralhealthchartbook-update.pdf

Bachrach, D., Boozang, P. M., & Davis, H. E. (2017). How Arizona Medicaid accelerated the integration of physical and behavioral health services. *Issue Brief (Commonwealth Fund), 14*, 1–11.

Bagalman, E., & Napili, A. (2018, January 19). *Prevalence of mental illness in the United States: Data sources and estimates*. Washington, DC: Congressional Research Service. Retrieved from http://www.fas.org/sgp/crs/misc/R43047.pdf

Bardach, S. H., Tarasenko, Y. N., & Schoenberg, N. E. (2011). The role of social support in multiple morbidity: Self-management among rural residents. *Journal of Health Care for the Poor and Underserved, 22*(3), 756–771. https://doi.org/10.1353/hpu.2011.0083

Barker, A. R., Londeree, J. K., McBride, T. D., Kemper, L. M., & Mueller, K. (2013). The uninsured: An analysis by income and geography. *Rural Policy Brief*(2013 6), 1–4.

Barnes, A. J., Hanoch, Y., & Rice, T. (2015). Determinants of coverage decisions in health insurance marketplaces: Consumers' decision-making abilities and the amount of information in their choice environment. *Health Services Research, 50*(1), 58–80. https://doi.org/10.1111/1475-6773.12181

Barnes, A. J., Hanoch, Y., & Rice, T. (2016). Can plan recommendations improve the coverage decisions of vulnerable populations in health insurance marketplaces? *PLoS One, 11*(3), e0151095. https://doi.org/10.1371/journal.pone.0151095

Bird, D. C., Lambert, D., Hartley, D., Beeson, P. G., & Coburn, A. F. (1998). Rural models for integrating primary care and mental health services. *Administration and Policy in Mental Health, 25*(3), 287–308.

Bolin, J. N., Bellamy, G. R., Ferdinand, A. O., Vuong, A. M., Kash, B. A., Schulze, A., & Helduser, J. W. (2015). Rural healthy people 2020: New decade, same challenges. *The Journal of Rural Health, 31*(3), 326–333. https://doi.org/10.1111/jrh.12116

Bureau of Health Workforce. (2018). *Designated health professional shortage areas statistics: Designated HPSA quarterly summary, as of December 31, 2017*. [Web page]. U.S. Department of Health & Human Services, Health Resources and Services Administration. Retrieved from https://ersrs.hrsa.gov/ReportServer?/HGDW_Reports/BCD_HPSA/BCD_HPSA_SCR50_Qtr_Smry_HTML&rc:Toolbar=false

Burholt, V., & Scharf, T. (2014). Poor health and loneliness in later life: The role of depressive symptoms, social resources, and rural environments. *The Journals of Gerontology. Series B, Psychological Sciences and Social Sciences, 69*(2), 311–324. https://doi.org/10.1093/geronb/gbt121

Burns, M. E., Dague, L., DeLeire, T., Dorsch, M., Friedsam, D., Leininger, L. J., … Voskuil, K. (2014). The effects of expanding public insurance to rural low-income childless adults. *Health Services Research, 49*(Suppl 2), 2173–2187. https://doi.org/10.1111/1475-6773.12233

Bushy, A. (1997). Mental health and substance abuse: Challenges in providing services to rural clients. In Center for Substance Abuse Treatment (Ed.), *Bringing excellence to substance abuse services in rural and frontier America* (pp. 45–54). Rockville, MD: U.S. Department of Health and Human Services, Rural Information Center Health Service.

California Rural Health Policy Council. (1998). 1998 report on collaboration and innovation in rural health: Part II. In *Annual report to the legislature and planned future actions*. Sacramento, CA: California Rural Health Policy Council.

Center for Behavioral Health Statistics and Quality. (2017, September 7). *Results from the 2016 National Survey on Drug Use and Health: Detailed tables: Prevalence estimates, standard errors, p values, and sample sizes*. Rockville, MD: Substance Abuse and Mental Health Services Administration. Retrieved from https://www.samhsa.gov/data/sites/default/files/NSDUH-DetTabs-2016/NSDUH-DetTabs-2016.pdf

Chavez, L. J., Kelleher, K. J., Matson, S. C., Wickizer, T. M., & Chisolm, D. J. (2018). Mental health and substance use care among young adults before and after Affordable Care Act (ACA) implementation: A rural and urban comparison. *The Journal of Rural Health, 34*(1), 42–47. https://doi.org/10.1111/jrh.12258

Cromartie, J. (2017, November). *Rural America at a glance, 2017 edition* (Economic Information Bulletin No. (EIB-182)). Washington, DC: U.S. Census Bureau, Economic Research Service. Retrieved from https://www.ers.usda.gov/webdocs/publications/85740/eib-182.pdf?v=43054

Cummings, N. A., O'Donohue, W. T., & Cummings, J. L. (2009). The financial dimension of integrated behavioral/primary care. *Journal of Clinical Psychology in Medical Settings, 16*(1), 31–39. https://doi.org/10.1007/s10880-008-9139-2

Cummings, J. R., Wen, H., Ko, M., & Druss, B. G. (2013). Geography and the Medicaid mental health care infrastructure: Implications for health care reform. *JAMA Psychiatry, 70*(10), 1084–1090. https://doi.org/10.1001/jamapsychiatry.2013.377

Cummings, J. R., Wen, H., Ko, M., & Druss, B. G. (2014). Race/ethnicity and geographic access to Medicaid substance use disorder treatment facilities in the United States. *JAMA Psychiatry, 71*(2), 190–196. https://doi.org/10.1001/jamapsychiatry.2013.3575

Derrett, S., Gunter, K. E., Nocon, R. S., Quinn, M. T., Coleman, K., Daniel, D. M., … Chin, M. H. (2014). How 3 rural safety net clinics integrate care for patients: A qualitative case study. *Medical Care, 52*(11 Suppl 4), S39–S47. https://doi.org/10.1097/mlr.0000000000000191

Dotson, J. A., Roll, J. M., Packer, R. R., Lewis, J. M., McPherson, S., & Howell, D. (2014). Urban and rural utilization of evidence-based practices for substance use and mental health disorders. *The Journal of Rural Health, 30*(3), 292–299. https://doi.org/10.1111/jrh.12068

Douglas, M. D., Xu, J., Heggs, A., Wrenn, G., Mack, D. H., & Rust, G. (2017). Assessing telemedicine utilization by using Medicaid claims data. *Psychiatric Services, 68*(2), 173–178. https://doi.org/10.1176/appi.ps.201500518

Druss, B. G., Hwang, I., Petukhova, M., Sampson, N. A., Wang, P. S., & Kessler, R. C. (2009). Impairment in role functioning in mental and chronic medical disorders in the United States: Results from the National Comorbidity Survey Replication. *Molecular Psychiatry, 14*(7), 728–737. https://doi.org/10.1038/mp.2008.13

Economic Research Service. (2017, August 9). *Frontier and remote area codes: Documentation*. [Web page]. Washington, DC: U. S. Department of Agriculture. Retrieved from https://www.ers.usda.gov/data-products/frontier-and-remote-area-codes/documentation/

Economic Research Service. (2018, April 18). *Rural poverty & well-being*. [Web page]. Washington, DC: U. S. Department of Agriculture. Retrieved from https://www.ers.usda.gov/topics/rural-economy-population/rural-poverty-well-being/

Epstein Becker Green. (2017). *50-state survey of telemental/telebehavioral health (2017 appendix)*. Washington, DC: Author. Retrieved from https://www.ebglaw.com/content/uploads/2017/10/EPSTEIN-BECKER-GREEN-2017-APPENDIX-50-STATE-TELEMENTAL-HEALTH-SURVEY.pdf

Foutz, J., Artiga, S., & Garfield, R. (2017, April). *The role of Medicaid in rural America: Issue brief*. Menlo Park, CA: Kaiser Family Foundation. Retrieved from http://files.kff.org/attachment/Issue-Brief-The-Role-of-Medicaid-in-Rural-America

Gong, G., Huey, C. C., Johnson, C., Curti, D., & Philips, B. U. (2016). Enrollment in health insurance through the marketplace after implementation of the Affordable Care Act in Texas. *Texas Medicine, 112*(10), e1.

Gong, G., Huey, C. C., Johnson, C., Curti, D., & Philips, B. U., Jr. (2017). The health insurance gap after implementation of the Affordable Care Act in Texas. *Texas Medicine, 113*(3), e1.

Harman, J. S., Fortney, J. C., Dong, F., & Xu, S. (2010, February). *Assessment of the mental health funding marketplace in urban vs. rural settings: Findings brief.* Boulder, CO: Western Interstate Commission for Higher Education. Retrieved from https://www.wiche.edu/info/publications/HarmanYear4Project3FindingsBrief.pdf

Harris, J. K., Beatty, K., Leider, J. P., Knudson, A., Anderson, B. L., & Meit, M. (2016). The double disparity facing rural local health departments. *Annual Review of Public Health, 37*, 167–184. https://doi.org/10.1146/annurev-publhealth-031914-122755

Ivey-Stephenson, A. Z., Crosby, A. E., Jack, S. P. D., Haileyesus, T., & Kresnow-Sedacca, M. J. (2017). Suicide trends among and within urbanization levels by sex, race/ethnicity, age group, and mechanism of death - United States, 2001-2015. *Morbidity and Mortality Weekly Report. Surveillance Summaries, 66*(18), 1–16. https://doi.org/10.15585/mmwr.ss6618a1

Kosteniuk, J., Morgan, D., Innes, A., Keady, J., Stewart, N., D'Arcy, C., & Kirk, A. (2014). Who steers the ship? Rural family physicians' views on collaborative care models for patients with dementia. *Primary Health Care Research & Development, 15*(1), 104–110. https://doi.org/10.1017/s146342361300011x

Larson, E. H., Patterson, D. G., Garberson, L. A., & Andrilla, C. H. A. (2016, September). *Supply and distribution of the behavioral health workforce in rural America* (Data Brief #160). Seattle, WA: WWAMI Rural Health Center, University of Washington. Retrieved from http://depts.washington.edu/fammed/rhrc/wp-content/uploads/sites/4/2016/09/RHRC_DB160_Larson.pdf

MacDonald-Wilson, K. L., Schuster, J. M., & Wasilchak, D. (2015). In managed behavioral health care, a seat at the table is not enough. *Psychiatric Rehabilitation Journal, 38*(4), 374–376. https://doi.org/10.1037/prj0000167

Mehrotra, A., Huskamp, H. A., Souza, J., Uscher-Pines, L., Rose, S., Landon, B. E., … Busch, A. B. (2017). Rapid growth in mental health telemedicine use among rural Medicare beneficiaries, wide variation across states. *Health Affairs, 36*(5), 909–917. https://doi.org/10.1377/hlthaff.2016.1461

Meit, M., Knudson, A., Gilbert, T., Yu, A. T.-C., Tanenbaum, E., Ormson, E., … NORC Walsh Center for Rural Health Analysis. (2014, October). *The 2014 update of the rural-urban chartbook.* Bethesda, MD: Rural Health Reform Policy Research Center. Retrieved from https://ruralhealth.und.edu/projects/health-reform-policy-research-center/pdf/2014-rural-urban-chartbookupdate.pdf

Miller, B. F., Petterson, S., Brown Levey, S. M., Payne-Murphy, J. C., Moore, M., & Bazemore, A. (2014). Primary care, behavioral health, provider colocation, and rurality. *Journal of the American Board of Family Medicine, 27*(3), 367–374. https://doi.org/10.3122/jabfm.2014.03.130260

Monnat, S. M., & Beeler Pickett, C. (2011). Rural/urban differences in self-rated health: Examining the roles of county size and metropolitan adjacency. *Health & Place, 17*(1), 311–319. https://doi.org/10.1016/j.healthplace.2010.11.008

Mowbray, O., McBeath, B., Bank, L., & Newell, S. (2016). Trajectories of health and behavioral health services use among community corrections-involved rural adults. *Social Work Research, 40*(1), 7–18. https://doi.org/10.1093/swr/svv048

National Advisory Committee on Rural Health and Human Services. (2017, January). *Social determinants of health* (Issue Brief). Washington, DC: Author. Retrieved from https://www.hrsa.gov/sites/default/files/hrsa/advisory-committees/rural/publications/2017-social-determinants.pdf

National Center for Frontier Communities. (2007). *The consensus definition - 2007 update.* Silver City, NM: Author. Retrieved from http://frontierus.org/wp-content/uploads/2007/01/consensus-definition-2007-update.pdf

Nelson, W. A., Barr, P. J., & Castaldo, M. G. (2015). The opportunities and challenges for shared decision-making in the rural United States. *HEC Forum, 27*(2), 157–170. https://doi.org/10.1007/s10730-015-9283-7

Newkirk, V., & Damico, A. (2014, May 29). *The Affordable Care Act and insurance coverage in rural areas: Issue brief.* San Francisco, CA: Kaiser Family Foundation. Retrieved from https://www.kff.org/uninsured/issue-brief/the-affordable-care-act-and-insurance-coverage-in-rural-areas/

Nover, C. H. (2014). Implementing a mental health and primary care partnership program in Placer County, California. *Social Work in Health Care, 53*(2), 156–182. https://doi.org/10.1080/00981389.2013.864378

Patient Protection and Affordable Care Act, U.S.C. 42 §18001, Pub. L. No. 111–148. (2010). Retrieved from https://www.congress.gov/111/plaws/publ148/PLAW-111publ148.pdf

Phillips, S., & Moylan, C. (2017). *Data shows rural hospitals at risk without special attention from lawmakers.* Nashville, TN: Healthcare Management Partners, LLC. Retrieved from https://hcmpllc.com/wp-content/uploads/2017/06/2017-6-28-CORRECTED-Rev.-HMP-Study-AHCA-Imperils-Rural-Hospitals.pdf

Ratcliffe, M., Burd, C., Holder, K., & Fields, A. (2016, December). *Defining rural at the U.S. Census Bureau* (ACSGEO-1). Washington, DC: U.S. Census Bureau. Retrieved from https://www2.census.gov/geo/pdfs/reference/ua/Defining_Rural.pdf

Roberts, L. W., Battaglia, J., & Epstein, R. S. (1999). Frontier ethics: Mental health care needs and ethical dilemmas in rural communities. *Psychiatric Services, 50*(4), 497–503. https://doi.org/10.1176/ps.50.4.497

Robohm, J. S. (2017). Training to reduce behavioral health disparities: How do we optimally prepare family medicine residents for practice in rural communities? *International Journal of Psychiatry in Medicine, 52*(3), 298–312. https://doi.org/10.1177/0091217417730294

Schroeder, S., & Leigh-Peterson, M. (2017, June). *Rural and urban utilization of the emergency department for mental health and substance abuse* (Rural Health Reform Policy Research Center Issue Brief). Grand Fork, ND; Bethesda, MD: Center for Rural Health; NORC Walsh Center for Rural Health Analysis. Retrieved from https://ruralhealth.und.edu/assets/355-922/rural-urban-utilization-emergency-department.pdf

Seigel, J. (2018, February 20). Rebuild rural: The importance of health care in infrastructure. *Rural Health Voices.* [Web page]. Washington, DC; Leawood, KS: National Rural Health Association. Retrieved from https://www.ruralhealthweb.org/blogs/ruralhealthvoices/february-2018/rebuild-rural-the-importance-of-health-care-in-in

Semega, J. L., Fontenot, K. R., & Kollar, M. A. (2017). *Income, poverty and health insurance coverage in the United States: 2016* (Current Population Reports, P60-259). Washington, DC: U.S. Census Bureau. Retrieved from https://www.census.gov/content/dam/Census/library/publications/2017/demo/P60-259.pdf

Somers, J. M., Moniruzzaman, A., Rezansoff, S. N., Brink, J., & Russolillo, A. (2016). The prevalence and geographic distribution of complex co-occurring disorders: A population study. *Epidemiology and Psychiatric Sciences, 25*(3), 267–277. https://doi.org/10.1017/s2045796015000347

Tjaden, K. (2015). Health disparities between rural and urban women in Minnesota. *Minnesota Medicine, 98*(10), 40–43.

van der Klauw, D., Molema, H., Grooten, L., & Vrijhoef, H. (2014). Identification of mechanisms enabling integrated care for patients with chronic diseases: A literature review. *International Journal of Integrated Care, 14*, e024. Retrieved from https://www.ncbi.nlm.nih.gov/pmc/articles/PMC4109400/pdf/IJIC-14-2014024.pdf

Weaver, A., Capobianco, J., & Ruffolo, M. (2015). Systematic review of EBPs for SMI in rural America. *Journal of Evidence-Informed Social Work, 12*(2), 155–165. https://doi.org/10.1080/15433714.2013.765815

Weinhold, I., & Gurtner, S. (2014). Understanding shortages of sufficient health care in rural areas. *Health Policy, 118*(2), 201–214. https://doi.org/10.1016/j.healthpol.2014.07.018

Wielen, L. M., Gilchrist, E. C., Nowels, M. A., Petterson, S. M., Rust, G., & Miller, B. F. (2015). Not near enough: Racial and ethnic disparities in access to nearby behavioral health care and primary care. *Journal of Health Care for the Poor and Underserved, 26*(3), 1032–1047. https://doi.org/10.1353/hpu.2015.0083

Williams, D., Eckstrom, J., Avery, M., & Unützer, J. (2015). Perspectives of behavioral health clinicians in a rural integrated primary care/mental health program. *The Journal of Rural Health, 31*(4), 346–353. https://doi.org/10.1111/jrh.12114

Wilson, W., Bangs, A., & Hatting, T. (2015, February). *Future of rural behavioral health* (National Rural Health Association Policy Brief). Washington, DC; Leawood, KS: National Rural Health Association. Retrieved from https://www.ruralhealthweb.org/NRHA/media/Emerge_NRHA/Advocacy/Policy%20documents/The-Future-of-Rural-Behavioral-Health_Feb-2015.pdf

Wright, B., Damiano, P. C., & Bentler, S. E. (2015). Implementation of the Affordable Care Act and rural health clinic capacity in Iowa. *Journal of Primary Care & Community Health, 6*(1), 61–65. https://doi.org/10.1177/2150131914542613

Reframing the Concept of Cultural Competence to Enhance Delivery of Behavioral Health Services to Culturally Diverse Populations

Linda M. Callejas and Mario Hernandez

This chapter presents readers with a practical framework for making behavioral health services and supports accessible and appropriate for culturally diverse populations. It begins with an overview of important concepts, particularly behavioral health disparities and health equity, which have shaped research and practice efforts aimed at ensuring that all people receive the services and supports they need. It follows with an examination of "cultural competence" as a concept and how it has evolved. An implementation-based conceptual model is also presented, which operationalizes cultural competence from an organizational perspective and discusses issues with regard to its implementation in service delivery settings, as well as implications for future research and practice.

Introduction

The latter half of the twentieth century witnessed a growing recognition that rapid changes in the cultural diversity of the population in the United States must be considered when designing and implementing behavioral health services. Following social movements that called for greater civic inclusion of minority groups during the Civil Rights era, social scientists and health practitioners in the 1970s and 1980s began highlighting persistent and troubling disparities in health status and access to services among historically underserved populations. With regard to behavioral health, research concerning the prevalence of mental illnesses among racial and ethnic minority groups has found little difference in rates of specific disorders but has documented differences in referral patterns, problem manifestations,

L. M. Callejas (✉) · M. Hernandez
Department of Child and Family Studies, College of Behavioral and Community Sciences, University of South Florida, Tampa, FL, USA
e-mail: callejas@usf.edu

© Springer Nature Switzerland AG 2020
B. L. Levin, A. Hanson (eds.), *Foundations of Behavioral Health*,
https://doi.org/10.1007/978-3-030-18435-3_15

321

applicability of assessment protocols, and diagnoses (Coard & Holden, 1998; Yeh, McCabe, Hough, Dupuis, & Hazen, 2003). In addition, researchers have found the burden of mental illness was higher for minority populations, who were found to be persistently underserved and/or inappropriately served in this country's behavioral health systems (Alegría et al., 2004; Chow, Jaffee, & Snowden, 2003; Hough et al., 2002; Kataoka, Zhang, & Wells, 2002; President's New Freedom Commission on Mental Health, 2003).

By 2005, the rapidly growing body of disparities research was focused more specifically on examining the underlying social causes for consistent and adverse behavioral health outcomes found in minority populations and more deliberately identified them as *health inequalities* or differences understood to be "avoidable, unnecessary, and unjust" (see Braveman, 2014, p. 7; see also Whitehead, 1990). In support of this position, researchers and policymakers in the United States are more explicitly concentrating their contemporary efforts achieving on *health equity*, defined at the federal level as:

> attainment of the highest level of health for all people. Achieving health equity requires valuing everyone equally with focused and ongoing societal efforts to address avoidable inequalities, historical and contemporary injustices, and the elimination of health and healthcare disparities (Rollins, 2011, p. 9)

The ongoing development of knowledge regarding health equity has benefitted from an examination of the complex roles that culture and society play with regard to behavioral health, mental illnesses, and the delivery of services (US Department of Health and Human Services [DHHS], 2001). Understanding the universality of culture within the human experience and its role in the formation of identity can prepare behavioral health practitioners to understand the underlying social conditions that are now thought to cause and/or exacerbate disparities.

What Is Culture?

As with most theoretical concepts, culture is a complex, multifaceted one. It has multiple definitions and aspects, used by a variety of professionals and disciplines, and many of these definitions are interrelated and therefore nuanced in their differences. Although there is no authoritative definition of culture, the most widely accepted definition of the term and many of its variants are derived from the definition first set forth in 1871, by Tyler (1923). More recent definitions include the importance of symbolic representation or the unique human ability to invent meanings for observable phenomena (also known as "cultural invention"), to act as if those meanings are true and to pass these meanings on to others (see Smedley & Smedley, 2005, p. 17). We use the following definition to frame this chapter's discussion of how culture shapes human experience and identity and thereby provide a foundation for the development of more responsive behavioral health service delivery processes for diverse populations:

The system of shared beliefs, values, customs, behaviors, and artifacts that the members of society use to cope with their world and with one another, and that are transmitted from generation to generation through learning. (Bates & Plog, 1990, p. 7)

Culture is therefore dynamic and changes over time, in response to ever-changing environmental conditions (see Guarnaccia & Rodriguez, 1996; Harris, 1968).

Reframing the concept of culture in this way allows behavioral health practitioners and other professionals to more fully appreciate how categories and identities that unify groups of people, such as "race," "ethnicity," "gender," "disability," "age," and "social class," are socially constructed and culturally reproduced over time. The concept of race provides a useful vehicle for exploring how difference is structured through the creation, development, and application of categories at a national level. Although a discussion of the creation and development of race and its application throughout the Americas is beyond the scope of this chapter, race has been a defining feature of the social fabric of this country for centuries. Further, although racial identity has largely been ascribed based on phenotypical characteristics, the ideology of race has emphasized the principle that racial differences are biologically rooted thereby allowing for the proliferation of widespread belief that differences between racial groups are genetically measurable (Fine, Ibrahim, & Thomas, 2005).

Examination of the socially rooted aspect of race in the United States, in particular, also allows behavioral health practitioners to understand how other identities, such as gender identity or sexual identity, are often understood as biologically based despite changing societal meanings associated with these categories (see Brooks & Bolzendahl, 2004; Diamond & Butterworth, 2008; Drescher, 2009). Disability, age, and social class may also be understood as cultures and, as such, are laden with meanings and identities. Any of these identities, singly or in combination, may influence the delivery and utilization of services.

Researchers and practitioners have recommended the provision of culturally competent services as a means of reducing behavioral health disparities and increasing health equity. However, the term has remained a largely philosophical concept that lacks clarity with regard to operationalization in research and implementation in practice. Operationalization of cultural competence is needed if behavioral health researchers and practitioners are to continue relying on this concept for guidance on how to reduce behavioral health disparities among diverse populations.

Review of the Literature

The concept of cultural competence in service delivery emerged in the late 1980s to address what providers and researchers were finding in their work with diverse communities: adverse outcomes in behavioral health among "minority" populations. Perhaps the most well-known definition is the one established by Cross, Bazron, Dennis, and Isaacs in 1989. However, a number of researchers have questioned the utility of relying on the cultural competence concept for establishing clear-cut implementation strategies that can direct behavioral health research and practice (see Hernandez, Nesman, Mowery, Acevedo-Polakovich, & Callejas, 2009; Kleinman & Benson, 2006; Saha et al., 2013). While the concept has gained widespread recognition and provoked changes in thinking about serving diverse communities, cultural competence has remained largely an ideology with a set of guiding principles that lack clear operationalization (Saha et al., 2013; Vega & Lopez, 2001). As Saha et al. (2013, p. 626) argue, the proliferation of the concept in behavioral health and beyond is "largely based on expert opinions about the theoretical benefits [of the concept]… rather than empirical research." Researchers have also been critical of the way in which the cultural competence philosophy has developed over time, often leading to training and workshops that focus on "teaching about the 'cultures' of non-white racial and ethnic groups" (Malat, 2013, p. 605).

Notwithstanding best intentions, Malat (2013) argues that such training serves to reinforce stereotypes as opposed to helping providers critically examine systemic issues, such as institutionalized racism, poverty, and, ultimately, persistent social inequality, and how these factors may create and/or exacerbate behavioral health disparities. In essence, this state of affairs can be seen as ensuring the continuous promotion of cultural generalizations and racial stereotypes and, potentially, lending support (inadvertent though it might be) to a larger social environment that can exacerbate negative differences in behavioral health outcomes among diverse groups. Cultural competence therefore has gained status as an ideology; yet, it has not resulted in a testable theory of its application or its ability to ameliorate racial disparities (Malat, 2013). Interestingly, despite its lack of operationalization and because it has achieved ideological status, the concept of cultural competence maintains a prominent position as a key concept in the behavioral health field.

In an effort to better operationalize the term, Hernandez et al. (2009, p. 1047) established a definition that focuses specifically on implementation:

> [A]n organization's cultural competence can be described as the degree of compatibility and adaptability between the cultural and linguistic characteristics of a community's population and the way the organization's combined policies, structures, and processes work together to impede and/or facilitate access, availability and utilization of needed services and supports.

Presentation of Critical Issues: Conceptualizing Cultural Competence as an Organizational Process

This section presents a conceptual model that illustrates how organizational cultural competence can be successfully implemented by focusing on the relationships between a community's population(s), organizational structures and processes, and direct services within a larger community context. The model was developed from research conducted to examine implementation of culturally competent service delivery on the part of behavioral health organizations across the country (Hernandez et al., 2009; Hernandez, Nesman, Isaacs, Callejas, & Mowery, 2006). It organizes the findings from a literature review that examined over 1100 articles on the topic of cultural competence in behavioral health services for racially and ethnically diverse populations in the United States. This review focused on identifying and describing measurable factors associated with cultural competence in behavioral health services and the relationships between the factors documented (Hernandez et al., 2006, 2009). The literature review was conducted as part of a larger study that focused on identifying organizational practices designed to implement culturally competent service delivery and reduce behavioral health disparities by improving service accessibility.

Figure 1 presents the conceptual model of organizational cultural competence, which illustrates the relationships between diverse populations of behavioral health service users and the key structures and processes of behavioral health organizations, including their direct service functions and processes, as presented in our definition established earlier. It further highlights the importance of the community contexts that shape the way in which behavioral health services are delivered by organizations (or systems) *and* received by the populations that need them. As Fig. 1

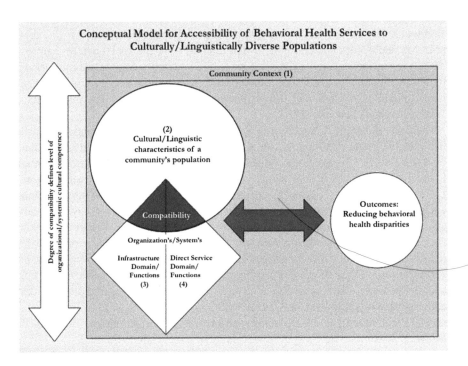

Fig. 1 Conceptual model for accessibility of behavioral health services to culturally/linguistically diverse population

indicates, the compatibility between an organization and the population(s) it serves determines the level of cultural competence and ultimately, a reduction in behavioral health disparities within a given community. The remainder of this section outlines key components of the model (numbered for clarity) and discusses how these components are thought to interact within a given community. Special attention is given to the concept of "culture," because of its central importance to an understanding of cultural competence.

Community Context

As noted earlier, community context is central to this model; it is the setting within which behavioral health organizations and the populations they serve exist and interact with one another. The model also highlights the premise that all individuals respond to their behavioral health issues within the context of a larger social environment. Community context can therefore affect the ways in which culturally diverse individuals reach the services and supports they may need. For instance, intrinsic characteristics generally associated with particular populations have been found to affect access to services and the utilization of these services. These include beliefs about disability, awareness of behavioral health needs, and understanding of available services, or knowledge of how service systems work (Bailey, Skinner, Rodriguez, Gut, & Correa, 1999). Context is also shaped by the underlying social, political, and economic conditions (often referred to as the social determinants of health) in particular neighborhoods within the community or communities served by an organization and which are understood by researchers as playing a critical role in overall health and well-being (Barten, Mitlin, Mulholland, Hardoy, & Stern, 2007; Shavers & Shavers, 2006).

Behavioral health organizations also operate within a larger context, which includes the larger city, county, state, and national environments that affect their efforts to serve diverse populations. One example is how implementation of Federal policy varies across states in the delivery and utilization of services. Different interpretation of the laws regarding mental health parity in benefits management by plans, providers, and governments (state and Federal) may adversely affect utilization of services based on severity of diagnoses (Busch et al., 2012). Behavioral health organizations can also shape their service delivery practices to respond to the direct lived experiences of the families they serve. For instance, an organization serving Black populations in the Midwest works with families to address issues of domestic violence and anger/aggression, through a program that addresses historical trauma in African American populations and positive emphasis on "Black Identity and the Black Experience" (Callejas, Hernandez, Nesman, & Mowery, 2010).

Cultural and Linguistic Characteristics of a Community's Populations

Before behavioral health organizations can implement culturally competent service delivery, they need to have information about the populations (and the conditions in which they live) within the neighborhood(s) that they serve. Understanding the population(s) that we serve includes awareness of the influences of culture, ethnicity, race, socioeconomic status, and related social factors on the provision of services and help-seeking. As Staudt (2003) points out, it is important to link interventions to the factors that contribute to a lack of engagement that we find within our service use population and to recognize that these factors will vary across groups and service types. Development of compatible service delivery strategies that are compatible with the populations that we serve will not be possible without this information.

Understanding culture includes identifying shared social norms, beliefs, and values, as well as languages of preference, and how institutions, such as marriage, family, or education, are viewed and practiced (Guerra & Jagers, 1998). Behavioral health practitioners should expect variability within a culture rather than considering certain characteristics to be consistent across all potential members. As noted earlier, consideration should also be given to how culture develops in response to specific contextual demands (Cauce et al., 2002) and the changes that may occur as the social environments change (Bernal & Sáez-Santiago, 2006). Our perspective on culture provides a way to work with populations despite situations where families and/or individuals maintain widely varying beliefs or attitudes about specific aspects of their identity (Dressler, 1993). Although we believe that culture impacts how families and providers think about seeking/providing help, defining/diagnosing problems, or understanding/treating mental health conditions, the way that culture impacts these perspectives may vary. Therefore, the way that we characterize the populations with which we work should be considered carefully (Akutsu, Snowden, & Organista, 1996; Alvidrez, 1999; Cauce et al., 2002).

Understanding how identity shapes the ways in which diverse populations interact with service systems can contribute to the development of more compatible service systems. For instance, although biological foundations or genetic roots for commonly accepted racial categories have been discounted (Bonham, Warshauer-Baker, & Collins, 2005), race continues to shape provider decision-making processes that result in disparities (Aronson, Burgess, Phelan, & Juarez, 2013). For example, health disparities have been linked to decreased willingness of doctors to interact with racially and ethnically diverse clients, different interpretations of symptoms, and stereotypes about health-related behaviors (Aronson et al., 2013; Institute of Medicine, 2002). Better understanding of the underlying causes of disparities linked to race can point to important organizational adaptations, such as whether to focus on information-based policies (e.g., provider and patient education) or rule-based policies (e.g., requirements aimed at equity) (Aronson et al., 2013).

Level of acculturation, migration history, and displacement experiences are also important for understanding how to serve diverse populations. Acculturation, or the adaptation to a host culture, may result in varying relationships for both the host society and immigrant or displaced populations (Gamst et al., 2002). Knowledge about the socioeconomic status (SES) of the populations that we serve is another important factor for practitioners to acknowledge. In the United States, the overlap between SES and culture/race/ethnicity can be significant (LaVeist, 2005). Socioeconomic status has been specifically tied to barriers such as lack of insurance, time, and transportation that impact utilization of mental health services (Alvidrez, 1999).

Organizational Implementation Domains

The conceptual model of organizational cultural competence also highlights two organizational domains that play a central role in the delivery of culturally competent services within a given community. Fig. 2 illustrates the importance of ensuring compatibility of functions and strategies within a given behavioral health organization, in addition to the degree of compatibility between an organization's service delivery and a given population within the community it serves.

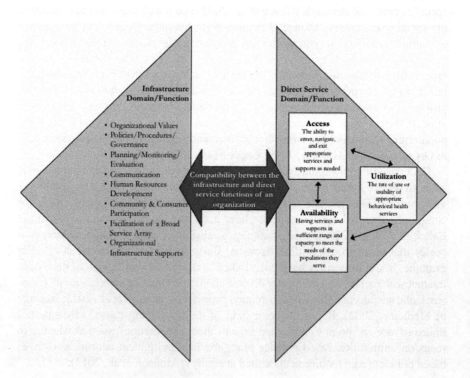

Fig. 2 Organizational implementation domains

Organizational Infrastructure

The first domain, organizational infrastructure, includes eight interrelated components that are typical of organizations, each of which must be adapted to achieve culturally competent service delivery. For example, organizational values, policies, procedures, and governance can be adapted to address a given population's unique characteristics or to address identified community issues, such as uneven rates of insurance coverage or immigration laws that might affect the ways in which service users interact with behavioral health organizations and service systems. Communication that supports cultural competence includes inclusive communication and learning within the organization, as well as between a given organization and the community it serves. Human resources and service array domains include strategies to increase bilingual/bicultural capacity, recruitment, and retention and availability of services that are appropriate and of high quality for the target population. Methods of outreach to communities and opportunities for community/consumer participation are important mechanisms that can lead to increased use of needed services by building trust between behavioral health organizations and the diverse populations that they serve. Likewise, planning and evaluation processes contribute to cultural competence when they include communities of color as fully contributing partners with shared responsibilities and when they collect data that reflects the diversity of the community (see SenGupta, Hopson, & Thompson-Robinson, 2004).

Organizational leadership can also promote cultural competence by working to increase an organization's technological resources, perhaps by adopting a more efficient database, for instance, or by securing diverse forms of funding. Organizational leadership may also work to advocate for changes in funding mechanisms by leveraging existing relationships with key policymakers and/or funding agencies (Callejas et al., 2010). Implementation of strategies within an organization's infrastructure can influence the ways in which it interacts with the diverse populations it serves and as the conceptual model illustrates.

Direct Service Functions

The direct service domain of an organization includes functions related to the availability, availability, and utilization of behavioral health services, which are conceptualized as three interrelated functions. Behavioral health organizations seeking to provide culturally competent service delivery can implement a number of strategies or direct service practices designed to increase service use by diverse populations. *Availability* is defined as having services and supports in sufficient range and capacity to meet the needs of the diverse populations served by a given behavioral health organization (or system). Direct service strategies designed to enhance or increase the availability of behavioral health services may include the implementation of ethnic specific services and/or the use of mental health interpreters or cultural brokers. Culturally competent service *accessibility* encompasses the mechanisms established by organizations that support individuals' entry, navigation, and exit of needed services and supports. Behavioral health organizations may choose to implement a number of strategies designed to increase accessibility to services, including providing services at times that accommodate the schedules of service users (e.g., evenings and weekends); providing transportation support or home visiting services; and/or increasing contacts with service users to maintain levels of engagement and retention in services. *Utilization* is defined as the rate of use of services or the degree of usability for populations served. To increase utilization of services behavioral health organizations may promote the use of available services within the community that they serve, as well as track service use patterns to more accurately understand service use patterns.

Figure 2 illustrates how behavioral health service delivery can be enhanced through the development of culturally responsive practices at both the organizational and direct service levels. Access is shown as influencing and being influenced by availability and utilization of services (shown as two-way arrows) indicating that compatibility with the population involves adaptations in all three service domains, which are understood as encompassing the continuum of service delivery from prevention to problem identification and help-seeking and to assessment, treatment, and follow-up.

Organizational Compatibility

As noted throughout this section, the conceptual model presented in this chapter emphasizes compatibility— between the organizational infrastructure and direct service, as well as between each of the direct service functions within that particular domain. Dynamic relationships (represented by two-way arrows) within the model emphasize that organizational components do not operate in isolation. That is, implementation of a direct service strategy designed to increase access to services for a particular population should be supported at the organizational level through specific governance procedures, creative and flexible funding of services, and other strategies that will support direct service personnel in their efforts. Further as this model seeks to make clear, compatibility between the organizational infrastructure and direct service domains supports, at a much broader level, supports compatibility between a behavioral health organization (or service system) and the target population(s) within a given community.

Research conducted with 12 behavioral health organizations around the country identified and documented a number of strategies used to increase service availability, accessibility, and utilization as a means for reducing disparities in behavioral health outcomes among ethnically and racially diverse populations and provided support for the importance of ensuring compatibility between organizational domains when developing and implementing culturally competent behavioral health services (Callejas et al., 2010). For instance, co-location of behavioral health services within a one-stop family services center may be used to increase accessibility to needed services and to reduce stigma associated with mental illness. However, a hypothetical lack of bilingual services available at the one-stop center engenders a lack of trust in the organization among local residents, who are limited English speakers and make up the majority of the residents in the immediate neighborhood where the center is located. The lack of trust on the part of residents and the center's limited bilingual capacity then results in low levels of service utilization and little improvement in mental health outcomes. Although hypothetical, this example highlights the dynamic relationship between organizational components. Changes in one area can affect service delivery processes, or lack of change in one area may cancel out efforts in other areas. Incorporating cultural competence into every aspect of a behavioral health organization or system requires careful consideration of compatibility between important organizational components.

Implications for Implementing Culturally Competent Behavioral Health Services

The conceptual model presented in this chapter provides a framework for operationalizing cultural competence as a means for reducing behavioral health disparities in diverse populations. This model expands previous theorizing on cultural competence which has often focused on the interpersonal relationship between a practitioner and a consumer or on efforts to culturally adapt interventions to encompass the role of organizations and systems in the service delivery process (Hernandez et al., 2009). Rather than focusing on memorizing the particular cultural values associated with a given population and working to accommodate them, our model emphasizes an organizational response to the contextual conditions of local communities, *as well as* the culturally influenced factors that may enable or constrain accessibility to needed services and supports on the part of diverse populations. Perhaps more importantly, this model presents cultural competence as an approach that can be implemented by all behavioral health organizations, not only those organizations focused on serving racial or ethnic minority groups. As such, it frames cultural competence as an active process to be undertaken by organizations in response to changing community conditions. Moreover, it provides an overview of the infrastructure elements that behavioral health organizations should address if they are to sustain cultural competence over time.

The continued attention to stark disparities in behavioral healthcare outcomes among diverse populations has led behavioral health and other practitioners to call for increase guidance on specific strategies that can be implemented to provide more culturally responsive services. In addition to the research referenced throughout this chapter, readers are encouraged to review the National Standards for Culturally and Linguistically Appropriate Services (CLAS) in healthcare to establish concrete strategies that address the cultural and linguistic needs of the populations that they serve (Betancourt, Green, Carrillo, & Park, 2005). Although a number of researchers have begun to examine whether implementation of such strategies leads to reduced disparities in behavioral health and general healthcare, more research is needed (see Betancourt et al., 2005; Bhui et al., 2007).

Discussion related to culturally competent service delivery has also engaged the question of culturally relevant interventions for diverse populations. The conceptual model presented in this chapter is similar to one proposed by Bernal and Sáez-Santiago (2006), which emphasizes the need for "cultural congruence" between client and therapist but is aimed solely at the treatment level. Dimensions of congruence in this case include language use, relationship between client and provider, use of metaphors (concepts and symbols) in therapy, cultural knowledge about the client, problem and treatment conceptualization, development of goals/methods/procedures for treatment, and awareness of the client's broader social/economic/political context (Bernal & Sáez-Santiago, 2006).

The question of cultural adaptation of interventions has generated some degree of controversy, especially between researchers that have called for a wider use of empirically supported treatments (ESTs) to reduce behavioral health disparities and those that have called for increased testing of interventions with racially and ethnically diverse populations, in particular (Bernal & Domenech-Rodriguez, 2012). Despite such contention, a number of studies have shown that culturally adapted treatments produce positive outcomes (Bernal & Domenech-Rodriguez, 2012; Huey & Polo, 2010). In addition, a number of practitioners and researchers have called for increased recognition of practice-based evidence and community-defined evidence as alternative paradigms that emphasize the "cultural fit" between interventions and its recipients (Isaacs et al., 2008; Martinez, Callejas, & Hernandez, 2010).

The prominence that the cultural competence concept has attained within the field of behavioral health continues to increase as researchers and practitioners seek to better understand how to address persistent disparities in behavioral health outcomes among diverse populations. As the organizational cultural competence model suggests, implementation of strategies in the interrelated infrastructure and direct service domains of an organization can increase compatibility with diverse populations in a given community. Despite research conducted with organizations around the country to identify implementation of such strategies, additional research is needed to test whether the implementation of culturally competent practice ultimately serves to reduce behavioral health disparities in the delivery of behavioral health services. Nevertheless, the model provides direction for behavioral health practitioners and researchers working to address the behavioral health needs of underserved populations and communities.

References

Akutsu, P. D., Snowden, L. R., & Organista, K. C. (1996). Referral patterns in ethnic specific and mainstream programs for ethnic minorities and whites. *Journal of Counseling Psychology, 43,* 56–64.

Alegría, M., Canino, G., Lai, S., Ramirez, R. R., Chavez, L., Rusch, D., & Shrout, P. E. (2004). Understanding caregivers' help-seeking for Latino children's mental health care use. *Medical Care, 42,* 447–455.

Alvidrez, J. (1999). Ethnic variations in mental health attitudes and service use among low-income African American, Latina, and European American young women. *Community Mental Health Journal, 35,* 515–530.

Bailey, D. B., Jr., Skinner, D., Rodriguez, P., Gut, D., & Correa, V. (1999). Awareness, use, and satisfaction with services for Latino parents of young children with disabilities. *Exceptional Children, 65,* 367–381.

Aronson, J., Burgess, D., Phelan, S. M., & Juarez, L. (2013). Unhealthy interactions: The role of stereotype threat in health disparities. *American Journal of Public Health, 103*(1), 50–56. https://doi.org/10.2105/AJPH.2012.300828

Bates, D. G., & Plog, F. (1990). Cultural anthropology. New York, NY, US: McGraw-Hill.

Barten, F., Mitlin, D., Mulholland, C., Hardoy, A., & Stern, R. (2007). Integrated approaches to address the social determinants of health for reducing health inequity. *Journal of Urban Health,* 84(3 Suppl), i164–173. http://doi.org/10.1007/s11524-007-9173-7

Bernal, G., & Domenech-Rodriguez, M. M. (Eds.). (2012). *Cultural adaptations: Tools for evidence-based practice with diverse populations.* Washington, DC: American Psychological Association.

Bernal, G., & Sáez-Santiago, E. (2006). Culturally centered psychosocial interventions. *Journal of Community Psychology, 34,* 121–132.

Betancourt, J. R., Green, A. R., Carrillo, J. E., & Park, E. R. (2005). Cultural competence and health care disparities: Key perspectives and trends. *Health Affairs, 24,* 499–505.

Bhui, K., Warfa, N., Edonya, P., McKenzie, K., & Bhugra, D. (2007). Cultural competence in mental health care: A review of model evaluations. *BMC Health Services Research, 7,* 1–10.

Bonham, V. L., Warshauer-Baker, E., & Collins, F. S. (2005). Race and ethnicity in the genome era. *American Psychologist, 60,* 9–15.

Braveman, P. (2014). What are health disparities and health equity? We need to be clear. Nursing in 3D: Diversity, disparities, and social determinants. *Public Health Reports, 129*(Suppl. 2), 5–8.

Brooks, C., & Bolzendahl, C. (2004). The transformation of US gender role attitudes: Cohort replacement, social-structural change, and ideological learning. *Social Science Research, 33,* 106–133.

Busch, A. B., Yoon, F., Barry, C. L., Azzone, V., Normand, S. L., Goldman, H. H., & Huskamp, H. A. (2012). The effects of mental health parity on spending and utilization for bipolar, major depression, and adjustment disorders. *American Journal of Psychiatry, 170,* 180–187.

Callejas, L. M., Hernandez, M., Nesman, T., & Mowery, D. (2010). Creating a front porch: Improving access to behavioral health services for diverse children and families. *Evaluation and Program Planning, 33,* 32–35.

Cauce, A. M., Domenech-Rodriguez, M., Paradise, M., Cochran, B. N., Shea, J. M., Srebnik, D., & Baydar, N. (2002). Cultural and contextual influences in mental health help seeking: A focus on ethnic minority youth. *Journal of Counsulting and Clinical Psychology, 70,* 44–55.

Coard, S. I., & Holden, E. W. (1998). The effect of racial and ethnic diversity on the delivery of mental health services in pediatric primary care. *Journal of Clinical Psychology in Medical Settings, 5,* 275–294.

Chow, J. C. C., Jaffee, K., & Snowden, L. (2003). Racial/ethnic disparities in the use of mental health services in poverty areas. *American Journal of Public Health, 93,* 792–797.

Cross, T. L., Bazron, B. J., Dennis, K. W., & Isaacs, M. R. (1989). *Towards a culturally competent system of care: Vol. I. A monograph on effective services for minority children who are severely emotionally disturbed.* Washington, DC: Georgetown University Child Development Center, CASSP Technical Assistance Center.

Diamond, L. M., & Butterworth, M. (2008). Questioning gender and sexual identity: Dynamic links over time. *Sex Roles, 59,* 365–376.

Drescher, J. (2009). Queer diagnoses: Parallels and contrasts in the history of homosexuality, gender variance, and the diagnostic and statistical manual. *Archives of Sexual Behavior, 39,* 427–460.

Dressler, W. W. (1993). Health in the African American community: Accounting for health inequalities. *Medical Anthropology Quarterly, 7,* 325–345.

Fine, M. J., Ibrahim, S. A., & Thomas, S. B. (2005). The role of race and genetics in health disparities research. *American Journal of Public Health, 95,* 2125–2128.

Gamst, G., Dana, R. H., Der-Karabetian, A., Aragon, M., Arellano, L., & Kramer, T. (2002). Effects of Latino acculturation and ethnic identity on mental health outcomes. *Hispanic Journal of Behavioral Sciences, 24,* 479–505.

Guarnaccia, P., & Rodriguez, O. (1996). Concepts of culture and their role in the development of culturally competent mental health services. *Hispanic Journal of Behavioral Sciences, 18,* 418–443.

Guerra, N. G., & Jagers, R. (1998). The importance of culture in the assessment of children and youth. In V. C. McLoyd & L. Steinberg (Eds.), *Studying minority adolescents: Conceptual, methodological, and theoretical issues* (pp. 167–181). Thousand Oaks, CA: Sage.

Harris, M. (1968). *The rise of anthropological theory.* New York, NY: Crowell.

Hernandez, M., Nesman, T., Mowery, D., Acevedo-Polakovich, I. D., & Callejas, L. M. (2009). Cultural competence: A literature review and conceptual model for mental health services. *Psychiatric Services, 60,* 1046–1050.

Hernandez, M., Nesman, T., Isaacs, M., Callejas, L. M., & Mowery, D. (Eds.). (2006). *Examining the research base supporting culturally competent children's mental health services.* (Making children's mental health services successful series, FMHI pub. no. 240-1). Tampa, FL: University of South Florida, Louis de la Parte Florida Mental Health Institute, Research & Training Center for Children's Mental Health.

Hough, R. L., Hazen, A. L., Soriano, F. I., Wood, P., McCabe, K., & Yeh, M. (2002). Mental health services for Latino adolescents with psychiatric disorders. *Psychiatric Services, 53,* 1556–1562.

Huey, S. J., Jr., & Polo, A. J. (2010). Assessing the effects of evidence-based psychotherapies with ethnic minority youths. In J. R. Weisz & A. E. Kazdin (Eds.), *Evidence-based psychotherapies for children and adolescents* (2nd ed., pp. 451–455). New York, NY: Guilford Press.

Institute of Medicine. (2002). *Unequal treatment: Confronting racial and ethnic disparities in health care.* Washington, DC: National Academy Press.

Isaacs, M. R., Huang, L. N., Hernandez, M., Echo-Hawk, H., Acevedo-Polakovich, I. D., & Martinez, K. (2008). Services for youth and their families in diverse communities. In B. A. Stroul & G. M. Blau (Eds.), *The system of care handbook: Transforming mental health services for children, youth, and families* (pp. 619–639). Baltimore, MD: Paul H. Brookes Publishing Co.

Kataoka, S. H., Zhang, L., & Wells, K. B. (2002). Unmet need for mental health care among U.S. children: Variation by ethnicity and insurance status. *American Journal of Psychiatry, 159,* 1548–1555.

Kleinman, A., & Benson, P. (2006). Anthropology in the clinic: The problem of cultural competency and how to fix it. *PLoS Medicine, 3,* 1673–1676.

LaVeist, T. A. (2005). Disentangling race and socioeconomic status: A key to understanding health inequalities. *Journal of Urban Health: Bulletin of the New York Academy of Medicine, 82,* iii26–iii34.

Malat, J. (2013). The appeal and problems of a cultural competence approach to reducing racial disparities. *Journal of General Internal Medicine, 28,* 605–607.

Martinez, K., Callejas, L. M., & Hernandez, M. (2010). Community-defined evidence: A "bottom up" behavioral health approach to measure "what works" in Latino communities. *Report on Emotional and Behavioral Disorders in Youth, 10*, 11–16.

President's New Freedom Commission on Mental Health. (2003). *Achieving the promise: Transforming mental health care in America* (Final report. DHHS Pub. No. SMA-03-3832). Rockville, MD: Author.

Rollins, R. (2011). *Building partnerships through the "National Stakeholder Strategy for achieving health equity"*. Paper presented at the annual meeting of the Health Outcomes among Children and Families Living in Rural Communities Conference, Bethesda, MD.

Saha, S., Korthuis, P. T., Cohn, J. A., Sharp, V. L., Moore, R. D., & Beach, M. C. (2013). Primary care provider cultural competence and racial disparities in HIV care and outcomes. *Journal of General Internal Medicine, 28*, 622–629.

SenGupta, S., Hopson, R., & Thompson-Robinson, M. (2004). Cultural competence in evaluation: An overview. *New Directions for Evaluation, 102*, 5–19.

Shavers, V. L., & Shavers, B. S. (2006). Racism and health inequity among Americans. *Journal of National Medical Association, 98*, 386–396.

Smedley, A., & Smedley, B. D. (2005). Race as biology is fiction, racism as a social problem is real: Anthropological and historical perspectives on the social construction of race. *American Psychologist, 60*, 16–26.

Staudt, M. M. (2003). Helping children access and use services: A review. *Journal of Child and Family Studies, 12*, 49–60.

Tyler, E. B. (1923). *Primitive culture: Researches into the development of mythology, philosophy, religion, language, art, and custom* (Vol. 1, 7th ed.). New York, NY: Brentano.

U.S. Department of Health and Human Services. (2001). *Mental health: Culture, race, and ethnicity – A supplement to mental health: A report of the Surgeon General*. Rockville, MD: U.S. Department of Health and Human Services, Substance Abuse and Mental Health Services Administration, Center for Mental Health Services.

Vega, W. A., & Lopez, S. R. (2001). Priority issues in Latino mental health services research. *Mental Health Services Research, 3*, 189–200.

Whitehead, M. (1990). *The concepts and principles of equity and health (EUR/ICP/RPD 414)*. Copenhagen, Denmark: WHO Regional Office for Europe. Retrieved from http://whqlibdoc. who.int/euro/-1993/EUR_ICP_RPD_414.pdf

Yeh, M., McCabe, K., Hough, R. L., Dupuis, D., & Hazen, A. (2003). Racial/ethnic differences in parental endorsement of barriers to mental health services for youth. *Mental Health Services Research, 5*, 65–77.

Pharmacy Services in Behavioral Health

Carol A. Ott

Introduction

Pharmacists have long been considered the most accessible healthcare professionals, from the days of the independent community pharmacy with the lunch counter and ice cream soda jerk to present day. Pharmacists traditionally have held a distributive role, filling prescriptions that are written by physicians and presented to the pharmacy counter, either in the community or hospital pharmacy. Until 2000, a pharmacist may have held a Bachelor of Science Degree in Pharmacy; in that year, the Doctor of Pharmacy Degree became the entry-level degree program for the practice of pharmacy. While the general public often sees pharmacists in the distributive "prescription filling" role, the profession of pharmacy has been pushing pharmacists to take a broader role in patient care, including rounding with patient care teams in the hospital setting to medication therapy management in community pharmacies. In the past decade, the role of the pharmacist in patient care had expanded to providing medication-related services in outpatient and primary care clinics for a variety of disease states. A newer important area of practice is in transitions of care, with the pharmacist helping the patient move from the inpatient hospital to home with a greater understanding of their medications and how to take them. Pharmacists who practice in a more clinical role, whether in an inpatient or outpatient setting, are often residency-trained and board-certified in their area of practice. Pharmacists may specialize in the treatment of patients with mental disorders in the distributive and clinical practice settings.

C. A. Ott (✉)
Purdue University College of Pharmacy, Indianapolis, IN, USA

Eskenazi Health/Midtown Community Mental Health, Indianapolis, IN, USA
e-mail: caott@iupui.edu

© Springer Nature Switzerland AG 2020
B. L. Levin, A. Hanson (eds.), *Foundations of Behavioral Health*,
https://doi.org/10.1007/978-3-030-18435-3_16

Community Pharmacies

As more Americans rely on prescriptions to manage their health issues, community pharmacists often are one of the first health points of contact for families. Hence, it is important to understand their role as key from a behavioral and public health perspective.

Health System Pharmacies

In addition to traditional independent and chain retail community pharmacies, there are pharmacies that are housed within outpatient clinics in health systems. These pharmacies generally fill prescriptions for patients who have appointments with providers within the health system or outpatient clinic and may also provide over-the-counter medications. These pharmacies are convenient for the patient, and the pharmacists and pharmacy technicians commonly have access to the patient medical records for the health system. This access to the medical record allows the pharmacist to see health conditions, laboratory monitoring, drug allergies, and prescription medications the patient is taking and is a more reliable way for the pharmacist to provide patient-centered care than asking the patient for this information in a traditional community pharmacy. It also permits the pharmacist to have easier access to the physician in case of questions about a prescription or need for refills.

Recent research has studied the role of the community pharmacy in providing earlier detection of mental disorders, specifically depression (Rubio-Valera, Chen, & O'Reilly, 2014). For the past few decades, pharmacists have been involved in screening for high blood pressure and diabetes, but few have ventured into screening for mental disorders. Stigma related to behavioral health conditions and discomfort in talking to patients about these disorders may be a significant reason. Studies of pharmacists and their comfort in providing medication counseling for various disease states have shown that pharmacists in general feel more confident in counseling about high blood pressure or diabetes medications than about behavioral disorders and medications (Phokeo, Sproule, & Raman-Wilms, 2004).

Improvement in didactic and experiential education in pharmacy school/college programs as well as redesigning community pharmacies to offer truly private patient counseling are areas of focus in the profession of pharmacy to impact these concerns (Calogero & Caley, 2017). Pharmacists who have been trained in the use of screening tools for depression feel more comfortable with patient interactions. They are accessible due to the lack of need for appointments and the opportunity in the community pharmacy to screen for depression, recognize patients who may be at-risk, and make appropriate referrals (Rubio-Valera et al., 2014). These screenings may be done in either traditional community pharmacies or in pharmacies within health systems. As noted previously, pharmacists within health systems may have greater access to medical records and physicians than other pharmacists.

Pharmacies in Community Mental Health Centers (CMHCs)

CMHCs may have pharmacies that are located within the clinic setting. Health systems may have a pharmacy in the outpatient clinic; some health systems also have an affiliated CMHC that has a pharmacy. Independent and chain retail pharmacies may partner with a CMHC to have a pharmacy located within the clinic. Pharmacy companies may specialize in placing a community pharmacy in a CMHC.

Genoa Healthcare is the most recognized of these pharmacy companies. In 2018, Genoa Healthcare had 418 pharmacies located in a CMHC, recorded about 650,000 patient encounters in their pharmacies, and had more than 250 psychiatrists working with their telepsychiatry services (www.genoahealthcare.com). Genoa Healthcare pharmacies can provide specialized packaging of medication, refill reminders, and medication delivery.

While the pharmacy is located in a CMHC, medications for primary care and other conditions are available in addition to behavioral health medications. A pharmacist is embedded in the outpatient treatment team to provide medication reviews and adherence information. A retrospective study comparing traditional community pharmacies and pharmacies integrated into CHMCs evaluated Medicaid claims and medication adherence. The results of the study showed that patients who filled medications in a CMHC integrated pharmacy had higher medication adherence, decreased rates of hospitalization, and decreased emergency department use, resulting in improved care and a decrease in the use and cost of acute care services (Wright, Gorman, Odorzynski, Peterson, & Clayton, 2016).

Insurance Coverage

The Mental Health Parity Act of 1996 (MHPA) required that large group health plans provide mental health (MH) benefits that are equal to medical benefits in annual and lifetime benefits. The Paul Wellstone and Pete Domenici Mental Health Parity and Addiction Equity Act of 2008 (MHPAEA) clarified the MHPA to include substance use disorder (SUD) treatment and smaller health plans and group insurance coverage (The Center for Consumer Information & Insurance Oversight, 2018). The Affordable Care Act (ACA) added these benefits to individual health insurance coverage. The MHPAEA did not require health insurers to cover MH/SUD treatment; the parity law requirement applies to those plans that choose to provide these benefits. The ACA built upon the MHPAEA in requiring MH/SUD coverage as one of the ten essential health benefits.

Commercial Insurance

Commercial insurance may come from employers or from the individual private insurance marketplace created by the ACA. Commercial insurance may be more likely than Medicaid and Medicare programs to be subject to more restrictive preferred drug lists, formularies, and prior authorizations for medications (covered in a later section). The Healthcare Marketplace is set up for individuals to obtain healthcare insurance that fits their needs and they can afford. Challenges exist for individuals in determining if their current healthcare provider is covered under a plan they may choose, which has resulted in patients not being able to keep their current provider or have the same medication coverage they may have had with previous insurance plans (www.cms.gov).

Medicare and Medicaid

President Lyndon B. Johnson signed the Social Security Act Amendments that created Medicare and Medicaid in 1965. The Medicare program is designed to provide insurance coverage and healthcare treatment for people who are over the age of 65, are disabled, or have end-stage renal disease. In 2003, the Medicare Part D Prescription Drug Improvement and Modernization Act added Medicare Part D, which provides prescription drug insurance coverage for Medicare recipients.

Medicaid is a healthcare coverage program for people who are low-income, pregnant women, people with disabilities, and those who need long-term care services. The federal government provides funding to the states to administer Medicaid programs based upon the state decisions. In addition to providing for the Health Insurance Marketplace, the ACA 2010 allowed states to choose to expand their Medicaid programs to cover more people by raising the maximum low-income standard to a higher wage (www.cms.gov).

Preferred Drug Lists

Preferred drug lists (PDLs) are employed by insurance programs to steer prescribers and patients toward lower-cost medications, including generic drugs. Insurance providers are often able to negotiate with drug manufacturers to obtain a lower price for their programs if a specific drug made by a manufacturer is considered to be preferred, even if it is not a generic. These are called "supplemental rebate programs". Commercial insurance programs, Medicare, Medicaid, and the Veterans' Administration each utilize this type of rebate program to lower costs. PDLs also decrease the cost of treatment per member of each insurance program. Managed care insurance programs, often utilized by state Medicaid insurers, are commonly paid a set rate per member per month. This leads managed care and pharmacy benefits managers to search for the lowest-cost medication or treatment for a disease state. Co-payments for medication that are paid by the patient at the pharmacy can also impact the cost to the insurer. Co-payments are either a set amount per prescription or a percentage of the cost of the prescription. Medications that are considered to be first-tier on PDLs have co-payments that are lower in percentage or set price than medications that are second- or third-tier.

A literature review by Ovsag, Hydery, and Mousa (2008) evaluated the impact of PDLs in Medicaid on cost and quality of care. Problems with PDLs identified by this review include the influence of PDLs on the use of other healthcare services, potentially increasing overall cost, and the concern that restricting access to medication can lead to a decreased quality of care for a patient. A retrospective cohort study evaluated the impact of a new PDL on adherence to medication for Medicaid patients in Alabama, specifically focused on medications used for heart disease and elevated cholesterol. The results of the study identified an 82% increased odds of Medicaid patients becoming non-adherent to statin medications used to treat elevated cholesterol after the implementation of the new PDL (Ridley & Axelsen, 2006).

Another study focused on changes to Medicaid evaluated how a decrease in days' supply per prescription and an increase in co-payment affected adherence to cholesterol and hypertension medication. For those Medicaid patients who took nearly all of their medications prior to the change, there was a significant decline in adherence to these medication after the change (Amin, Farley, Maciejewski, & Domino, 2017). Overall, while PDLs are perceived by insurers to decrease short-term cost, a growing body of evidence suggests that quality of life and healthcare outcomes are negatively impacted by PDL programs.

Patient Assistance/Co-Payment Assistance Programs

Drug manufacturers will often make patient assistance programs (PAPs) that provide either free or reduced cost medications available to patients who meet eligibility criteria. Patients who do not have insurance, are not eligible for Medicaid or other insurance programs, are low-income, or have insurance that does not cover certain medications may benefit from enrolling in a PAP program. PAP programs require an application, as well as proof of income, and occasionally citizenship, which can limit their widespread use. Pharmacists are in a position to be aware of PAPs and to aid patients in applying for them. Manufacturer websites generally provide information about available PAPs for their medications, and there are groups/websites that list more general PAP information. These groups/websites include RxAssist (www.rxassist.org), NeedyMeds (https://www.needymeds.org/pap), Paying for Senior Care (www.payingforseniorcare.com), and a list of pharmaceutical manufacturers at www.cms.gov.

One manufacturer, Janssen, provides a comprehensive assistance program known as Janssen Connect® for patients diagnosed with schizophrenia and prescribed a long-acting injection (LAI) made by the company. A recent evaluation of the program noted that nearly 80% of patients enrolled did not miss receiving their injection for more than 7 weeks and 87% were fully adherent with an every-4-week injection regimen (Benson, Joshi, Lapane, & Fastenau, 2015). The cost of co-payments can be a burden to patients, especially those who have co-payments based upon a percentage of the drug cost and those who are receiving expensive brand-name medications.

One study evaluated patients diagnosed with schizophrenia and the impact of Medicaid prescription co-payments on their use of antipsychotics as well as other medications for medical conditions. The study included fee-for-service Medicaid patients in 42 states and the District of Columbia. The study results suggested that as the co-payment cost increased, the number of medication refills decreased in a small, but statistically significant, way for antipsychotics. For medications for medical conditions, patients were 4–11 times less likely to fill prescriptions (Doshi, Li, Desai, & Marcus, 2017). Co-payments for prescriptions have risen significantly for the past several years and have become a significant burden for patients. The use of PAPs and co-pay assistance programs can help to decrease this burden and increase medication adherence.

Clinical Pharmacy Services

The Clinical Pharmacist in the Inpatient Mental Health Setting

For several decades, clinical pharmacists have been working in the inpatient treatment setting in mental health, rounding with prescribers, evaluating medication regimens, providing medication groups, and making recommendations for treatment changes and monitoring needs. Clinical pharmacists may have collaborative practice agreements (CPAs) with physicians in the inpatient setting to make medication adjustments and order laboratory monitoring under protocols. Most psychiatric clinical pharmacists have completed both a postgraduate year 1 residency in pharmacy practice and a postgraduate year 2 residency in psychiatric pharmacy. Board Certification in Psychiatric Pharmacy (BCPP) is available through the Board of Pharmacy Specialties, and this certification is held by most psychiatric clinical pharmacists.

In the past decade, research in this area has focused on improvement in medication adherence and cost-savings realized by utilizing a clinical pharmacist in the inpatient setting. An economic analysis reviewed clinical pharmacist interventions to evaluate cost-savings from the addition of a clinical pharmacist. The study results indicated that inpatient clinical pharmacists have a positive impact on hospital budgets, especially in the areas of prevention of adverse drug reactions, discontinuation of unnecessary drugs, and a positive effect in high-cost environments, such as intensive care units (Dalton & Byrne, 2017; Gallagher, McCarthy, & Byrne, 2014). A comprehensive review of clinical pharmacy services in mental health noted that there is a significant potential for these services to improve clinical and quality of life outcomes through review of medication charts and laboratory monitoring, evaluation of physician prescribing, and the provision of education to patients and other healthcare professionals (Richardson, O'Reilly, & Chen, 2014).

Clinical Pharmacists in the Community Mental Health Setting

More recently, psychiatric clinical pharmacists have taken roles as healthcare providers in outpatient clinic treatment settings. These pharmacists have also generally completed two postgraduate residency years and are BCPP certified. Outpatient psychiatric clinical pharmacists have CPAs with physicians that can range from focused medication management via protocol to independent medication management. Outpatient CPAs can be limited to seeing patients for medication regimen reviews, adherence, prescription refills, laboratory monitoring, and side effect evaluation. The outpatient clinical pharmacist CPA can also have a broad focus with independent medication management, including the ability to do the tasks in the limited CPA in addition to seeing patients for mental status assessments and addition, discontinuation, and adjustment of medications.

Outpatient psychiatric clinical pharmacists can also play a role in PAPs and co-payment assistance programs. A recent Cochrane review of the effect of non-dispensing roles for outpatient pharmacy concluded that the pharmacist role has expanded and the evidence supports medication management, patient counseling, patient education, and education outreach to physicians regarding prescribing practices (Nkansah et al., 2010). A retrospective study that evaluated 10 years of medication therapy management in an integrated healthcare system reviewed the medical records of more than 9000 patients for clinical pharmacist intervention. Cost-savings to the health system over 10 years from pharmacist intervention was approximately $700,000 (Ramalho de Oliveira, Brummel, & Miller, 2010).

Transitions of Care

Increased hospital readmissions within 30 days has prompted health systems to evaluate their discharge practice and implement policies and practices that improve patient education about medications and treatment, improve follow-up treatment interactions, and reduce readmission rates. Pharmacists play a role on teams for transitions of care by providing discharge counseling on medications for clear patient understanding, ensuring that there are no duplicate prescription orders at the pharmacy, and evaluating insurance coverage and the patient's ability to pay for medications in the outpatient pharmacy prior to discharge.

Some health systems have piloted transitions of care teams that are run by pharmacists and include communication between the inpatient and outpatient clinical pharmacists so that the outpatient treatment team is aware of the need for follow-up for the patient. A prospective study of 98 patients who had physician-initiated outpatient follow-up with pharmacist intervention compared 236 patients who had outpatient follow-up without pharmacist intervention. The patients who received pharmacist intervention had a hospital readmission rate within 30 days of 9.2% compared to a 19.4% 30-day readmission rate for those patients who did not have a pharmacist intervention (Arnold, Buys, & Fullas, 2015).

Cavanaugh, Lindsey, Shilliday, and Ratner (2015) studied patient outcomes for a pharmacist-coordinated multidisciplinary follow-up team that included a total of 140 patient visits. The 30-day readmission rate for the multidisciplinary team was 14.3% compared to 34.3% for patients who were followed up by the physician-only team (Cavanaugh et al., 2015). The implementation of services that are coordinated between inpatient and outpatient services can include an evaluation of the patient medication regimen prior to admission, performance of medication reconciliation, patient education on medications initiated during the hospitalization, and the initiation of affordable medication regimens that the patient would be counseled on and receive prior to discharge (Gilmore et al., 2015).

Medication Factors for Successful Treatment

The term "adherence to treatment" assumes the patient and the healthcare provider have developed a plan for treatment and it is agreed upon by both parties. "Compliance with treatment" is a term often used interchangeably with adherence to treatment but assumes that the provider had determined a plan and the patient will follow it. Adherence implies a partnership and is a patient-centered approach, while compliance is following a plan for which the patient did not have input. Healthcare providers can use several tools to ensure that the patient understands and agrees to the plan and that the plan includes decisions made by the patient.

Motivational Interviewing (MI)

MI is a tool that is collaborative, patient-centered, and relies on the provider to discover what will lead to behavioral change based upon the needs of the individual patient. MI uses the "OARS" approach to behavioral change: (1) open-ended questions, (2) affirmations, (3) reflective listening, and (4) summaries. Pharmacists are accessible healthcare professionals who are positioned to identify patient nonadherence and can use the techniques of MI in any patient care setting, including the community pharmacy. Pharmacists who use MI can discuss the patient's understanding of their disease and medications, determine how the treatment plan includes patient goals, and engage the patient in communication about any resistance to the plan (Salvo & Cannon-Breland, 2015). In the past, pharmacists gave advice to patients based upon specific questions asked with drug or dosing information. The practice of MI is now taught in schools and colleges of pharmacy to enhance pharmacist communication and include patient-centered aspects of care.

A study by Luetsch and Burrows (2018) evaluated 89 pharmacists and their reflective journal entries after training and implementation of MI. The pharmacists were asked to reflect on their perceptions of practice changes related to emotional aspects of communication and success in difficult situations. Prior to the training and implementation, none of the reflections indicated transformative changes in their frame of reference toward patient-centered care. After the training, 38% of the journal reflections were considered to be transformational, indicating that MI techniques can be learned and are successful in improving communication in the pharmacy setting (Luetsch & Burrows, 2018).

Shared Decision-Making (SDM)

In addition to MI, SDM is a communication tool that empowers patients to be active participants in treatment decisions. It is considered an important concept in mental health and a recovery-oriented system of care. SDM considers both the healthcare provider and the patient to be "experts" in the care of the patient. Each "expert" must share information, assess the advantages and disadvantages of a proposed treatment, and use collaboration to choose the intervention. In a study that evaluated 22 adults with mental health disorders, semi-structured focus groups evaluated how these patients perceived SDM (Grim, Rosenberg, Svedberg, & Schon, 2016). The focus group participants appreciated being included in discussion of their choices for treatment, the specifics of options, and the ability to be included in the decisions, especially related to their personal needs. The area for improvement noted by the participants was feeling prepared for this type of communication. Most participants did not feel prepared and felt that their choices were not trusted by the healthcare provider because they were not informed (Grim et al., 2016).

Psychiatric medication management is a specific area where SDM is useful. Mental health medications are a mainstay of treatment but often have significant adverse effects and less effectiveness than is hoped for by patients. Treatment with medications may be coerced, and patients may feel that they are being pressured to take medications in general or to agree to LAIs if they are not adherent to oral medications. SDM in the context of medication use may be subject to loss of true collaboration if the healthcare provider feels that the patient does not have insight or is not able to make fully informed treatment decisions. This may lead to the patient feeling a lack of respect for their input and not initiating treatment or discontinuing a medication. SDM related to psychiatric medication use should include a discussion of all possible adverse effects, the risk versus benefit of taking the medication, an allowance for the patient to "test" a treatment regimen by adjusting doses to times that fit their schedule, and clear information about the risks of not taking medication (Morant, Kaminskiy, & Ramon, 2016).

While the technique of MI is a part of the curriculum in schools and colleges of pharmacy, the concept of SDM is not common. Younas, Bradley, Holmes, Sud, and Maidment (2016) studied the perception of SDM by mental health pharmacists in the United Kingdom, where national guidelines encourage the use of SDM in antipsychotic prescribing. Semi-structured interviews were performed with 13 mental health pharmacists who were currently in psychiatric practice settings. The results of the study suggest that the pharmacists considered SDM regarding antipsychotic medications to improve clinical outcomes and relationships with patients; barriers to implementation of more widespread SDM included a lack of training, staff time constraints, and the ability of the patient to participate in SDM (Younas et al., 2016).

Long-Acting Injectable (LAI) Antipsychotic Medication

LAI antipsychotic medications are depot intramuscular injections that last from 2 weeks to 12 weeks depending on the medication and the formulation. Guidelines for the treatment of schizophrenia and bipolar disorder state that oral formulations should be tried first but that LAI antipsychotic formulations may be considered either after failure of oral medication or if the patient would benefit and agree to the LAI for convenience. The history of LAI antipsychotic use has often included coercion or pressure on the patient to agree to a LAI after not being adherent to oral medications, which has led to a lack of trust in healthcare providers who suggest these medications. More recently, healthcare providers have introduced the idea of LAI antipsychotics earlier in a course of treatment as a convenience to the patient, resulting in an increased use of LAI antipsychotics.

There is clinical evidence that LAI antipsychotics do improve adherence to medication and decrease the rate of hospitalization during a symptom relapse. A study by Marcus, Zummo, Pettit, Stoddard, and Doshi (2015) compared oral and LAI antipsychotic adherence and outcomes after release from a psychiatric hospitalization. Adherence to medication was better in the LAI group (adherence = 48.2%) versus the oral group (adherence = 32.3%). LAI participants also were less likely to be rehospitalized for relapse (19.1% vs. 25.3%) (Marcus et al., 2015). Research is lacking that compares the use of communication techniques such as MI and SDM with rates of adherence with oral or LAI antipsychotics.

Barriers to Treatment

Dual Diagnosis Treatment

Dual diagnosis in the context of mental health care includes the evaluation and treatment of both mental and substance use disorders in the same clinic setting. Historically, treatment for these disorders has been differentiated into separate clinical settings as if they are unrelated to each other or that one condition cannot be successfully treated without first addressing the other disease state. Despite evidence and awareness that integrated services for dual diagnosis are beneficial for the patient, there are a significant lack of healthcare providers who have taken this approach. A 2012 study assessed the availability of dual diagnosis capability in the United States using a sample of 256 programs. Only about 18% of the addiction treatment services and 9% of mental health programs met the criteria for dual diagnosis treatment services (McGovern, Lambert-Harris, Gotham, Claus, & Xie, 2014).

Dual diagnosis is very common; one study noted that people with drug dependence presented with a mental health disorder 4.9 times more frequently than individuals without an addiction diagnosis (Di Lorenzo, Galliani, Guicciardi, Landi, & Ferri, 2014). A retrospective analysis of demographic and other factors related to dual diagnosis found that the participants in this study more often suffered from a personality disorder, had a family history of mental health or substance use disorders, and had suffered trauma (Di Lorenzo et al., 2014). Dual diagnosis patients may have more chronic, disabling, and severe disease, requiring longer and more intensive treatment. Mental health and addiction programs often have different structures, assessment procedures, continuity of care, and treatment plans that may not meet the needs of dual diagnosis patients; collaboration of care between mental health and addiction providers is challenged by treatment access and coordination of care (Padwa, Guerrero, Braslow, & Fenwick, 2015). Pharmacists may bridge the gap in treatment by providing coordination of care related to medication use and access to treatment.

Lack of Mental Health Providers

A significant concern for adequate mental health services is the lack of providers in rural and underserved patient populations. Starting in 2009, states enacted significant budget cuts to CMHCs, who are often the only provider of mental health services in rural areas. In addition, the MHPAEA of 2008 and the ACA 2010 required mental healthcare reform and parity that increased the number of persons able to afford treatment services. This increase in insured patients seeking services further stressed a mental health system with decreasing budgets (Larrison et al., 2011). In a study evaluating racial and ethnic disparities in mental health care, the results showed a significant difference in access to care for Black and Latino patients relative to White patients. Minorities lived in counties with greater poverty and unemployment rates compared to Whites. The availability of insurance, CMHC treatment, and density of specialty providers benefited Black individuals. Increased racial and ethnic residential segregation is associated with shortages of psychiatrists for Latino patients (Lê Cook, Doksum, Chen, Carle, & Alegria, 2013).

Community pharmacies are present in nearly every community, providing an opportunity for community pharmacists to bridge the gap in access to mental health services. Barriers to the provision of this service exist, including heavy dispensing workloads, negative attitudes about individuals experiencing mental health disorders, and stigma (Calogero & Caley, 2017). Clinical pharmacists in outpatient mental health treatment settings can provide medication regimen review; interview patients about medication adherence, side effects, and effectiveness; and work under collaborative practice agreements to provide mental health medication management services to increase the time available to both primary care and mental health providers for mental health treatment (Rubio-Valera et al., 2014).

Implications for Behavioral Health

Clinical psychiatric pharmacists have been practicing in the area of mental health for many years and are vital members of the treatment team. While inpatient clinical psychiatric pharmacists have been found in this practice area for some time, outpatient clinical psychiatric pharmacists have, for the past decade, begun to create roles within the clinic setting. Inpatient psychiatric pharmacists perform tasks related to medication regimen review, patient rounds, and transitions of care; outpatient psychiatric pharmacists provide medication management, adherence and side effect reviews, decreased medication overlap, and application for patient assistance programs under collaborative practice agreements with physicians. Because of a lack of mental health providers and decreased funding for CMHCs in rural areas, clinical pharmacists are filling the role of mental health provider in outpatient primary care settings.

Community pharmacists are the most accessible healthcare professionals and can provide evaluation of medication adherence, patient counseling, insurance assessments, and mental health screenings with referral to mental health providers. Education in schools and colleges of pharmacy has focused on decreasing pharmacist stigma and negative images of people with mental disorders and increasing the comfort level of the pharmacist for interacting with patients through the use of motivational interviewing and shared decision-making. Pharmacists are uniquely positioned to fill the gap in available mental health providers, both in the community pharmacy and clinical practice setting.

References

Amin, K., Farley, J. F., Maciejewski, M. L., & Domino, M. E. (2017). Effect of Medicaid policy changes on medication adherence: Differences by baseline adherence. *Journal of Managed Care & Specialty Pharmacy, 23*(3), 337–345. https://doi.org/10.18553/jmcp.2017.23.3.337

Arnold, M. E., Buys, L., & Fullas, F. (2015). Impact of pharmacist intervention in conjunction with outpatient physician follow-up visits after hospital discharge on readmission rate. *American Journal of Health-System Pharmacy, 72*(11 Suppl 1), S36–S42. https://doi.org/10.2146/sp150011

Benson, C. J., Joshi, K., Lapane, K. L., & Fastenau, J. (2015). Evaluation of a comprehensive information and assistance program for patients with schizophrenia treated with long-acting injectable antipsychotics. *Current Medical Research and Opinion, 31*(7), 1437–1448. https://doi.org/10.1185/03007995.2015.1050365

Calogero, S., & Caley, C. F. (2017). Supporting patients with mental illness: Deconstructing barriers to community pharmacist access. *Journal of the American Pharmacists Association, 57*(2), 248–255. https://doi.org/10.1016/j.japh.2016.12.066

Cavanaugh, J. J., Lindsey, K. N., Shilliday, B. B., & Ratner, S. P. (2015). Pharmacist-coordinated multidisciplinary hospital follow-up visits improve patient outcomes. *Journal of Managed Care & Specialty Pharmacy, 21*(3), 256–260. https://doi.org/10.18553/jmcp.2015.21.3.256

Dalton, K., & Byrne, S. (2017). Role of the pharmacist in reducing healthcare costs: Current insights. *Integrated Pharmacy Research & Practice, 6*, 37–46. https://doi.org/10.2147/iprp.S108047

Di Lorenzo, R., Galliani, A., Guicciardi, A., Landi, G., & Ferri, P. (2014). A retrospective analysis focusing on a group of patients with dual diagnosis treated by both mental health and substance use services. *Neuropsychiatric Disease and Treatment, 10*, 1479–1488. https://doi.org/10.2147/ndt.S65896

Doshi, J. A., Li, P., Desai, S., & Marcus, S. C. (2017). Impact of Medicaid prescription copayments on use of antipsychotics and other medications in patients with schizophrenia. *Journal of Medical Economics, 20*(12), 1252–1260. https://doi.org/10.1080/13696998.2017.1365720

Gallagher, J., McCarthy, S., & Byrne, S. (2014). Economic evaluations of clinical pharmacist interventions on hospital inpatients: A systematic review of recent literature. *International Journal of Clinical Pharmacy, 36*(6), 1101–1114. https://doi.org/10.1007/s11096-014-0008-9

Gilmore, V., Efird, L., Fu, D., LeBlanc, Y., Nesbit, T., & Swarthout, M. (2015). Implementation of transitions-of-care services through acute care and outpatient pharmacy collaboration. *American Journal of Health-System Pharmacy, 72*(9), 737–744. https://doi.org/10.2146/ajhp140504

Grim, K., Rosenberg, D., Svedberg, P., & Schon, U. K. (2016). Shared decision-making in mental health care-a user perspective on decisional needs in community-based services. *International Journal of Qualitative Studies on Health and Well-Being, 11*, 30563. https://doi.org/10.3402/qhw.v11.30563

Larrison, C. R., Hack-Ritzo, S., Koerner, B. D., Schoppelrey, S. L., Ackerson, B. J., & Korr, W. S. (2011). State budget cuts, health care reform, and a crisis in rural community mental health agencies. *Psychiatric Services, 62*(11), 1255–1257. https://doi.org/10.1176/ps.62.11.pss6211_1255

Lê Cook, B., Doksum, T., Chen, C. N., Carle, A., & Alegria, M. (2013). The role of provider supply and organization in reducing racial/ethnic disparities in mental health care in the U.S. *Social Science & Medicine, 84*, 102–109. https://doi.org/10.1016/j.socscimed.2013.02.006

Luetsch, K., & Burrows, J. (2018). From transitions to transformation: A study of pharmacists developing patient-centered communication skills. *Research in Social & Administrative Pharmacy, 14*(7), 686–694. https://doi.org/10.1016/j.sapharm.2017.08.003

Marcus, S. C., Zummo, J., Pettit, A. R., Stoddard, J., & Doshi, J. A. (2015). Antipsychotic adherence and rehospitalization in schizophrenia patients receiving oral versus long-acting injectable antipsychotics following hospital discharge. *Journal of Managed Care & Specialty Pharmacy, 21*(9), 754–768. https://doi.org/10.18553/jmcp.2015.21.9.754

McGovern, M. P., Lambert-Harris, C., Gotham, H. J., Claus, R. E., & Xie, H. (2014). Dual diagnosis capability in mental health and addiction treatment services: An assessment of programs across multiple state systems. *Administration and Policy in Mental Health, 41*(2), 205–214. https://doi.org/10.1007/s10488-012-0449-1

Morant, N., Kaminskiy, E., & Ramon, S. (2016). Shared decision making for psychiatric medication management: Beyond the micro-social. *Health Expectations, 19*(5), 1002–1014. https://doi.org/10.1111/hex.12392

Nkansah, N., Mostovetsky, O., Yu, C., Chheng, T., Beney, J., Bond, C. M., & Bero, L. (2010). Effect of outpatient pharmacists' non-dispensing roles on patient outcomes and prescribing patterns. *The Cochrane Database of Systematic Reviews, 7*, Cd000336. https://doi.org/10.1002/14651858.CD000336.pub2

Ovsag, K., Hydery, S., & Mousa, S. A. (2008). Preferred drug lists: Potential impact on healthcare economics. *Vascular Health and Risk Management, 4*(2), 403–413.

Padwa, H., Guerrero, E. G., Braslow, J. T., & Fenwick, K. M. (2015). Barriers to serving clients with co-occurring disorders in a transformed mental health system. *Psychiatric Services, 66*(5), 547–550. https://doi.org/10.1176/appi.ps.201400190

Phokeo, V., Sproule, B., & Raman-Wilms, L. (2004). Community pharmacists' attitudes toward and professional interactions with users of psychiatric medication. *Psychiatric Services, 55*(12), 1434–1436. https://doi.org/10.1176/appi.ps.55.12.1434

Ramalho de Oliveira, D., Brummel, A. R., & Miller, D. B. (2010). Medication therapy management: 10 years of experience in a large integrated health care system. *Journal of Managed Care Pharmacy, 16*(3), 185–195. https://doi.org/10.18553/jmcp.2010.16.3.185

Richardson, T. E., O'Reilly, C. L., & Chen, T. F. (2014). A comprehensive review of the impact of clinical pharmacy services on patient outcomes in mental health. *International Journal of Clinical Pharmacy, 36*(2), 222–232. https://doi.org/10.1007/s11096-013-9900-y

Ridley, D. B., & Axelsen, K. J. (2006). Impact of Medicaid preferred drug lists on therapeutic adherence. *PharmacoEconomics, 24*(Suppl 3), 65–78.

Rubio-Valera, M., Chen, T. F., & O'Reilly, C. L. (2014). New roles for pharmacists in community mental health care: A narrative review. *International Journal of Environmental Research and Public Health, 11*(10), 10967–10990. https://doi.org/10.3390/ijerph111010967

Salvo, M. C., & Cannon-Breland, M. L. (2015). Motivational interviewing for medication adherence. *Journal of the American Pharmacists Association, 55*(4), e354–e361.; quiz e362-353. https://doi.org/10.1331/JAPhA.2015.15532

The Center for Consumer Information & Insurance Oversight. (2018). *The mental health parity and addiction equality act (MHPAEA). [web page].* Baltimore, MD: Centers for Medicare & Medicaid Services. https://www.cms.gov/cciio/programs-and-initiatives/other-insurance-protections/mhpaea_factsheet.html

Wright, W. A., Gorman, J. M., Odorzynski, M., Peterson, M. J., & Clayton, C. (2016). Integrated pharmacies at community mental health centers: Medication adherence and outcomes. *Journal of Managed Care & Specialty Pharmacy, 22*(11), 1330–1336. https://doi.org/10.18553/jmcp.2016.16004

Younas, M., Bradley, E., Holmes, N., Sud, D., & Maidment, I. D. (2016). Mental health pharmacists views on shared decision-making for antipsychotics in serious mental illness. *International Journal of Clinical Pharmacy, 38*(5), 1191–1199. https://doi.org/10.1007/s11096-016-0352-z

Global Services, Systems, and Policy

Ardis Hanson and Bruce Lubotsky Levin

Introduction

Public policymaking begins with an official acknowledgment of an identified issue or concern (Hanson, 2014). This begins a series of practical actions to resolve the issue; an issue is identified and a multilayered process begins to seek a solution that attempts to address problems at an individual (micro)level as well as at the meso- and macro-levels. The policymaking process includes the selection of a "working group" (i.e., an individual, a group of individuals, or an institution to examine the problem and to generate recommendations). To do so, the working group requests one or more policy analyses, depending upon the complexity of the problem and the scope of its mandate.

These policy analyses review the identified problems from numerous perspectives, including economic, political, or social, to define and describe the problem and recommend possible solutions. Social, statistical, and epidemiologic data regarding behavioral health are gathered, as is the evidence on best practices. After the recommendations, an external agency or the executive, judicial, or legislative branch of a state or federal government then takes over to initiate the designated actions. This process, or variants of the process, occurs daily across the world as we seek to find best solutions to address behavioral disorders, improve quality of life and outcomes for persons with these disorders, and to improve population health (Hanson, 2014).

A. Hanson
Research and Education Unit, Shimberg Health Sciences Library,
University of South Florida, Tampa, FL, USA

B. L. Levin (✉)
Department of Child and Family Studies, College of Behavioral and Community Sciences,
University of South Florida, Tampa, FL, USA

Behavioral Health Concentration, College of Public Health, University of South Florida,
Tampa, FL, USA
e-mail: Levin@usf.edu

© Springer Nature Switzerland AG 2020   351
B. L. Levin, A. Hanson (eds.), *Foundations of Behavioral Health*,
https://doi.org/10.1007/978-3-030-18435-3_17

In this chapter, we attempt to integrate current trends in global behavioral health policy, systems, and services, examining the magnitude of the problem, from definitional and operational perspectives, with a focus on child and adolescent behavioral health. This includes a look at the ambiguity of behavioral health policymaking, as a policy problem, from numerous frames, perspectives, populations, and disciplines to the difficulties in integrating global and national priorities across disparate cultures, economies, and infrastructures.

Framing the Magnitude of a Public Policy Problem

Defining significant problems as policy actions in behavioral health are not only harder to define but also more open to dispute as to what constitutes a problem and what is the most effective solution to the problem. Public policy problems often are "wicked problems" (Rittel & Martin, 1973). Such problems are dependent upon how an issue is framed, the language used by stakeholders, and time and resource constraints, but more importantly, there is seldom a definitive solution. Such significant problems essentially are unique and do not have an exhaustively describable set of potential solutions.

Almost anything of an economic, social, or political nature can influence policy, particularly behavioral health policy. In almost any policy analysis in behavioral health, there are overlapping issues, including financing; organization of services; promotion, prevention, treatment, and rehabilitation; intersectoral collaboration; advocacy; legislation and human rights; workforce development; quality improvement; information systems; program evaluation; and research that can affect the continuation, revision, and development of policies that affect services delivery. Finally, any number of economic, social, and/or political factors (determinants) can affect each and every one of the issues identified above and may only reveal themselves during the policy process.

The measures of morbidity, mortality, and disability create a consistent narrative about behavioral health across age, gender, regions, and economies. Global, regional, and national studies that examine the global burden of disease (GBD), disability-adjusted life years (DALYS), and the social determinants of health (SDH) have different frames, but all are central to understand how best to address behavioral health services inequities from a policy perspective.

Behavioral health problems are a leading cause of health-related disability across all age groups (GBD 2016 Disease and Injury Incidence and Prevalence Collaborators, 2017; Maselko, 2017; Murray & Lopez, 1996; Whiteford et al., 2013). Further, the World Health Organization (WHO) estimates that nearly 35% of the global burden of disease (GDB) has its roots in childhood (Baranne & Falissard, 2018; Erskine et al., 2015; World Health Organization, 2014). Children and adolescents constitute almost a third (1.2 billion individuals) of the world's population (UNICEF, 2012).

National and global research estimates suggest behavioral health problems affect between 10% and 20% of children and adolescents worldwide (Kieling et al., 2011; National Research Council & Institute of Medicine, 2009; Waddell, Hua, Garland,

Peters, & McEwan, 2007). Nearly 90% of children and adolescents live in low-income and middle-income countries (LMIC), where they form up to 50% of the population (Kieling et al., 2011). In the United States, studies report a 22–24% increase in inpatient behavioral health admissions among children and adolescents and 80% increase in hospital stays for children for mood disorders (Health Care Cost Institute, 2012; Pfuntner, Wier, & Stocks, 2013).

Systematic reviews of mental health promotion and preventive interventions show there are long-lasting positive effects on levels of functioning (e.g., activities of daily living) and social and economic benefits (Barry, Clarke, Jenkins, & Patel, 2013; Durlak & Wells, 1997; Jané-Llopis, Barry, Hosman, & Patel, 2005; Patel et al., 2010).

Such interventions can mitigate the often "poor fit" that occurs when traditional clinical training and practice models fail to address the clinically and socially complex presentations of children and adolescents with behavioral disorders. The success of evidence-based decision-making, particularly in secondary prevention initiatives (Aldrich et al., 2015; Rith-Najarian, Daleiden, & Chorpita, 2016), is based on making decisions using the best available peer-reviewed quantitative and qualitative evidence and the systematic use of data and information systems (Brownson, Fielding, & Maylahn, 2009). However, only about 10% of randomized clinical mental health trials for children and adolescents come from an LMIC (Kieling et al., 2011).

There is ample evidence that behavioral disorders in childhood and adolescence adversely affect young adult and adult outcomes (Almuneef et al., 2016; Bellis, Lowey, Leckenby, Hughes, & Harrison, 2014; Crouch, Strompolis, Bennett, Morse, & Radcliff, 2017; Hughes et al., 2017; Hunt, Slack, & Berger, 2017; Ismayilova, Gaveras, Blum, To-Camier, & Nanema, 2016; Luby, Barch, Whalen, Tillman, & Belden, 2017; McGrath et al., 2017; Oh et al., 2018; Reuben et al., 2016; Sterling et al., 2018; Trotta, Murray, & Fisher, 2015). Hence, a developmental or life span approach is essential. Such a course incorporates universal actions, includes all social strata, and is proportionate to the level of disadvantage (World Health Organization & Calouste Gulbenkian Foundation, 2014). This approach will help "level the social gradient and successfully reduce inequalities in mental disorders" (WHO & Calouste, 2014, p. 10). By focusing on the relationships between and among macro-level context, systems, society, and life-course stages, nations can improve population behavioral health and reduce the risk of those mental disorders exacerbated by social inequalities.

Measuring and Developing Expert Evidence

Social, statistical, and epidemiologic data regarding populations, health, and illness have implications for global behavioral health policy, systems, and services across the developmental life span. The data illustrate the magnitude of the relationships among health, behavioral health, suicide, substance/alcohol use, intentional and unintentional injuries, interpersonal and community violence, war and disasters, and environmental factors across the life span.

Table 1 The World Health Organization's frames on social determinants of health

Action items	Themes
Adopt improved governance for health and development	Employment
Promote participation in policymaking and implementation	Social exclusion
Promote participation in policymaking and implementation	Priority public health conditions
Strengthen global governance and collaboration	Women and gender equity
Monitor progress and increase accountability	Early child development
	Globalization
	Health systems
	Measurements and evidence
	Urbanization

Excerpted from the Rio Political Declaration on Social Determinants of Health (World General Assembly, 2011)

There are numerous ways to frame the necessary evidence necessary to change policy. The World Health Organization, for example, drives the types of evidence for addressing SDH (Kelly et al., 2007). Divided into two components, the five "action areas" and nine themes focus on the conditions in which people are born, grow, live, work and age (World Health Assembly, 2011). Shaped by the distribution of money, power, and resources at global, national, and local levels, the SDH identifies health inequities, that is, the differences in health status seen within and between countries (see Table 1).

In 2015, all United Nations (UN) member states adopted the 2030 Agenda for Sustainable Development, with 17 Sustainable Development Goals (SDGs) and 169 associated targets. The Agenda commits the UN member states "… to the prevention and treatment of non-communicable diseases, including behavioural, developmental and neurological disorders, which constitute a major challenge for sustainable development" (United Nations General Assembly, 2015, p. 8).

Building upon the adoption of the Comprehensive Mental Health Action Plan (WHO, 2013) and the Global Strategy to Reduce the Harmful Use of Alcohol (WHO, 2010) by the World Health Assembly, Goal 3, Targets 3.4 and 3.5 include behavioral health as an integral element of national health policy, infrastructures, and services delivery plans. "Goal 3: Ensure healthy lives and promote well-being for all at all ages" (aka "Good Health and Well-Being") has two targets directly related to behavioral health. Target 3.4 aims to reduce premature mortality from NCDs by one-third with a three-legged approach: promotion of mental health and well-being, prevention, and treatment. Target 3.5 focuses on the prevention and treatment of substance abuse.

In the United States, plans are underway to develop a new set of 10-year national objectives as *Healthy People 2020* ends and *Healthy People 2030* begins. Like the SDH and SDGs, two of the foundational principles of *Healthy People*

2030 are health promotion and disease prevention for physical, mental, and social health while achieving health equity and reducing health disparities (Office of Disease Prevention and Health Promotion, 2018). *Healthy People 2030* continues the SDH, life-course, and population-based perspectives from *Healthy People 2020*, with an additional emphasis on community capacity (Secretary's Advisory Committee on National Health Promotion and Disease Prevention Objectives for 2030, 2018).

Community-based and community-driven initiatives are necessary to change the multiple determinants of health that inhibit health equity to those determinants that build and promote health equity, strengthening the integration of health systems, services, and policies (National Academies of Sciences, Engineering,, & Medicine, 2017).

Indicators

Policymakers use a number of indicators to describe countries and their ability to implement health policy priority initiatives successfully. The public policy issue often establishes the framework and indicators, helped by national and international stakeholders, policies, and legislation. Since we are dealing with numerous countries, regions, naming authorities, and languages, there will be differences in terminologies and challenges in identifying which issues need to be addressed and if/how services will be delivered.

Economic Indicators

One major indicator is the level of economic development in a country. The World Bank (2018a, 2018b) categorizes countries by economies (low-, low-middle, upper-middle, and high-income) and geographies (East Asia and Pacific, Europe and Central Asia, Latin America and the Caribbean, Middle East and North Africa, South Asia, and sub-Saharan Africa). The WHO follows the World Bank designations and separates out high-income countries within each of these regions as a seventh group.

Why is economy such an important consideration? A country's financial status affects how much it can or is able to allocate to identified, strategic concerns. Much of the literature establishes individual and national poverty as a significant factor that affects morbidity and mortality rates, infrastructure, employment, standard of living, political/social stability, health provision, population health, and resiliency to natural and man-made disasters (Balabanova et al., 2013; Bloom et al., 2011; Forouzanfar et al., 2015; Maselko, 2017; Stubbs et al., 2016).

Poverty

Considered a measurement of deprivation, the poverty level of a nation is linked intrinsically with the SDH and to the ability of a country to provide basic health services. Most policy measures have two elements: (1) a measure of need (poverty threshold) and (2) a measure of the resources and goods available to meet those needs. The most common poverty measures are income-based poverty measures, in which measures of need and the available resources are expressed in monetary terms. The World Bank (2018a, 2018b) reports that, in 2015, 10% (736 million) of people in the developing world lived on less than US $1.90 a day.

However, the relative measure used in international comparisons and the official poverty measure may not gauge the effect of non-income programs or resources, so an alternative is to use multidimensional poverty tools that measure non-income-based poverty dimensions. The preferred tool for measuring the SDGs is the United Nations Development Programme (UNDP, 2018) Multidimensional Poverty Index (MPI). Approximately 1.3 billion individuals across 105 developing countries live in multidimensional poverty, of which 1.1 billion people live in rural areas and 0.2 billion live in urban areas (Oxford Poverty and Human Development Initiative, 2018). Eighty-three percent of all multidimensionally poor people live in sub-Saharan Africa and South Asia (India, Nigeria, Ethiopia, Pakistan, and Bangladesh). Two-thirds (889 million) of all multidimensionally poor people live in middle-income countries. Almost 50% (665 million children) live in multidimensional poverty (Oxford Poverty and Human Development Initiative, 2018).

The UNDP MPI captures three dimensions and ten indicators of poverty (Alkire & Jahan, 2018). The three dimensions and ten indicators are health (nutrition, child mortality), education (years of school attendance and years of school), and standard of living (cooking fuel, sanitation, drinking water, electricity, housing, and assets). These dimensions and indicators have been shown to be influential in child and adolescent behavioral health.

Frames

Framing involves the definition or scope of a policy problem or image, that is, how issues are categorized or portrayed. Policy often is linked to accepted national, social, or cultural values; however, core values differ widely from country to country and may or may not change over time. Further, policy issues are complex and multifaceted. Behavioral health can be framed in terms of health, mental health, population mental health, substance abuse, addiction, and more, often related to disciplines (philosophies, epistemologies, and ontologies) and current social, political, and cultural frames.

Currently, a number of global and national anchor frames are used. Anchor frames are a tool to make sense of complex social issues that have many interrelationships or interdependent components. Simply stated, how we interpret, communicate, and understand goals and values in policy is based upon the frame or frames we base our understanding, and these frames underscore the importance of language and symbolic action in policymaking (Edelman, 1988; Fischer, 2003; Stone, 2012; Yanow, 1996).

"Health as a Human Right"

The importance of health, and its definition, from a global perspective, changed over seven decades. In 1946, the Constitution of the WHO defined health as "a state of complete physical, mental, and social well-being and not merely the absence of disease or infirmity." In 1948, Article 25 of the Universal Declaration of Human Rights (UDHR) also mentioned health as part of the right to have an adequate standard of living. In 1966, the International Covenant of Economic, Social, and Cultural Rights (ICESCR) codified health as a "human right" and first addressed the "underlying determinants of health." In 1989, the UN Convention on the Rights of the Child specifically framed health as a human right that is universally applicable to all children, regardless of the culture of a society (United Nations General Assembly, 1989).

Since that time, numerous international human rights treaties have recognized or referred to the right to health and codified health as a human right in international and domestic declarations, legislation, and policies. These treaties argue fundamental human needs create human rights obligations on the part of both the public and private sectors. However, studies on indicators that tease out the political determinants of health are rare. For their analysis of health policy performance in 43 European countries, Mackenbach and McKee (2013) developed a set of process and outcome indicators that may affect the implementation of effective health policies at a national level. Process indicators measured the degree of implementation of policies that had proved effective, while outcome indicators measured the impact of these policies on the exposure of the population to health risks (prevalence) and the impact on population health. They concluded that various levels of implementation of preventive health policy measures were caused by both the "will and the means" of national governments to implement policies. Stuckler and Basu (2013) suggest there is correlation between decreased health care and failed government austerity programs.

Social Determinants of Health

In 2008, the Commission on Social Determinants of Health defined the social determinants of health (SDH) as "These inequities in health, avoidable health inequalities, arise because of the circumstances in which people grow, live, work, and age, and the systems put in place to deal with illness. The conditions in which people live and die are, in turn, shaped by political, social, and economic forces"(Commission on Social Determinants of Health, 2008, [i]). The World Health Assembly urged the adoption of the SDH, especially for priority public health programs and research on effective policies and interventions (World Health Assembly, 2009, May 22). Hence, an individual's right to health must also address how to reduce these social (societal) determinants of health. Common nomenclature for SDH includes "health inequities," "health inequalities," or "disparities."

Global frames are re-anchored or reframed to meet the needs of local, regional, or national entities. Although the concept of SDH recently has broadened to encompass both the social and *behavioral* determinants of health (SBDs), a 2004 WHO summary report on the prevention of mental disorders listed the social, environmental, and economic determinants of mental health (p. 21). A decade later, the US Institute of Medicine (IOM, 2014, 2015) and the UN/WHO Sustainable Development Goals specifically addressed the social and behavioral determinants of health (SBDs).

Millennium Development Goals/Sustainable Development Goals

In 2000, the UN/WHO Millennium Development Goals (MDGs) committed world leaders to eight global goals that would reduce poverty, hunger, disease, illiteracy, environmental degradation, and discrimination against women. In 2015, the MDGs were recast within the 2030 Agenda for Sustainable Development as Sustainable Development Goals (SDGs). The 17 new SDGs (aka Global Goals), building upon the original MDGs, seek to eliminate rather than reduce poverty and have specific targets to achieve for health, education, and gender equality. Goal 3 of the SDGs clearly place mental (behavioral) health within the framework of health.

The European Framework for Action on Mental Health and Well-Being

The European Pact for Mental Health and Well-being, formed in 2008, resulted in the EU Joint Action for Mental Health and Well-being: Mental Health in All Policies initiative in 2013 (EU Joint Action on Mental Health and Wellbeing, 2016). The objective of the EU Joint Action is threefold: (1) the promotion of mental health and well-being, (2) prevention of mental disorders, and (3) social inclusion of persons with serious mental disorders. It focuses across five areas: (1) workplace mental health; (2) school mental health; (3) community-based mental health care; (4) e-health initiatives targeted to depression and suicide; and (5) the integration of mental health in all policies (EU Joint Action on Mental Health and Wellbeing, 2016).

To accomplish this, the EU JA MH-WB involved its 28 member states, the EU, pertinent stakeholders, and international organizations, using national working groups, to inform the EU (multi-country) working groups on national situations, capacity building, and commitments among stakeholders. The *European Framework* is the culmination of an EU Green Paper (European Communities, 2005), earlier works by the European Pact for Mental Health and Wellbeing, and the WHO's Global and European Mental Health Strategies and Action Plans.

Mental Health in All Policies (MHiAP)

The UN/WHO focus on health in all policies (HiAP) requires governments to examine the consequences of public policies that do not address the social determinants of health and to better prioritize efforts and capacity building to improve population health (Pena et al., 2013). The specific mention of mental health promotion and prevention as a critical NCD target within the larger global health and sustainable development agendas shows how the reframing of mental illnesses as noncommunicable diseases may be a first step to reducing the stigma attached to mental illnesses and the integration of mental health and physical health promotion and prevention efforts and initiatives. The EU Joint Action for Mental Health and Wellbeing: Mental Health in All Policies initiative has 14 points of discussion, of which two, measuring and monitoring MHiAP and translating MHiAP into practice, are of especial importance for implementation and assessment.

Projects, such as the European Commission's Mapping NCD project (Berg Brigham et al., 2016), and studies on issues surrounding policy, implementation, and governance (Bauman, King, & Nutbeam, 2014; Oneka et al., 2017; Stahl, 2018; Storm, Harting, Stronks, & Schuit, 2014; Synnevag, Amdam, & Fosse, 2018; Van Vliet-Brown, Shahram, & Oelke, 2018) hopefully will provide information to ensure that we do reach the goal of mental health in all policies.

Data from a Policy, Systems, and Services Perspective

How can we best monitor and measure actions to address the SDGs that can inform policymaking, evaluate implementation, and ensure accountability? What data do we collect? How do we normalize the data so we know we are comparing apples with apples, specifically red apples with red apples? How do we disaggregate data to understand better baseline levels and potential impacts of policies? While these are important questions, the answers and the processes necessary to produce the answers and the system in which to collect and use the data are complex.

The typical data sources are data generated through civil registries, vital statistics, economic and labor force statistics, educational systems, administrative systems of governments, utilities, geospatial and environmental agencies, and central banks. These include, but are not limited to, population and housing censuses, agricultural censuses, economic surveys and censuses, and periodic household surveys. If the data are collected, there is no guarantee the available data are current. There often are considerable time lags between data collection and data analysis, not to mention publication and dissemination. Most government data are at least 1–2 years out of date and, in the case of behavioral health data in the United States, for example, often 2–3 years older than year of publication.

There are challenges surrounding the use of interdependent data. Census data is central to calculating per capita economic data, civil registries and vital statistics track access to services, and administrative data and household surveys address safety net and other social programs usage by population. Administrative data in behavioral health captures service performance and population data, but may not capture more qualitative data collected in household surveillance sampling surveys.

Explaining the differences in data availability across countries requires us to examine a number of factors. These include variation in policy priorities, statistical capacities, overall development statuses, institutional/infrastructure, and whether the country sees the applicability or relevance of the indicators in its review of the SDGs and its own policy focal areas. In addition, when looking at regional or subregional policy priorities, there is more data collection on economic goal indicators than on environmental indicators. Further, targets under social goal indicators are more likely to be linked to economic indicators, particularly those which address the multidimensional aspects of poverty.

Of the 161 SDG indicators, there are 20 core objectives, measurement concepts, and indicators for the proposed monitoring system for action on the SDH (World Health Organization, 2016). Approximately one-third of the indicators (6 out of 20) are SDG indicators. A little over one-third of the indicators (8 out of 20) come from existing WHO program assessment initiatives. The remaining third are already part of routine information reported by WHO. At national levels, proposed indicators for monitoring action on the SDH will come from numerous sectors, including health, social protection, education, labor, and human rights.

The availability of data on social determinants, however, is poor. Not all governments collect the same type of data consistently over a period of years within the same region or among a specific population. Something as simple as registering all children who are born into a national registry does not happen in every country. UNICEF estimates the births of nearly 230 million children under the age of five have never been recorded (United Nations Children's Fund, 2014). For example, 39% of the children born in South Asia were unregistered and 44% of all births in sub-Saharan Africa were unregistered. Children are less likely to be registered if they come in poor households or from remote or rural areas, have uneducated mothers, or are female (United Nations Children's Fund, 2014). Lack of a birth certificate or registration may deny child access to basic education and health care. Without documentation, that child does not exist; hence, the child is not counted. When children are not counted, it is difficult to determine incidence or to estimate prevalence of disease.

Establishing Prevalence to Show the Need for Services

Prevalence is defined as a proportion of persons in a population in a given location and at a particular time, e.g., a count of the number of people affected. Counts are used to help determine need for resources, workforce requirements, scope of services, and other elements important to the delivery of behavioral health-care services. Prevalence estimates adjust the counts of the affected individuals to the size of a source population. Prevalence data is critical for child and adolescent health, as almost 75% of the cumulative prevalence of many behavioral health problems, including but not limited to substance abuse, anorexia nervosa, major depressive disorder, bipolar disorder, and schizophrenia, have their onset before age 25.

Reporting prevalence over a region or country can be problematic, as in the case of the European Union and the United States. The Child and Adolescent Mental Health in Enlarged European Union (CAMHEE) report provided a snapshot of child and adolescent behavioral health policies and practices across 15 European countries (Belgium, Bulgaria, Estonia, Finland, Germany (Heidelberg), Greece, Hungary, Latvia, Lithuania, Norway, Poland, Romania, Slovenia, Spain (Catalonia), and the United Kingdom (England)) (Braddick, Carral, Jenkins, & Jané-Lopis, 2009). About 50% of countries reported prevalence rates on positive mental health in children. More specifically, 13 of 15 countries reported the existence of information about the prevalence of mental disorders, whereas just 8 of 15 reported collecting the prevalence of some indicator of positive mental health (e.g., well-being, self-esteem, quality of life, and resilience). Budgets dedicated to CAMH issues, however, were rarely clearly identifiable and were often mixed with other funds (Braddick et al., 2009).

Within the United States, estimating prevalence is extremely difficult due to the lack of a "standard" inclusive definition for a minimum functional level of impairment for an agreed-upon duration in determining prevalence of disorders among children and adolescents (Brauner & Stephens, 2006). The term "serious emotional disturbance" (SED), for example, is not a formal DSM-IV diagnosis. State and federal agencies use that term to identify a population of children who have significant emotional and behavioral problems, who have a high need for services, and who may have a range of functional limitations (Center for Mental Health Services, 1998).

Therefore, estimates of the prevalence of behavioral disorders in children and adolescents in the United States vary widely. While some researchers estimate that between 13 and 20% of children and adolescents in the general population of the United States experience a DSM mental disorder in a given year (National Research Council & Institute of Medicine, 2009), others differentiate the lifetime and current prevalence of mental disorders among children and adolescents in the United States, that is, 21% and 14.8%, respectively (Lu, 2017).

Children and adolescents in specialty care systems, such as child welfare or juvenile justice, have a much higher prevalence of mental disorders (Underwood & Washington, 2016; Yampolskaya, Sharrock, Clark, & Hanson, 2017). However, the estimated prevalence of SEDs was 8.0% (Kessler et al., 2012). More than half (54.5%) of the SEDs were due to behavior disorders, and almost a third of SEDs (31.4%) were attributed to mood disorders (Kessler et al., 2012). Another interesting finding was that just under a third (29%) of respondents with complex (3 or more) disorders from the 12-month DSM-IV/Composite International Diagnostic

Interview disorders constituted more than 60% (63.5%) of children and adolescents with SEDs (Kessler et al., 2012).

Increasingly, in the United States and globally, comorbidity is seen as an index of burden of disease, with more severe courses and outcomes for children and adolescents with mental disorders. These findings then beg the question of how granular definitions should be, how to map between disorder differences effectively, and how to determine risk and effect of high comorbidity with DSM disorders, as well as with SED. This is another of the "wicked" problems in determining policy priorities for addressing global behavioral health problems in children and adolescents.

Overview of Child and Adolescent Behavioral Health Policies Globally

In 2003, the WHO first identified treatment gaps, promoted training, addressed evidence-based treatment, and promulgated a model national policy. Priority disorders were determined by higher frequency of occurrence, degree of associated impairment, therapeutic possibilities, and long-term care consequences (WHO, 2003). The WHO also emphasized the diagnosis of children and adolescents cannot be considered solely from a Western perspective. Presentation of a disorder would vary across countries and cultural/societal subgroups within a country. It also emphasized the importance of determining the degree of impairment and/or disability associated with a diagnosis. The specific diagnosis may be less important than the degree of impairment of the disorder and what supports the individual will need to participate in his or her society (WHO, 2003).

Finally, the WHO stressed the importance of a continuum of care to ensure good quality of care, compliance with best practices, and the ability to maintain children and adolescents in the least-restrictive environments. Establishing guidelines for a continuum of care can help in determining benchmarks and the collection of epidemiological and/or surveillance data to address treatment and services delivery (WHO, 2003).

In 2011, the WHO reported that spending on behavioral health was less than two (US) dollars per person per year, less than 25 cents per person in low-income countries (WHO, 2011). Further, only 36% of people who live in low-income countries overall were covered by behavioral health legislation.

In its 2013–2020 mental health action plan, the WHO defined mental health as "a state of well-being in which the individual realizes his or her own abilities, can cope with the normal stresses of life, can work productively and fruitfully, and is able to make a contribution to his or her community" (World Health Assembly, 2013, p. 3). In that report, mental health for children emphasized the developmental aspect of mental health. The definition included for adolescents "having a positive sense of identity, the ability to manage thoughts, emotions, and to build social relationships, as well as the aptitude to learn and acquire an education, ultimately enabling their full active participation in society" (World Health Assembly, 2013, p. 3).

North America

Both Canada and the United States lack a strong national strategy on behavioral health for children, a national framework for indicators, and a national organization to do the measuring. The systems of care in the United States and Canada also have difficulty in assessing prevalence and are underfunded to address the need for services in an increasingly larger child and adolescent population.

In the United States, the fragmented systems of care and difficulty normalizing data across multiple reporting agencies are still problematic. Integrated cross-referral social services and health-care data systems are rare. National studies suggest future surveillance should include standard case definitions of disorders to reliably categorize and count disorders, as well as to ensure comparability and reliability of estimates across surveillance systems (Perou et al., 2013). However, the continued lack of national health care and the inevitable federal vs. state's rights issues result in "best-guess" analysis from numerous sampling surveys and longitudinal studies.

In Canada, there was a concerted effort to address data collection about the behavioral health of children (Junek, 2012). The provincial and national governments wanted the data for policymaking, program construction, priority setting, and resource allocation. The most requested data concerned baseline information about children, specific groups of children, social determinants, characteristics of the user and general population, comparisons of regions and years, and indicators of child functioning, population health, and early identification data. However, across the reports, there were no standard criteria used which would allow comparison across governments (Junek, 2012). Hence, none of the published 64 reports could be considered effective monitoring reports.

South America

The 2011 WHO-AIMS report covers 10 of the 12 countries in South America. Six of the ten reporting countries in South America reported having a document that explicitly stated a national mental health policy (Pan American Health Organization, 2013). However, it is important to note that, similar to the Latin American, Caribbean, and Mexico group, governments in power often did not draft new policies or implement current policies. In addition, 9 of 10 countries reported having a national health plan. Only two countries have specific behavioral health legislation

(Brazil and Uruguay). In the eight reporting countries, the mental health budget as a percentage of the total health budget had a median of 2.05%. Eight countries reported having some coordinating structure (Pan American Health Organization, 2013). Eight countries reported the percentage of children treated ranges from 12% to 38%, with an average of 23% of children and adolescents receiving services (Pan American Health Organization, 2013).

Brazil

Children and adolescents comprise approximately 37% of the population of the Northeast of Brazil (Januário et al., 2017). The prevalence of child and adolescent mental disorders were similar to global estimates (10–20%) with 3–4% of children and adolescents classed with serious, chronic mental illnesses (Januário et al., 2017). Mental health indicators started to be part of the group of national basic health-care indicators after 2005 when Brazil increased their ambulatory care centers. In addition, the number of Psychosocial Healthcare Centers (CAPS) overall has increased dramatically. In Bahia State, CAPS increased from 14 in 2002 to 89 by 2011; Pernambuco State almost tripled its number of CAPS facilities within the last 4 years. More importantly, Brazil formally recognized child and adolescent mental health as a significant public health issue, which should be integrated into the larger Brazilian mental health system, not just limited to educational and social support systems (Januário et al., 2017).

Asia and the Pacific Island Region

Like the other regional reports, Asia and the Pacific Island region are difficult to compile as a single view (OECD & World Health Organization, 2012). Often divided into five regions (North and Central Asia, South and Southwest Asia, Southeast Asia, East and Northeast Asia, and the Pacific), the national, economic, and ethnic complexity of the region make it difficult to provide country comparisons (UNESCAP, 2017), especially when conducting SDG trend analyses. Only 64 of the 244 global SDG indicators, with two or more data points, are collected in fifty percent or more of the countries in the region. Although 89% of Tier 1 indicators have some data, less than 90% of Tier 1 indicators are collected on a regular basis (UNESCAP, 2017). In addition, data availability across the 17 goals is uneven. For SDG Goal 3: Good health and well-being, one or more data points are available for many of the indicators; however, a little over a quarter of indicators are unavailable (48 indicators are available for trend analysis, 22 indicators have an OK status, 4 have limited status, and 26 are unavailable) (UNESCAP, 2017).

Southeast Asia Region (SEAR)

In 2011, seven of the ten countries in the WHO Southeast Asia region (SEAR) reported a dedicated mental health policy (World Health Organization, 2011). In 2017, nine countries had a stand-alone mental health plan or policy, and eight countries had updated their plans or policies since 2013 (World Health Organization, 2018).

Australia

The Australian mental health "system" is a complex system comprised of cross-sector and inter-jurisdictional initiatives, with governments at federal and state levels that influence policy, strategy, funding, laws and legislation, regulations, and public and private services delivery entities (DeLoitte Australia, 2017). In addition to its National Mental Health Strategy and National Mental Health Commission, its *Roadmap for National Mental Health Reform 2012–2022* places an emphasis on "prevention and intervention activities appropriate to each person's life-stage and circumstances" (Council of Australian Governments, 2012, p. 15). This life span/developmental perspective is particularly key for child and adolescent behavioral health.

The second Australian Child and Adolescent Survey of Mental Health and Wellbeing determined the prevalence of mental disorders among children and adolescents in Australia was almost 14% (13.9%, or 1 in 7) (Lawrence et al., 2016). Almost 60% (59.8%) of children were diagnosed with mild mental disorders, a little over a quarter (25.4%) of the children were diagnosed with moderate mental disorders, and almost 15% (14.7%) were diagnosed with severe mental disorders (Lawrence et al., 2016). The Survey also showed a significant association between the presence of a mental disorder and suicidal behavior (Zubrick et al., 2016).

In the national *Young Minds Matter* survey, Johnson et al. (2016) found that 17% of all 4- to 17-year-olds used services for emotional or behavioral problems. Of those children with mental disorders, a little over 50% (56.0%) used available services.

More recently, Wave 6 of the K-cohort of the Longitudinal Study of Australian Children of adolescents who experienced bullying determined there was a marked increased incidence of mental disorders and heightened risk of poor mental health outcomes, self-harm, and suicidal ideation and behaviors (Ford, King, Priest, & Kavanagh, 2017).

Over $9 billion annually is spent on mental health-related services in Australia to serve the approximately 8.6 million, or 45% of Australians aged 16–85 will experience a common mental health-related condition such as depression, anxiety, or a substance use disorder in their lifetime, with an annual prevalence rate of 20% (1 in 5) (Australian Institute of Health and Welfare, 2018). Behavioral health problems are estimated to be responsible for 12% of the total burden of disease in Australia, with 1 in 4 years lived with a disability due to behavioral health disorders the leading cause of non-fatal burden (Australian Institute of Health and Welfare, 2018).

Africa

Africa is often broken into sub-Saharan Africa and North Africa. Sub-Saharan Africa includes all countries that are fully or partially located south of the Sahara, also referred to as East Africa, West Africa, and South Africa. North Africa covers Algeria, Egypt, Libya, Morocco, and Tunisia. There are 55 recognized countries in Africa. Africa is also one of the most diverse continents; the sub-Saharan region of Africa contains over 1000 languages, which is around one-sixth of the world's total number of languages.

Behavioral health issues generally are a very low priority in health services policies. In Africa, the majority of morbidity and mortality occurs from communicable diseases and malnutrition, and the armed conflicts and/or natural disasters in Africa have resulted in burgeoning refugee and displaced populations.

Of the 45 African member states surveyed in the WHO's 2011 *Mental Health Atlas project*, 30 reported they have an existing mental health plan and 20 reported they have existing mental health policies (World Health Organization, 2011). Seventy percent of African countries allocate less than 1% of the total health budget to mental health (Bird et al., 2011). Africa also has the lowest rate of mental health outpatient facilities, at 0.06 per 100,000 people (World Health Organization, 2011). Of the five countries in Africa which are reported in the *Atlas* survey, none had any prevention or promotion programs in schools.

South Africa

Children and adolescents may represent up to 50% of the population in low- and middle-income countries in Africa. However, even upper-middle-income countries may not have a vibrant child and adolescent mental health policy. In 2003, South Africa developed a national child and adolescent mental health policy as a policy and implementation framework for its nine provinces. A policy review by Mokitimi, Schneider, and de Vries (2018) found neither provincial child and adolescent mental health policies nor specific implementation plans supporting the 2003 national policy. Plans that did address child and adolescent mental health did so in a tangential manner and within the context of communicable diseases (e.g., HIV/AIDS and tuberculosis), maternal and child mortality, and the Millennium/Sustainable Development Goals (Mokitimi et al., 2018). However, specific goals for child and adolescent behavioral health can address family disadvantage, abusive parenting, and violence reduction, which in turn can reduce at-risk behaviors by adolescents, thereby improving developmental (psychological, behavioral, and physical health) outcomes across the life span (Meinck et al., 2017).

Central America and the Caribbean

The countries and territories of Central America and the Caribbean often are organized into two groups: (1) Central America, Mexico, and Latin Caribbean, who are comprised of the Spanish-speaking countries, and (2) the non-Latin Caribbean, who are comprised of the Dutch, English, and French-speaking countries. The subregions of the two groups are very different from each other. Each subregion includes countries of different sizes; different population sizes, from 5000 to 2.5 million inhabitants; different socioeconomic statuses; and different geographical locations, on the continent or on islands. The languages spoken also vary widely, including Dutch, English, French, Papiamento, Spanish, Caribbean Hindustani, and Antillean, Haitïan, and English Creoles.

However, the region is epidemiologically heterogeneous; many countries must deal with the double burden of communicable and chronic noncommunicable diseases. Like North America, a major policy emphasis is to integrate behavioral health into primary health care. A second policy emphasis is a universal health strategy (PAHO & WHO, 2017), approved by the PAHO member states in October 2014 (53rd Directing Council, 2014). Universal coverage and access would reduce inequities by strengthening health systems and services and decrease morbidity, disability, injuries, premature mortality, and risk for other health conditions (PAHO & WHO, 2017).

In Central America, Mexico, and the Latin Caribbean, eight countries currently have a national mental health policy (Pan American Health Organization, 2013). In the non-Latin Caribbean, 8 of 16 countries or territories have an explicit policy, Haiti had recently begun preparing one, and the remaining 7 had no specific policy (Pan American Health Organization, 2013). However, only three countries in the Central America, Mexico, and the Latin Caribbean area had specific behavioral health legislation, i.e., Dominican Republic, Mexico, and Cuba. In the non-Latin Caribbean area, only one country, Belize, did not have specific behavioral health legislation.

Behavioral health funding is also problematic. In the countries of the Central America, Mexico, and the Latin Caribbean, the median behavioral health budget was 0.9%. In the non-Latin Caribbean, the median was 3.5%.

All the countries in Central America, Mexico, and the Latin Caribbean have some central coordinating structure. In the non-Latin Caribbean, only five countries and territories have a coordinating entity at the Ministry of Health.

The percentage of children and adolescents receiving treatment in the Central America, Mexico, and the Latin Caribbean area ranges from 8% to 40%, with a median of 23%. In contrast, in the non-Latin Caribbean, the average number of children and adolescents receiving treatment is just 7.5%, making it the lowest in the region. So, within even the Caribbean, there are major differences among the Latin and non-Latin Caribbean. However, as with North America, the lack of a standard definition for surveillance makes it more difficult to determine prevalence, need, and services for children and adolescents with behavioral health problems.

Implications for Behavioral Health

Major gaps in data on adolescents pose one of the biggest challenges for behavioral health policy and services. Not only are data on early adolescents aged 10–14 scarce, data on pre-adolescence/middle childhood (ages 5–9) is practically unknown. Much of this has to do with the fact that fewer international indicators are disaggregated for children aged 5–9 than for early childhood or adolescence. Further, there are few internationally agreed-upon and collected indicators on adolescent mental health, disability, level of disability, and quality of life. Worse, for many developing countries, these data are simply not collected.

Further, disaggregation of data and causal analyses are critical to gain a better understanding of children and adolescents with behavioral disorders as well as the effects of the social determinants of health on this population, need for services, level of disability, and outcomes. Internationally accepted indicators disaggregated by age, disability, sex, ethnicity, caste, and religion are essential to provide for culturally and societally appropriate programs and policies.

There is a lack of numbers to address care in behavioral health services. Determining prevalence and having a 360° view for incidence reporting across public and private sectors are problematic. Two issues surrounding prevalence are definition and standardization. Since there are no consistent national or international criteria for the definition or standardization of prevalence data, the numbers are incomplete and inaccurate.

At a national level (United States), Brauner and Stephens (2006) offer the following recommendations to address the definitional issues surrounding prevalence as an argument for improving behavioral health services. The first steps are to expand the research and establish the use of valid and reliable screening measures, define levels of impairment in ranges, and update the standard definition (Brauner & Stephens, 2006). The next steps would be to create a standard "Developmental At-Risk Profile," remove barriers to treatment, and create and implement a new "Early Childhood Mental Health Plan" (Brauner & Stephens, 2006).

The use of standardized, fully structured, self-administered epidemiologic questionnaires and standardized screening measures designed for families would assist in the collection of data to help in the diagnosis and early treatment of a disorder and complex, multi-morbid disorders. As noted earlier, there is little consensus on how minimum functional impairment should be defined or measured. Without a clear definition or guideline, children and adolescents will not receive the appropriate levels of treatment and supports they need based upon level of impairment.

Misclassification of disorder results in skewed statistics as well as in inappropriate diagnosis and treatment.

As with any disease, the earlier practitioners diagnose and treat disorders, the better responses patients have. With lifelong chronic diseases, this maxim becomes even more important. Measures, such as the DALYS, clearly show the lifelong impact of behavioral disorders on individual levels of functioning and disability as well as larger societal concerns of morbidity and mortality. Creating family-focused measures also allows us to approach the prevention, identification, and treatment of behavioral disorders and accompanying morbid disorders from a generational, holistic public health perspective. If the definition of health from a global perspective is "state of complete physical, mental and social well-being and not merely the absence of disease or infirmity" (WHO, 1948), then clearly we have a formidable challenge ahead of us.

Governments, NGOs, and professional associations can all play a role in helping to push a global agenda for behavioral health across the life span (Remschmidt & Belfer, 2005). Each stakeholder has a role, whether it is in raising awareness through public health prevention and promotion campaigns to help establish facilities to provide services, to provide training programs for behavioral health-care workers, or to advocate and ensure global conventions are followed internationally.

Working with governments and NGOs to change behavioral health policy, services, and systems at global and national levels require intersectoral actions that are, by definition, highly collaborative and voluntary. Creating a conducive policy framework and approach to health brings together many of the issues touched upon in this chapter, starting with effective communication and a common language. Forming partnerships, creating a shared framework regarding visions and missions, determining "implementable" and sustainable goals, garnering political support, and ensuring transparency and accountability are all important elements in creating consensus on policy priorities.

An important consideration in global health policy is that "one size does not fit all." "The one size" should be addressed by a specific country due to its income, of infrastructure, and/or political stability. However, all countries can agree in principle that prevention and early intervention in child and adolescent behavioral health is a critical issue, and they can support it as an actionable item. By using SDH and SBD approaches in global behavioral health policymaking, we are looking at an extremely complex issue that is compounded since SDH and SBD affect the very fabric of society and the rationale of government. Nevertheless, with foresight, planning, and adherence to a global agenda, such an objective may be achievable.

References

53rd Directing Council, & 66th Session of the Regional Committee of WHO for the Americas. (2014, October 2). *Strategy for universal access to health and universal health coverage* (CD53/5, Rev. 2). Washington, DC: Pan American Health Organization & World Health

Organization. https://www.paho.org/uhexchange/index.php/en/uhexchange-documents/technical-information/26-strategy-for-universal-access-to-health-and-universal-health-coverage/file

Aldrich, M. C., Hidalgo, B., Widome, R., Briss, P., Brownson, R. C., & Teutsch, S. M. (2015). The role of epidemiology in evidence-based policy making: A case study of tobacco use in youth. *Annals of Epidemiology, 25*(5), 360–365. https://doi.org/10.1016/j.annepidem.2014.03.005

Alkire, S., & Jahan, S. (2018, September). *The New Global MPI 2018: Aligning with the Sustainable Development Goals* (UNDP HDRO occasional paper). New York, NY: United Nations Development Programme (UNDP) Human Development Report Office (HDRO). http://hdr.undp.org/sites/default/files/2018_mpi_jahan_alkire.pdfr

Almuneef, M., Hollinshead, D., Saleheen, H., AlMadani, S., Derkash, B., AlBuhairan, F., … Fluke, J. (2016). Adverse childhood experiences and association with health, mental health, and risky behavior in the kingdom of Saudi Arabia. *Child Abuse and Neglect, 60*, 10–17. https://doi.org/10.1016/j.chiabu.2016.09.003

Australian Institute of Health and Welfare. (2018). *Mental health services: In brief 2018*. Canberra, AT: Author. https://www.aihw.gov.au/getmedia/0e102c2f-694b-4949-84fb-e5db1c941a58/aihw-hse-211.pdf.aspx?inline=true

Balabanova, D., Mills, A., Conteh, L., Akkazieva, B., Banteyerga, H., Dash, U., … McKee, M. (2013). Good Health at Low Cost 25 years on: Lessons for the future of health systems strengthening. *Lancet, 381*(9883), 2118–2133. https://doi.org/10.1016/s0140-6736(12)62000-5

Baranne, M. L., & Falissard, B. (2018). Global burden of mental disorders among children aged 5-14 years. *Child and Adolescent Psychiatry and Mental Health, 12*, 19. https://doi.org/10.1186/s13034-018-0225-4

Barry, M. M., Clarke, A. M., Jenkins, R., & Patel, V. (2013). A systematic review of the effectiveness of mental health promotion interventions for young people in low and middle income countries. *BMC Public Health, 13*, 835. https://doi.org/10.1186/1471-2458-13-835

Bauman, A. E., King, L., & Nutbeam, D. (2014). Rethinking the evaluation and measurement of Health in all policies. *Health Promotion International, 29*(Suppl 1), i143–i151. https://doi.org/10.1093/heapro/dau049

Bellis, M. A., Lowey, H., Leckenby, N., Hughes, K., & Harrison, D. (2014). Adverse childhood experiences: Retrospective study to determine their impact on adult health behaviours and health outcomes in a UK population. *Journal of Public Health (Oxford, England), 36*(1), 81–91. https://doi.org/10.1093/pubmed/fdt038

Berg Brigham, K., Darlington, M., Wright, J. S., Lewison, G., Kanavos, P., & Durand-Zaleski, I. (2016). Mapping research activity on mental health disorders in Europe: Study protocol for the Mapping_NCD project. *Health Research Policy and Systems, 14*(1), 39. https://doi.org/10.1186/s12961-016-0111-6

Bird, P., Omar, M., Doku, V., Lund, C., Nsereko, J. R., & Mwanza, J. (2011). Increasing the priority of mental health in Africa: Findings from qualitative research in Ghana, South Africa, Uganda and Zambia. *Health Policy and Planning, 26*(5), 357–365. https://doi.org/10.1093/heapol/czq078

Bloom, D. E., Cafiero, E. T., Jané-Llopis, E., Abrahams-Gessel, S., Bloom, L. R., Fathima, S., … Weinstein, C. (2011). The global economic burden of non-communicable diseases: A report by the World Economic Forum and the Harvard School of Public Health. Geneva, Switzerland. http://www3.weforum.org/docs/WEF_Harvard_HE_GlobalEconomicBurdenNonCommunicableDiseases_2011.pdf

Braddick, F., Carral, V., Jenkins, R., & Jané-Lopis, E. (2009). *Child and adolescent mental health in europe: Infrastructures, policy and programs*. Luxembourg, Europe: European Communities.

Brauner, C. B., & Stephens, C. B. (2006). Estimating the prevalence of early childhood serious emotional/behavioral disorders: Challenges and recommendations. *Public Health Reports, 121*(3), 303–310. http://www.ncbi.nlm.nih.gov/pmc/articles/PMC1525276/

Brownson, R. C., Fielding, J. E., & Maylahn, C. M. (2009). Evidence-based public health: A fundamental concept for public health practice. *Annual Review of Public Health, 30*, 175–201.

Center for Mental Health Services. (1998). Children with serious emotional disturbance; estimation methodology. *Federal Register, 63*(137), 38861–38865. https://www.govinfo.gov/content/pkg/FR-1998-07-17/pdf/98-19039.pdf

Commission on Social Determinants of Health. (2008). *Closing the gap in a generation: Health equity through action on the social determinants of health*. Geneva, Switzerland: WHO.

Council of Australian Governments. (2012). *Roadmap for national mental health reform 2012–2022*. Melbourne, AT: Author. https://www.coag.gov.au/sites/default/files/communique/The%20Roadmap%20for%20National%20Mental%20Health%20Reform%202012-2022.pdf

Crouch, E., Strompolis, M., Bennett, K. J., Morse, M., & Radcliff, E. (2017). Assessing the interrelatedness of multiple types of adverse childhood experiences and odds for poor health in South Carolina adults. *Child Abuse and Neglect, 65*, 204–211. https://doi.org/10.1016/j.chiabu.2017.02.007

DeLoitte Australia. (2017). *Review of the National Mental Health Commission: Final report*. Melbourne, AT: Author. http://www.health.gov.au/internet/main/publishing.nsf/content/D015B02A481D8BC8CA2581D000014AC7/$File/Strengthening%20the%20National%20Mental%20Health%20Commission.pdf

Durlak, J. A., & Wells, A. M. (1997). Primary prevention mental health programs for children and adolescents: A meta-analytic review. *American Journal of Community Psychology, 25*(2), 115–152.

Edelman, M. J. (1988). *Constructing the political spectacle*. Chicago, IL: University Of Chicago Press.

Erskine, H. E., Moffitt, T. E., Copeland, W. E., Costello, E. J., Ferrari, A. J., Patton, G., … Scott, J. G. (2015). A heavy burden on young minds: The global burden of mental and substance use disorders in children and youth. *Psychological Medicine, 45*(7), 1551–1563. https://doi.org/10.1017/s0033291714002888

EU Joint Action on Mental Health and Wellbeing. (2016). *European framework for action on mental health and wellbeing*. Brussels, Belgium: Author. https://ec.europa.eu/research/participants/data/ref/h2020/other/guides_for_applicants/h2020-SC1-BHC-22-2019-framework-for-action_en.pdf

European Communities. (2005). *Green Paper: Improving the mental health of the population: Towards a strategy on mental health for the European Union*. Brussels, Belgium. https://ec.europa.eu/health/ph_determinants/life_style/mental/green_paper/mental_gp_en.pdf

Fischer, F. (2003). *Reframing public policy: Discursive politics and deliberative practices*. Oxford, UK: Oxford Unviersity Press.

Ford, R., King, T., Priest, N., & Kavanagh, A. (2017). Bullying and mental health and suicidal behaviour among 14- to 15-year-olds in a representative sample of Australian children. *Australian and New Zealand Journal of Psychiatry, 51*(9), 897–908. https://doi.org/10.1177/0004867417700275

Forouzanfar, M. H., Alexander, L., Anderson, H. R., Bachman, V. F., Biryukov, S., Brauer, M., … Murray, C. J. (2015). Global, regional, and national comparative risk assessment of 79 behavioural, environmental and occupational, and metabolic risks or clusters of risks in 188 countries, 1990-2013: A systematic analysis for the Global Burden of Disease Study 2013. *Lancet, 386*(10010), 2287–2323. https://doi.org/10.1016/s0140-6736(15)00128-2

GBD 2016 Disease and Injury Incidence and Prevalence Collaborators. (2017). Global, regional, and national disability-adjusted life-years (DALYs) for 333 diseases and injuries and healthy life expectancy (HALE) for 195 countries and territories, 1990-2016: A systematic analysis for the Global Burden of Disease Study 2016. *Lancet, 390*(10100), 1260–1344. https://doi.org/10.1016/s0140-6736(17)32130-x

Hanson, A. (2014). Illuminating the invisible voices in mental health policymaking. *Journal of Medicine and the Person, 12*(1), 13–18. https://doi.org/10.1007/s12682-014-0170-9

Health Care Cost Institute. (2012). *2007–2011 children's health care spending report*. Washington, DC: Author. https://www.healthcostinstitute.org/images/pdfs/HCCI_CHCSR20072010.pdf

Hughes, K., Bellis, M. A., Hardcastle, K. A., Sethi, D., Butchart, A., Mikton, C., … Dunne, M. P. (2017). The effect of multiple adverse childhood experiences on health: A systematic review and meta-analysis. *The Lancet Public Health, 2*(8), e356–e366. https://doi.org/10.1016/s2468-2667(17)30118-4

Hunt, T. K. A., Slack, K. S., & Berger, L. M. (2017). Adverse childhood experiences and behavioral problems in middle childhood. *Child Abuse and Neglect, 67*, 391–402. https://doi.org/10.1016/j.chiabu.2016.11.005

Institute of Medicine. (2014). *Capturing social and behavioral domains in electronic health records: Phase 1* (Vol. 1). Washington, DC: National Academies Press.

Institute of Medicine. (2015). *Capturing social and behavioral domains and measures in electronic health records: Phase 2* (Vol. 2). Washington, DC: National Academies Press.

Ismayilova, L., Gaveras, E., Blum, A., To-Camier, A., & Nanema, R. (2016). Maltreatment and Mental Health Outcomes among Ultra-Poor Children in Burkina Faso: A latent class analysis. *PLoS One, 11*(10), e0164790. https://doi.org/10.1371/journal.pone.0164790

Jané-Llopis, E., Barry, M., Hosman, C., & Patel, V. (2005). Mental health promotion works: A review. *Promotion et Education, 12*, 9–25, 61, 67. https://doi.org/10.1177/10253823050120020103x

Januário, S. S., das Neves Peixoto, F. S., Lima, N. N., do Nascimento, V. B., de Sousa, D. F., Pereira Luz, D. C., … Rolim Neto, M. L. (2017). Mental health and public policies implemented in the Northeast of Brazil: A systematic review with meta-analysis. *International Journal of Social Psychiatry, 63*(1), 21–32. https://doi.org/10.1177/0020764016677557

Johnson, S. E., Lawrence, D., Hafekost, J., Saw, S., Buckingham, W. J., Sawyer, M., … Zubrick, S. R. (2016). Service use by Australian children for emotional and behavioural problems: Findings from the second Australian Child and Adolescent Survey of Mental Health and Wellbeing. *Australian and New Zealand Journal of Psychiatry, 50*(9), 887–898. https://doi.org/10.1177/0004867415622562

Junek, W. (2012). Government monitoring of the mental health of children in Canada: Five surveys (Part II). *Journal of the Canadian Academy of Child and Adolescent Psychiatry, 21*(1), 37–44. http://www.ncbi.nlm.nih.gov/pmc/articles/PMC3269247/

Kelly, M. P., Morgan, A., Bonnefoy, J., Butt, J., Bergman, V., Mackenbach, J., … Florezano, F. (2007). *Final report of the Measurement and Evidence Knowledge Network: The social determinants of health: Developing an evidence base for political action.* Geneva, Switzerland: World Health Organization (WHO) Commission on the Social Determinants of Health, Measurement and Evidence Knowledge Network.

Kessler, R. C., Avenevoli, S., Costello, J., Green, J. G., Gruber, M. J., McLaughlin, K. A., … Merikangas, K. R. (2012). Severity of 12-month DSM-IV disorders in the National Comorbidity Survey Replication Adolescent Supplement. *Archives of General Psychiatry, 69*(4), 381–389. https://doi.org/10.1001/archgenpsychiatry.2011.1603

Kieling, C., Baker-Henningham, H., Belfer, M., Conti, G., Ertem, I., Omigbodun, O., … Rahman, A. (2011). Child and adolescent mental health worldwide: Evidence for action. *Lancet, 378*(9801), 1515–1525. https://doi.org/10.1016/s0140-6736(11)60827-1

Lawrence, D., Hafekost, J., Johnson, S. E., Saw, S., Buckingham, W. J., Sawyer, M. G., … Zubrick, S. R. (2016). Key findings from the second Australian Child and Adolescent Survey of Mental Health and Wellbeing. *Australian and New Zealand Journal of Psychiatry, 50*(9), 876–886. https://doi.org/10.1177/0004867415617836

Lu, W. (2017). Child and adolescent mental disorders and health care disparities: Results from the National Survey of Children's Health, 2011-2012. *Journal of Health Care for the Poor and Underserved, 28*(3), 988–1011. https://doi.org/10.1353/hpu.2017.0092

Luby, J. L., Barch, D., Whalen, D., Tillman, R., & Belden, A. (2017). Association between early life adversity and risk for poor emotional and physical health in adolescence: A putative mechanistic neurodevelopmental pathway. *JAMA Pediatrics, 171*(12), 1168–1175. https://doi.org/10.1001/jamapediatrics.2017.3009

Mackenbach, J. P., & McKee, M. (2013). A comparative analysis of health policy performance in 43 European countries. *European Journal of Public Health, 23*(2), 195–201. https://doi.org/10.1093/eurpub/cks192

Maselko, J. (2017). Social epidemiology and global mental health: Expanding the evidence from high-income to low- and middle-income countries. *Current Epidemiology Reports, 4*(2), 166–173. https://doi.org/10.1007/s40471-017-0107-y

McGrath, J. J., McLaughlin, K. A., Saha, S., Aguilar-Gaxiola, S., Al-Hamzawi, A., Alonso, J., … Kessler, R. C. (2017). The association between childhood adversities and subsequent first onset of psychotic experiences: A cross-national analysis of 23 998 respondents from 17 countries. *Psychological Medicine, 47*(7), 1230–1245. https://doi.org/10.1017/s0033291716003263

Meinck, F., Cluver, L. D., Orkin, F. M., Kuo, C., Sharma, A. D., Hensels, I. S., & Sherr, L. (2017). Pathways from family disadvantage via abusive parenting and caregiver mental health to adolescent health risks in South Africa. *Journal of Adolescent Health, 60*(1), 57–64. https://doi.org/10.1016/j.jadohealth.2016.08.016

Mokitimi, S., Schneider, M., & de Vries, P. J. (2018). Child and adolescent mental health policy in South Africa: History, current policy development and implementation, and policy analysis. *International Journal of Mental Health Systems, 12*(36). https://doi.org/10.1186/s13033-018-0213-3

Murray, C. J. L., & Lopez, A. D. (1996). *The global burden of disease: A comprehensive assessment of mortality and disability from diseases, injuries, and risk factors in 1990 and projected to 2020*. Cambridge, MA: Harvard School of Public Health on behalf of the World Health Organization and the World Bank.

National Academies of Sciences, Engineering, & Medicine. (2017). *Communities in action: Pathways to health equity*. Washington, DC: The National Academies Press.

National Research Council, & Institute of Medicine. (2009). *Preventing mental, emotional, and behavioral disorders among young people: Progress and possibilities*. Washington, DC: The National Academies Press. https://www.nap.edu/catalog/12480/preventing-mental-emotional-and-behavioral-disorders-among-young-people-progress

OECD, & World Health Organization. (2012). *Health at a glance: Asia/Pacific 2012*. Paris, France: OECD. https://www.oecd-ilibrary.org/docserver/9789264183902-en.pdf?expires=1548265880&id=id&accname=oid006180&checksum=BA49C97C5DE9ADEE882000034D78A3DA

Office of Disease Prevention and Health Promotion. (2018). *Healthy People 2030 framework*. [Web page]. Washington, DC: U.S. Department of Health and Human Services. https://www.healthypeople.gov/2020/About-Healthy-People/Development-Healthy-People-2030/Framework

Oh, D. L., Jerman, P., Silverio Marques, S., Koita, K., Purewal Boparai, S. K., Burke Harris, N., & Bucci, M. (2018). Systematic review of pediatric health outcomes associated with childhood adversity. *BMC Pediatrics, 18*(1), 83. https://doi.org/10.1186/s12887-018-1037-7

Oneka, G., Vahid Shahidi, F., Muntaner, C., Bayoumi, A. M., Mahabir, D. F., Freiler, A., … Shankardass, K. (2017). A glossary of terms for understanding political aspects in the implementation of Health in All Policies (HiAP). *Journal of Epidemiology and Community Health, 71*(8), 835–838. https://doi.org/10.1136/jech-2017-208979

Oxford Poverty and Human Development Initiative. (2018). *Global Multidimensional Poverty Index 2018: The most detailed picture to date of the world's poorest people*. Oxford, UK: Oxford University. https://ophi.org.uk/wp-content/uploads/G-MPI_2018_2ed_web.pdf

Pan American Health Organization. (2013). *WHO-AIMS: Report on mental health systems in Latin America and the Caribbean*. Washington, DC: PAHO. http://www.paho.org/hq/index.php?option=com_docman&task=doc_view&gid=21325&Itemid=

Pan American Health Organization, & World Health Organization. (2017). *Health in the Americas: Summary: Regional outlook and country profiles*. Washington, DC: Pan American Health Organization & World Health Organization. https://www.paho.org/salud-en-las-americas-2017/wp-content/uploads/2017/09/Print-Version-English.pdf

Patel, V., Lund, C., Hatjeril, S., Plagerson, S., Corrigall, J., Funk, M. K., & Flisher, A. J. (2010). Mental disorders: Equity and social determinants. In E. Blas & A. S. Kurup (Eds.), *Equity, social determinants and public health programmes* (pp. 115–134). Geneva, Switzerland: World Health Organization. http://apps.who.int/iris/bitstream/handle/10665/44289/9789241563970_eng.pdf?sequence=1

Pena, S., Cook, S., Leppo, M., Ollila, E., Wismar, M., & United Nations Research Institute for Social Development. (2013). *Health in all policies: Seizing opportunities, implementing policies*. Helsinki, Finland: Ministry of Social Affairs and Health.

Perou, R., Bitsko, R. H., Blumberg, S. J., Pastor, P., Ghandour, R. M., Gfroerer, J. C., ... Huang, L. N. (2013). Mental health surveillance among children: United States, 2005-2011. *Morbidity and Mortality Weekly Report. Surveillance Summaries, 62*(Suppl 2), 1–35. https://www.cdc.gov/mmwr/preview/mmwrhtml/su6202a1.htm

Pfuntner, A., Wier, L. M., & Stocks, C. (2013). *Most frequent conditions in U.S. hospitals, 2010* (Healthcare Cost and Utilization Project (HCUP) Statistical Briefs, #148). Rockville, MD: Agency for Healthcare Research and Quality.

Remschmidt, H., & Belfer, M. (2005). Mental health care for children and adolescents worldwide: A review. *World Psychiatry, 4*(3), 147–153. http://www.ncbi.nlm.nih.gov/pmc/articles/PMC1414760/

Reuben, A., Moffitt, T. E., Caspi, A., Belsky, D. W., Harrington, H., Schroeder, F., ... Danese, A. (2016). Lest we forget: Comparing retrospective and prospective assessments of adverse childhood experiences in the prediction of adult health. *Journal of Child Psychology and Psychiatry and Allied Disciplines, 57*(10), 1103–1112. https://doi.org/10.1111/jcpp.12621

Rith-Najarian, L. R., Daleiden, E. L., & Chorpita, B. F. (2016). Evidence-based decision making in youth mental health prevention. *American Journal of Preventive Medicine, 51*(4 Suppl 2), S132–S139. https://doi.org/10.1016/j.amepre.2016.05.018

Rittel, H., & Martin, W. (1973). Dilemmas in a general theory of planning. *Policy Sciences, 4*, 155–169.

Secretary's Advisory Committee on National Health Promotion and Disease Prevention Objectives for 2030. (2018). *Report #2: Recommendations for developing objectives, setting priorities, identifying data needs, and involving stakeholders for Healthy People 2030*. Washington, DC: Author. https://www.healthypeople.gov/sites/default/files/Advisory_Committee_Objectives_for_HP2030_Report.pdf

Stahl, T. (2018). Health in all policies: From rhetoric to implementation and evaluation - the finnish experience. *Scandinavian Journal of Public Health, 46*(20_suppl), 38–46. https://doi.org/10.1177/1403494817743895

Sterling, S., Chi, F., Weisner, C., Grant, R., Pruzansky, A., Bui, S., ... Pearl, R. (2018). Association of behavioral health factors and social determinants of health with high and persistently high healthcare costs. *Preventive Medical Reports, 11*, 154–159. https://doi.org/10.1016/j.pmedr.2018.06.017

Stone, D. (2012). *Policy paradox: The art of political decision making* (3rd ed.). London, UK: W.W. Norton & Company Ltd.

Storm, I., Harting, J., Stronks, K., & Schuit, A. J. (2014). Measuring stages of health in all policies on a local level: The applicability of a maturity model. *Health Policy, 114*(2–3), 183–191. https://doi.org/10.1016/j.healthpol.2013.05.006

Stubbs, B., Koyanagi, A., Veronese, N., Vancampfort, D., Solmi, M., Gaughran, F., ... Correll, C. U. (2016). Physical multimorbidity and psychosis: Comprehensive cross sectional analysis including 242,952 people across 48 low- and middle-income countries. *BMC Medicine, 14*(1), 189. https://doi.org/10.1186/s12916-016-0734-z

Stuckler, D., & Basu, S. (2013). *The body economic: Why austerity kills, and what we can do about it*. London, UK: Allen Lane.

Synnevag, E. S., Amdam, R., & Fosse, E. (2018). Public health terminology: Hindrance to a Health in All Policies approach? *Scandinavian Journal of Public Health, 46*(1), 68–73. https://doi.org/10.1177/1403494817729921

Trotta, A., Murray, R. M., & Fisher, H. L. (2015). The impact of childhood adversity on the persistence of psychotic symptoms: A systematic review and meta-analysis. *Psychological Medicine, 45*(12), 2481–2498. https://doi.org/10.1017/s0033291715000574

Underwood, L. A., & Washington, A. (2016). Mental illness and juvenile offenders. *International Journal of Environmental Research and Public Health, 13*(2), 228. https://doi.org/10.3390/ijerph13020228

UNICEF. (2012). *Progress for children: A report card on adolescents.* New York, NY: United Nations Children's Fund (UNICEF).

United Nations Children's Fund. (2014). *Every child's birth right: Inequities and trends in birth registration.* New York, NY: UNICEF. http://www.data.unicef.org/corecode/uploads/document6/uploaded_pdfs/corecode/Birth_Registration_lores_final_24.pdf

United Nations Development Programme. (2018). *The 2018 Global Multidimensional Poverty Index (MPI).* [Web page]. New York, NY: Author. http://hdr.undp.org/en/2018-MPI

United Nations Economic and Social Conditions for Asia and the Pacific. (2017). *Statistical yearbook for Asia and the Pacific 2017: Measuring SDG progress in Asia and the Pacific: Is there enough data?* Bangkok, Thailand: Author. https://www.unescap.org/sites/default/files/publications/ESCAP-SYB2017.pdf

United Nations General Assembly. (1989). *Convention on the Rights of the Child. United Nations Office of the High Commissioner for Human Rights.* New York, NY: United Nations. http://www.ohchr.org/en/professionalinterest/pages/crc.aspx

United Nations General Assembly. (2015, October 21). *Resolution adopted by the General Assembly on 25 September 2015: 70/1. Transforming our world: The 2030 Agenda for Sustainable Development* (A/RES/70/1). New Yok, NY: United Nations. http://www.un.org/ga/search/view_doc.asp?symbol=A/RES/70/1&Lang=E

Van Vliet-Brown, C. E., Shahram, S., & Oelke, N. D. (2018). Health in All Policies utilization by municipal governments: Scoping review. *Health Promotion International, 33*(4), 713–722. https://doi.org/10.1093/heapro/dax008

Waddell, C., Hua, J. M., Garland, O. M., Peters, R. D., & McEwan, K. (2007). Preventing mental disorders in children: A systematic review to inform policy-making. *Canadian Journal of Public Health. Revue Canadienne de Santé Publique, 98*(3), 166–173.

Whiteford, H. A., Degenhardt, L., Rehm, J., Baxter, A. J., Ferrari, A. J., Erskine, H. E., … Vos, T. (2013). Global burden of disease attributable to mental and substance use disorders: Findings from the Global Burden of Disease Study 2010. *Lancet, 382*(9904), 1575–1586. https://doi.org/10.1016/s0140-6736(13)61611-6

World Bank. (2018a). *Data: World Bank country and lending groups.* [Web page]. Washington, DC: The World Bank Group. https://datahelpdesk.worldbank.org/knowledgebase/articles/906519

World Bank. (2018b). *Poverty overview.* Washington, DC: World Bank Group. http://www.worldbank.org/en/topic/poverty/overview

World Health Assembly. (2009). *Reducing health inequities through action on the social determinants of health* (WHA62.14). Geneva, Switzerland. http://apps.who.int/gb/ebwha/pdf_files/WHA62-REC1/WHA62_REC1-en-P2.pdf

World Health Assembly. (2011). *Rio Political Declaration on Social Determinants of Health.* Rio de Janiero, Brasil: World Health Organization. https://www.who.int/sdhconference/declaration/Rio_political_declaration.pdf

World Health Assembly. (2013). *Comprehensive mental health action plan 2013–2020.* Geneva, Switzerland: WHO. http://apps.who.int/gb/ebwha/pdf_files/WHA66/A66_R8-en.pdf?ua=1

World Health Organisation. (2010). *Global strategy to reduce the harmful use of alcohol.* Geneva, Switzerland: Author. http://apps.who.int/iris/bitstream/handle/10665/44395/9789241599931_eng.pdf?sequence=1

World Health Organization. (1948). *Official records of the World Health Organization, no. 2.* Geneva, Switzerland: WHO.

World Health Organization. (2003). *Caring for children and adolescents with mental disorders.* Geneva, Switzerland: WHO. http://www.who.int/mental_health/media/en/785.pdf

World Health Organization. (2004). *Prevention of mental disorders. Effective interventions and policy options: Summary report: A report of the World Health Organization Dept. of Mental Health and Substance Abuse; in collaboration with the Prevention Research Centre of the Universities of Nijmegen and Maastricht.* Geneva, Switzerland: Author.

World Health Organization. (2011). *Mental health atlas*. Geneva, Switzerland: WHO. http://whqlibdoc.who.int/publications/2011/9799241564359_eng.pdf?ua=1

World Health Organization. (2013). *Comprehensive mental health action plan 2013–2020*. Geneva, Switzerland: Author. http://apps.who.int/iris/bitstream/handle/10665/89966/9789241506021_eng.pdf?sequence=1

World Health Organization. (2014). *Adolescent health epidemiology*. Geneva, Switzerland: WHO. http://www.who.int/maternal_child_adolescent/epidemiology/adolescence/en/

World Health Organization. (2016). *Global monitoring of action on the social determinants of health: A proposed framework and basket of core indicators [consultation paper]*. Geneva, Switzerland: Author. https://www.who.int/social_determinants/consultation-paper-SDH-Action-Monitoring.pdf?ua=1

World Health Organization. (2018). *Mental health atlas 2017*. Geneva, Switzerland: Author. http://apps.who.int/iris/bitstream/handle/10665/272735/9789241514019-eng.pdf?ua=1

World Health Organization, & Calouste Gulbenkian Foundation. (2014). *Social determinants of mental health*. Geneva, Switzerland: Author. http://apps.who.int/iris/bitstream/handle/10665/112828/9789241506809_eng.pdf;jsessionid=95F6342ABB84737B1E3A4B22BBEBE83F?sequence=1

Yampolskaya, S., Sharrock, P. J., Clark, C., & Hanson, A. (2017). Utilization of mental health services and mental health status among children placed in out-of-home care: A parallel process latent growth modeling approach. *Child Psychiatry and Human Development, 48*(5), 728–740. https://doi.org/10.1007/s10578-016-0699-3

Yanow, D. (1996). *How does a policy mean? Interpreting policy and organizational actions*. Washington, DC: Georgetown University Press.

Zubrick, S. R., Hafekost, J., Johnson, S. E., Lawrence, D., Saw, S., Sawyer, M., … Buckingham, W. J. (2016). Suicidal behaviours: Prevalence estimates from the second Australian Child and Adolescent Survey of Mental Health and Wellbeing. *Australian and New Zealand Journal of Psychiatry, 50*(9), 899–910. https://doi.org/10.1177/0004867415622563

Correction to: Foundations of Behavioral Health

Bruce Lubotsky Levin and Ardis Hanson

Correction to:
B. L. Levin, A. Hanson (eds.), *Foundations of Behavioral Health*, https://doi.org/10.1007/978-3-030-18435-3

1. The original version of the opening page of chapter 8 and contributors section in FM were inadvertently published with incorrect affiliation (city) information of author "Ralph J. DiClemente". This has been updated as "New York, NY, USA".

2. An email ID of the author "Kevin C. Heslin" has been also updated as "kevin_heslin@gwu.edu" in chapter 2 (**The Global Epidemiology of Mental and Substance Use Disorders**).

3. The below mentioned content in chapter 9 has been printed twice and the duplicate occurrence has been deleted.

"While there have been some policy changes to improve health services delivery, outcomes have not been sufficient in meeting the health needs of this population. Clearly, developing amended and updated policies must address the needs of underserved populations."

The updated online versions of these chapters can be found at
https://doi.org/10.1007/978-3-030-18435-3_2
https://doi.org/10.1007/978-3-030-18435-3_8
https://doi.org/10.1007/978-3-030-18435-3_9
https://doi.org/10.1007/978-3-030-18435-3

Index

© Springer Nature Switzerland AG 2020
B. L. Levin, A. Hanson (eds.), *Foundations of Behavioral Health*,
https://doi.org/10.1007/978-3-030-18435-3

CPSIA information can be obtained
at www.ICGtesting.com
Printed in the USA
LVHW081109151219
640572LV00002B/98/P